ETHICS & ISSUES
IN CONTEMPORARY NURSING

First Canadian Edition

Margaret A. Burkhardt

PhD, RN, CS, FNP

Alvita K. Nathaniel

MSN, RN, CS, FNP

Nancy Walton

RN, PhD (Collaborative Program in Bioethics),
Associate Director; Daphne Cockwell School of Nursing,
Faculty of Community Services,
Chair, Research Ethics Board,
Ryerson University

NELSON / EDUCATION

NELSON / EDUCATION

Ethics and Issues In Contemporary Nursing, First Canadian Edition

by Margaret A. Burkhardt, Alvita K. Nathaniel, and Nancy A. Walton

Vice President, Editorial Director:
Evelyn Veitch

Editor-in-Chief, Higher Education:
Anne Williams

Executive Editor:
Paul Fam

Marketing Manager:
Amanda Henry

Developmental Editor:
Mark Grzeskowiak

Photo Researcher and Permissions Coordinator:
Daniela Glass

Content Production Manager:
Susan Wong

Production Service:
Macmillan Publishing Solutions

Copy Editor:
Karen Rolfe

Proofreader:
Dianne Fowlie

Indexer:
David Luljak

Production Coordinator:
Ferial Suleman

Design Director:
Ken Phipps

Managing Designer:
Franca Amore

Cover Design:
Peter Papayanakis

Cover Image:
Shaun Egan/The Image Bank/ Getty Images

Compositor:
Macmillan Publishing Solutions

Printer:
Webcom

Library and Archives Canada Cataloguing in Publication

Burkhardt, Margaret A
Ethics and issues in contemporary nursing / Margaret A. Burkhardt, Alvita K. Nathaniel, Nancy A. Walton.— 1st Canadian ed.

ISBN 978-0-17-610528-0
1. Nursing ethics--Textbooks.
I. Nathaniel, Alvita K. II. Walton, Nancy A., 1967-III. Title.

RT85.B872 2009 174.2 C2009-900328-7

ISBN-13: 978-0-17-610528-0
ISBN-10: 0-17-610528-X

Contents

Preface

*We who lived in the concentration camps can remember the men
who walked through the huts comforting others, giving away their last
piece of bread. They may have been few in number, but they offer
sufficient proof that everything can be taken from a man but one
thing: The last of his freedoms—to choose one's attitude in any given
set of circumstances, to choose one's own way.*
—V. E. Frankl, *Man's Search for Meaning*

As contemporary nurses, we face complex and challenging personal, interpersonal, professional, institutional, and social issues. Appropriate responses to these issues are seldom clear. Ethical dilemmas, in particular, involve choices with no clearly correct solutions. We believe that declaring that there is one correct approach to solving ethical problems risks imposing personal values on others. We must be sensitive to that possibility and recognize that our responses to dilemmas depend on such variables as contextual factors, patient and family values, relationships, moral development, religious beliefs, spiritual perspective, cultural orientation, and legal constraints.

It is our intention in this book to (1) acknowledge that each person is a moral agent, (2) raise awareness of the myriad factors that need to be considered when dealing with ethical decisions, (3) present a decision-making model to help individuals learn to process information and move toward action, and (4) affirm nursing as an ethically responsible profession. We present ethical issues from the perspective of nursing, recognizing that relationships and the authority to make decisions are affected by contextual factors such as professional status; gender; the development of the profession; personal ethical stance; social, economic, institutional, and political climate; and personal and professional empowerment.

Dealing with ethical issues requires skill in the processes of values clarification, ethical decision making, self-awareness, empowerment, transcultural sensitivity, and challenging injustice. The text poses questions about contemporary issues and provides processes for the development of sensitivity and skill in resolving ethical problems. Highlighting nurses in a variety of settings and roles, exercises and activities are intended to facilitate self-reflection and awareness of personal approaches to issues and decision making. Our goal is that you will become engaged in active learning throughout the text through the use of *Case Presentations* based on real-life situations, *Ask Yourself* and *Think About It* exercises derived from thought-provoking material and case presentations, and *Discussion Questions and Activities*.

Although acknowledging the rich and divergent history of nursing in other cultures, we have chosen to write primarily from the Western perspective. The background that we give explains the many factors that lead to social systems which either encourage or prohibit certain people from critically examining issues and making authoritative decisions. The book begins with a chapter that explores the impact of historical factors, particularly religion and gender, on the profession of nursing in Western culture. We hope that this will help you to understand more fully the context of nursing and question arbitrary and artificial barriers to ethical decision making.

With a strong groundwork of ethical theories and principles in Part I, subsequent chapters deal with various issues as they pertain to ethics and ethical decision making. As you explore political, professional, legal, social, and gender issues, we encourage you to look at the related ethical questions and to continually move back and forth from the concrete to the abstract, from the general to the specific, from the global to the personal, and from issue to principle—recognizing the interrelatedness of many factors.

While continuing to discuss ethical issues from the perspective of nursing, in this second edition we have attempted to strengthen the thematic layer of holistic caring. Because we feel it is essential to the study of ethics, we have continued to incorporate classical and older philosophical thought, as well as the perspectives of contemporary philosophers and ethicists as we expand our exploration of complex contemporary issues. Overall improvements from the first edition include a change in language and voice to make the content more personal and accessible to students of all levels, and the addition of a second colour to highlight various features and make the text more visually appealing. We updated and expanded the text to include a more thorough discussion of modern and contemporary influences on the profession, virtue ethics, the ethics of care, ethics and the law, nurse practice acts, and the responsibilities of boards of nursing, palliative care, self-determination, managed care, and complementary therapies. We also added some recent noteworthy cases to our discussions of palliative care, legal issues, and protection of human subjects.

Principled behaviour in personal and professional situations is the organizing theme of this text. Beginning with a brief descriptive history of nursing as it relates to ethics, Part I, *Guides for Principled Behavior,* presents ethical theories, models, and principles that serve as guides for principled behaviour. Part II, *Developing Principled Behavior,* discusses personal issues, including values clarification, moral development, and ethical decision making. Part III, *Principled Behavior in the Professional Domain,* presents professional and legal overviews and chapters related to specific issues important to contemporary nursing. This section includes discussion about autonomy, authority, accountability, codes of practice, scholarship issues, practice issues related to health care providers, systems within which nurses work, technology, and patient self-determination. Part IV, *Global Issues That Impinge on Nursing Practice,* addresses health care changes and challenges as a background for understanding issues that nurses encounter in the contemporary health care system. Considerations related to political, economic, social, gender, transcultural, and spirituality issues are discussed in light of nursing role, potential dilemmas, and professional practice. Part V, *The Power to Make a Difference,* focuses on developing skills to empower both nurses and patients to make principled choices and act with courage.

Throughout this book, we have chosen to refer to the recipient of nursing care as *patient* rather than *client*. Since nurses function as members of interdisciplinary health care teams and the term *patient* is commonly used by other health providers, using a common language fosters better communication, understanding, and collegiality. In addition, the American Nurses Association (1996) *Nursing's Social Policy Statement* notes that although the term *client* is preferred by some nurses, it implies that the recipient of care is able to choose one nurse from among many, a choice that typically does not occur. We recognize that the term *client, person,* or *individual* may be the better choice in some circumstances and encourage the reader to make that distinction if needed.

Although we have written from the Western perspective, we recognize that our culture is a melding of traditions and people from many other cultures. We have attempted to be sensitive in reflecting transcultural situations and issues. In that vein, you will notice that when referring to the dates of historical events, we have used the designation B.C.E. (Before the Common Era) rather than the more familiar B.C.

This book is meant to be very personal. You should become engaged, examining and questioning your options and values as they relate to real-life situations. As learning is demonstrated by changed behaviour, we hope that you will become a more sensitive, capable, courageous, and responsible decision maker and citizen. We believe with Phyllis Kritek (1994) that "the measure of [one's] character and worth is not whether [one has] avoided making poor choices, but how willing [one is] to learn from these errors in an effort to not repeat them, and how [one elects] to attend to their consequences. . . . Finding meaning, discovering that which is of worth, becomes a searching process where everyone's help is welcome" (pp. 21, 33). This book is offered as a guide to help in the process of learning to make sound choices and act in principled ways in both personal and professional realms. As you use this book, we echo the same sentiment voiced by Florence Nightingale in the preface to her *Notes on Nursing:* "I do not pretend to teach her how, I ask her to teach herself, and for this purpose I venture to give her some hints" (1859, preface).

REFERENCES

American Nurses Association. (1996). *Nursing's social policy statement*. Washington, DC: Author.

Frankl, V. E. (1984). *Man's search for meaning* (Rev. ed.). New York: Washington Square Press.

Kritek, P. B. (1994). *Negotiating at an uneven table: A practical approach to working with difference and diversity*. San Francisco: Jossey-Bass.

Nightingale, F. (1859). *Notes on nursing: What it is, and what it is not*. London: Harrison & Sons.

NOTES FOR THE CANADIAN EDITION

In this first Canadian edition of *Ethics and Issues in Contemporary Nursing*, we have made a number of changes throughout the book to ensure that the content and cases reflect the realities of nursing and health care in Canada. The chapter on legal issues has been completely revised to reflect the Canadian legal system, both at a federal and at provincial levels. We have also included landmark legal-ethical cases from Canada. The newest revisions of the *Canadian Nurses Association Code of Ethics for Registered Nurses,* the *International Council of Nurses Code of Ethics* and the *Canadian Charter of Rights and Freedoms* appear as appendices.

In our discussions of nursing as a regulated profession, we have ensured that the provincial regulatory bodies are noted. We have also taken care to ensure that the kinds of issues reflected in our cases and discussions of the practice of nursing reflect the diversity of practice across our country.

In our discussions of integrity, we have included definitions of academic integrity from a number of prominent Canadian university nursing programs. We have also ensured that the discussions of research integrity refer to the newest draft of Canada's Tri-Council Policy Statement (2008).

Finally, throughout the book, we have included more life cases and made certain that they include modern Canadian health care issues and challenges as well as the realities of nursing in Canada.

INSTRUCTOR'S RESOURCES

Instructor's Resource CD (ISBN: 0-17-647540-0)

The Instructor's Resource CD-ROM contains the Instructor's Manual, Test Bank, Computerized Test Bank, and PowerPoint® presentation. Details about each supplement are provided below.

Instructor's Manual

Adapted by Paula Crawford-Dickinson of George Brown College, the Instructor's Resource Manual to accompany the first Canadian edition of *Ethics and Issues in Contemporary Nursing* provides instructors with additional instructional strategies, teaching aids and resources, ideas for critical reflection exercises, Web links, and test questions.

For each chapter in the text, this manual provides (1) an overview, which briefly describes the importance of the content for nurses; (2) instructional strategies; (3) selected teaching aids and resources; and (4) a critical reflection exercise.

Test Bank

Adapted by Monique Bacher of George Brown College, the test bank includes 200 multiple choice questions to test your students' knowledge of the concepts and issues addressed in each chapter.

Computerized Test Bank in Exam View®

This computerized testing software helps instructors create and customize exams in minutes. Instructors can easily edit and import their own questions and graphics, change test layouts, and reorganize questions. The Computerized Test Bank is available for both Windows and Macintosh.

Microsoft® PowerPoint® Presentation

Adapted by Carrie Mines of Mohawk College, this presentation features important concepts and key points from the textbook, and is provided for classroom use to enhance your lectures. The PowerPoint® presentation is available on CD and on the website.

U.S. Acknowledgments

The journey of writing a book requires solitude and the companionship and support of many people. We express gratitude to the many friends and colleagues who have encouraged us along the way. Special thanks are due to Mary Jo Butler and Cynthia Persily, who have encouraged scholarship and principled behavior. We are grateful to Barbara C. Banonis, Mary Jo Butler, Sandra L. Cotton, Sr., Barbara Kupchak, Robin Shirley, and Mary Gail Nagai-Jacobson for their chapter contributions, and to Anna Nicoloudakis for secretarial assistance and general support in innumerable ways. Thanks go to all those who gave the time and care to review the manuscript at various stages in the writing process, providing us with helpful comments and guidance.

Finally, we are eternally grateful to our families, Joe Golden and Tim, Josh, and Maggie Nathaniel, for their loving patience, humor, caretaking, and encouragement throughout this challenging and growthful journey.

Canadian Acknowledgments

The author and Nelson Education Ltd. would like to thank the following reviewers for their help in the development of the First Canadian Edition of *Ethics and Issues in Contemporary Nursing*:

Heather McIntosh	Algonquin College
Pasquale Fiore	Camosun College
Sandra McDonald	Memorial University
Carrie J. Mines	Mohawk College
Donna Romyn	Athabasca College
Donna Daines	Thomson Rivers University

I would like to thank Nelson Education, and the following people in particular for making the project enjoyable and possible and for their seemingly endless patience and efforts: Mark Grzeskowiak, Paul Fam, Kevin Smulan, and Susan Wong. I would also like to thank Karen Rolfe and Ruma Khurana for their valuable help in the preparation of this text as well as Dr. Chris MacDonald for his ongoing advice, proofreading and support. I would like to acknowledge the original authors for an already strong and thoughtful text with which to work. Many people supported me in many kinds of ways while I revised and "Canadianized" this textbook. My parents, family and friends were there for me, patiently understanding my frequent absences, work schedules and need for child care on long writing days. Finally, I would like to thank my colleagues and students, who were understanding and supportive of the time I have needed to do this work and who have dropped by my office to offer words of support and encouragement. Without all of these people, the work I have contributed to this textbook would not have been possible. Thank you all.

Contributors

Barbara C. Banonis, MSN, RN
Well-Being Consultant
LifeQuest International
Charleston, WV

Mary Jo Butler, EdD, RN
Former Associate Professor and Director
West Virginia University
School of Nursing, Charleston Division
Charleston, WV

Sandra L. Cotton, MS, RN, C-ANP
Instructor
West Virginia University
School of Nursing
Morgantown, WV

Sr. Barbara Kupchak, PhD, RN-C
Associate Professor
West Virginia University
School of Nursing
Morgantown, WV

Mary Gail Nagai-Jacobson, MSN, RN
Director, Healing Matters
San Marcos, TX

GUIDES FOR PRINCIPLED BEHAVIOUR

Part I lays a foundation for nurses to begin critically examining issues and systematically participating in ethical decision making. Examining the history and context of nursing in Western cultures, Chapter 1 gives nurses insight into the profession of nursing as part of an overall social system—focusing specifically on the influence of the practice of religion and the status of women in society on the profession. Recognizing that knowledge of ethical theories and principles can help the nurse to develop a cohesive and logical system for making individual decisions, Chapters 2 and 3 describe philosophical stance, various classic ethical theories, and ethical principles.

CHAPTER 1

Social, Philosophical, and Other Historical Forces Influencing the Development of Nursing

OBJECTIVES

After completing this chapter, the reader should be able to:

1. Discuss the relationship between social need and the origin of the profession of nursing.

2. Briefly discuss the relationship between moral reasoning and the origin of nursing.

3. Describe the mutually beneficial relationship between the broader society and its professions.

4. Explain the effect of a culture's prevailing belief system on the practice of nursing.

5. Identify how issues such as gender, spiritual beliefs, and religious practices have influenced the evolution of nursing.

6. Discuss how the historical background of the status of women in various cultures is related to the practice of nursing.

7. Make plausible inferences relating the evolution of the practice of nursing to the current state of the profession.

INTRODUCTION

Nursing has been called the "morally central health care profession" (Jameton, 1984, p. xvi). Although the development of the profession is difficult to trace, moral action is the historical basis for the creation, evolution, and practice of nursing. The spirit and substance of nursing are based on social and individual moral codes. In this chapter, we look at three historical influences on nursing as a moral discipline— social need, spirituality/religion, and the role of women.

Morals and ethics affect nursing on different levels. As nurses, our motivation to care for others is underpinned by moral reasoning. Collectively, moral beliefs of groups of people produce rules of action, or ethics. These culturally accepted rules are an integral part of both the experience and the profession of nursing. Expressions of ideals, discussions of moral issues, statements of moral principles, and codes of ethics are found throughout the history of nursing. In addition, Jameton (1984) says nursing is morally worthy work since "caring for and treating the sick, and comforting and protecting the suffering, are basic benefits of human culture" (p. 1). As our modern health care technology extends the boundaries of what is possible, all of society is challenged to examine emerging ethical issues. We are faced with ethical tension in a health care system that requires moral decision making, yet sometimes restricts us from legitimate decision-making roles. We examine the history of nursing to help understand our position within the contemporary health care system and the evolution of nursing as a moral profession.

One of our purposes in writing this text is to present nursing ethics in a manner that will encourage empowered decision making. In an examination of nursing empowerment, Fulton (1997) proposes that nurses' perspectives are distorted and constrained by historical forces that impart negative messages. According to Stevens, these distortions and constraints "impede free, equal and uncoerced participation in society" (1989, p. 58). Struggling to cope with impossible situations, nurses continue to believe negative messages about themselves and behave in ways that are neither constructive nor empowered (Roberts, 1983; Hedin, 1986). In other words, we can understand our present situation only in relation to our social and professional history (Harden, 1996). These ideas are related to critical social theory as proposed by Habermas (1971) and Freire (1972). The basic principle of critical social theory is that we can understand each aspect of a social phenomenon only in relation to the history and structure in which it is found. The significance of ideas can be grasped only when we remove ourselves and objectively view them in the context of historical and social practices and entanglements of power and interest (McCarthy, 1990). Habermas (1971) proposes that as individuals we can assess the evidence and fully participate only when we are aware of, and free from, the hidden oppressions that are working on our lives. Insights gained from the study of nursing history enable us to see these conditions for what they are and find ways of interpreting and releasing them in order to move forward. To this end, we present some selected historical and social forces that have shaped the contours of our profession.

It is difficult to establish a clear picture of the development of the profession of nursing through history. Medicine and nursing both emerged from a long history of healers. It is not possible for us to know the exact origin of either profession, since the earliest stages of each are so closely interwoven (Donahue, 1996). Even so, we know that the history of nursing is one in which people—usually women—have attempted to relieve suffering. Selanders writes, "Nursing's history is one of people, both ancient and modern. It has not evolved solely because of one individual or one event or with directed purpose. Rather, nursing's current status represents a collective picture of societal evolution in a health care framework" (Selanders, 1998a, p. 227). From the beginning, the motivation of nurses to care for others came from practical, moral, or spiritual influences. Our history is also the story of a profession inescapably linked to the status of women and changing notions of gender and power. The history of healers, and subsequently that of nurses, has gone through many phases and has been an important part of social movements. Ours is a narrative of a professional group whose status has always been affected by the prevalent standards of society (Donahue, 1996).

THE INFLUENCE OF SOCIAL NEED

Helping professions find their origin, purpose, and meaning within the context of culturally accepted moral norms, individual values, and perceived social need. By serving others, and responding to their need, we express moral belief. The term **moral thought** relates to the thoughtful examination of right and wrong, good and bad. Moral reasoning includes any level of this type of thinking. It may be complex and well developed, or it may be rudimentary. Why do we care about moral issues? Some moral philosophers propose that empathy is a motive for moral reasoning and action. For example, if we visualize the suffering of another person, we begin to imagine ourselves suffering. Some describe the desire to help others as a natural outcome of social consciousness and motivation similar to the golden rule, "Do unto others as you would have them do unto you." A universally popular precept, the "Golden Rule" is found in some form in most major moral traditions (Honderich, 1995). Some say that we follow the "Golden Rule" both to help someone in need and, to some degree, in the hope that someone will show us consideration if we are unfortunate enough to find ourselves in similar circumstances. Whatever our original motivation, ethical action is based on a desire to help others and the desired outcome of the action is the same: meeting the health needs of others. As the morally central health care profession, nursing has historically responded to human suffering.

It is likely that at least some members of the hypothetical community described in the *Ask Yourself* exercise below will recognize the importance of helping those in need. These people will begin to exercise moral thinking as they examine their beliefs. Ethics will emerge in the form of rules of action that are specifically related to solving the moral problem. Those committed to helping the ill will devise methods to utilize individual abilities to the best advantage, and fairly distribute the burden of providing services and resources. As this example implies, nursing can be described as a profession that exists to meet certain needs of individuals and groups, and thus is a product of the moral reasoning of people in society.

Ask Yourself

What Is the Motivation for Helping?

Imagine a utopian world in which all people are happy and healthy, and have satisfying relationships. There is neither illness nor death. Each person's needs are entirely met without the help of other people. Within this model society, because everyone is satisfied, healthy, and happy, there is no social disorder and no need for any helping profession: no police, doctors, nurses, lawyers, or social workers. Neither is there need for moral discernment. Now, imagine the social disorder that would follow the introduction of serious disease. Individuals who become ill are unable to care for themselves and to meet their own basic needs.

- How should society deal with this problem?
- Are the ill entirely responsible for themselves?
- Should unaffected members of society continue to live the utopian existence, ignoring the suffering of others, or is the whole of society responsible for helping those in need?
- Should society allow the diseased members to suffer, or do healthy members act to help those afflicted, thus altering their own "perfect" lives—and in turn the prevailing social order?

As we will see in later chapters, the needs of society at a given time combined with the technological capabilities and knowledge base determine the existence and parameters of a profession. Societies establish dynamic boundaries of a profession that move and change as needs change. Our profession is a part of society and, to continue to exist, our professional interest must continue to aim to serve interests of individuals, families, groups and communities (International Council of Nurses, 2006).

Think About It

What Makes People Service Oriented?

- Why do you think people are motivated to help those who are in need?
- The actions of those who choose to help others in specific situations might be described as based on self-interest, altruism, or a combination of other motives. How would you describe the motivation to care for others within the healing professions today?
- Think about your own reasons for entering nursing. What were they? Are they the same today?

The nursing profession was created by society for the purpose of meeting specific health needs. In response, the profession has made an implicit promise to ensure, by various means, that members are competent to provide the service, and further, that these are the *only* members of society who can qualify to provide the service. The relationship of social need and our motivation to care for others is complementary. It is fortunate that human nature is such that some of us, for whatever reason, are interested in serving others.

GENDER AND SPIRITUAL INFLUENCES

Gender Influences. One of the most critical factors that influences nursing practice is the role of women in society. In every culture women have traditionally been healers. Because nursing has generally been a profession of women (from the beginning, the majority of nurses have been women), women's status in society is central to determining the extent of freedom and respect granted to nurses. Contours of the profession have been shaped, in large part, by social forces that determine gender roles in society. As a result of the perception that women are more humane and more caring by nature, they have been viewed as naturally endowed with nursing talents. Even Florence Nightingale wrote, "Every woman . . . has, at one time or another of her life, charge of the personal health of somebody, whether child or invalid—in other words, every woman is a nurse" (Nightingale, 1859, preface). Gender stereotyping has been both a blessing and a curse to nursing.

It has also created discouragement and, at times, barriers for males wishing to enter the nursing profession. Because nursing is labelled by some as a calling that is inherently female instead of a legitimate and highly skilled profession, male nurses often find themselves ridiculed or challenged. As well, even in today's world, society may allow or fail to allow women to assume roles of knowledge and authority, roles that allow independent decision making or even limited participation in decision-making processes. One would hope that today, in a world with both an increased awareness of the unique skills and knowledge of nursing alongside more progressive notions of gender, these would no longer be issues. Unfortunately, they are.

Spiritual/Religious Influences. The spiritual and religious foundation of past and present cultures has influenced many aspects of health care. Spiritual belief and religious practice have made major contributions to the moral foundation of nursing and other healing professions; they have also influenced both the gender and, to some degree, much of the activity of healers. Spirituality and religious doctrine have also influenced beliefs about the value of individuals, life, death, and health. Historically, many of the dominant religious institutions have made judgments about the origin and essence of healing and endorsed (and sometimes certified) those who would hold positions as legitimate healers. The path that nursing has taken since ancient times has not been smooth. There have been advances and setbacks; libraries have been destroyed; widely diverse groups have held the title of nurse; and those who were the nurses in some early cultures left few records. Nevertheless, nursing in some form has existed in every culture, and has been influenced by spiritual beliefs, religious practices, and related cultural values.

There are documented periods in history in which women were the honoured sole practitioners of the healing arts, and there were periods in which women were forced into submissive and subservient healing roles. It remains that the status of women and the role of nurses in society have always been intertwined. This is sometimes referred to as the feminization of nursing. Although there are more males in nursing and recognition of nursing as a profession not necessarily tied to gender in the modern world, some of these more archaic beliefs still persist.

Ancient Times

To examine nursing from a historical perspective, we must keep in mind that, throughout history, the sociological view of gender and the historical connection between spirituality and healing have both influenced the evolution of health care and nursing. While we can and must separate Church and state in the modern view of health care and health care ethics, throughout history, religion and spirituality have played greater roles in how nursing care is considered and delivered and how moral dilemmas in health care have been approached and solved.

We will begin by looking at nursing and health in the Middle Ages, a significantly large expanse of time from the fall of the Roman Empire in the fifth century until approximately the sixteenth century, the dawn of the early Modern Age. While there is much to document about ancient times and the early Middle Ages in terms of healing and views of illness, we see more evidence of direct influence on nursing in Canada from the later Middle Ages onward. Trends such as the translation of important writings by Aristotle, the rise of Islamic science (in which we find the first public hospitals and lending libraries, for example) urbanization and the establishment of universities are all fundamentally important in how we view and experience health care and nursing today.

The Middle Ages

The Middle Ages was a time of great change and growth for the scientific and political landscape of Western Europe. During this time, the urbanization of much of Northern and Western Europe occurred, and many political geographical boundaries that persist today were established. But most of all, this millennium was a period of significant scientific change, with great influence from the Islamic Golden Age, a period from approximately the eighth century to the twelfth or the sixteenth century, according to different scholars. While Western Europe was concerned with spreading urbanization and heading toward the Crusades, much of the Islamic world was making advances in science and technology, including astronomy, medicine, and research, as well as the establishment of degree-granting universities. Obviously, some of these key events have influenced European and modern global history.

As the early Middle Ages began, many people believed that the world was falling into ruin. During this time, disease, large-scale food shortages, and war interacted to produce a predictable sequence: war drove farmers from their fields and destroyed their crops; destruction of the crops led to famine; and the starved and weakened people were easy victims to the onslaught of disease (Cartwright, 1972). The established social structure was deteriorating, and disorganized communities turned to feudalism and monasticism. During this time, monasticism and other religious groups offered the only opportunities for men and women to pursue careers in nursing. Much of hospital nursing was carried out by repentant women and widows called sisters and by male nurses called brothers. Deaconesses, matrons, and secular nursing orders were among the organized groups that had religious foundations and offered nursing services.

According to Dolan, these early nurses, mainly in Western Europe, believed they were following the command of God to imitate Jesus, who spent his life ministering to those in need. For many, this service was viewed as a means of securing salvation. Dolan quotes the Sisters of Charity founder Saint Louise De Marillac, who wrote in a letter dated 1633, "We do not want those who have no desire to work at their spiritual perfection in the service of God. They should have no motive in coming except the one of serving God and their neighbor" (1973, p. 100). Women who entered nursing orders donated their property and wealth to the Christian Church and devoted their lives to service. Believing that "charity" was synonymous with "love," they sold their possessions and gave everything to the Church or the poor. Although in many cases "nursing" care was given by slaves or servants, religious orders offered the only route through which respectable women and men could serve as nurses.

The overall belief system of a culture influences the extent to which members accept various healing methods and health care practices. An example of this can be seen in historical accounts of the healing arts in the Middle Ages. The term **empirical** relates to knowledge gained through the processes of observation and experience. Many people, especially those involved with the Christian Church, had deeply anti-empirical beliefs. Consequently, people were more likely to seek healing through religious intervention, touching of religious relics, visiting of sacred places, chanting, and other methods approved by the Church. Because of religious fervour at the time in Christian Europe, empirical treatment (particularly if provided by anyone not explicitly sanctioned by the

Church), even if it was successful, was thought to be produced by the devil, since the position of the Church was that only God and the devil had the power to either cause illness or promote healing.

Beginning in 1096 the Crusades were military campaigns driven by mostly Christian Western Europe against opponents, such as the Muslims, Jews, those identified as pagans, the Greek Orthodox church, and anyone else viewed as a political or ideological enemy of the papal legacy. Much has been written about the Crusades and, while they are seen as religious wars, they were very much about ideologies, beliefs, and political power associated with religion. During these times, religion was very much the mechanism with which political power was sought and gained. The Crusades lasted nearly two hundred years and brought many changes in the health of the population. The effects of the crusades were long lasting and far reaching, and include religious, social, and political consequences and divides, some of which can be seen still today. The Crusades engendered much resentment against Christianity and isolation of other religious sects. Many scientific, technological, and philosophical advances were claimed, without legitimacy, in the name of Christianity. Many groups joined and fought together, either alongside the Christians, or against the Christian crusaders. Some of these alliances created historical bonds while deep crevasses were created between fighting groups, many of which persist today.

As well, the holy wars led to deplorable sanitary conditions, fatigue, poor nutrition, diarrhea, and the spread of communicable diseases. These health problems led to a need for more hospitals and greater numbers of health care providers. In response to the compelling need, military nursing orders were formed. These orders drew large numbers of men into the field of nursing (Dolan, 1973).

Another direct result of the Crusades was the collection of relics by the Christian Church. Believed to offer the potential of healing miracles, the spoils of war included body parts of Crusade martyrs. Through their sale the Church obtained significant wealth and power. Achterberg (1990) compares this time to an earlier Roman mythology in which large numbers of deities or sainted mortals, their relics, and pilgrimages to their sacred sites were believed to hold the key to health.

For most of the Middle Ages, the Roman Catholic Church held tremendous influence over the people and governments of European countries. Powerful leaders within the Church determined the appropriateness of various healing practices. Official credentialling of physicians, nurses, and midwives was left in the hands of the Church. Even after civic legislation became common, the Church continued to enforce the law and monitor practitioners (Achterberg, 1990). As we will see in the following section, this power was also used to enforce religious doctrine related to the status of women in society.

Accounts of the actual treatment of patients in early times vary. In some hospitals operated by religious orders, patients were treated as welcome guests. People sometimes pretended to be ill to be admitted. In contrast, there are reports that some groups of patients were treated inhumanely, even by members of nursing orders. If these nurses believed their duty was to God and to the spiritual rather than physical needs of the patients, they may have been less attentive to physical, emotional, and comfort needs.

For centuries the treatment of persons with mental illnesses was based on the idea that they were possessed by devils or that they were being punished for their sins (Dolan, 1973). They were often put in chains, starved, and kept under filthy conditions. There was even a time when it was thought that torture was useful in driving out what was labelled at that time as "madness." Because the public perception of mental illness was based on religious beliefs related to demon possession and punishment for sin, the mentally ill were treated inhumanely.

During the Middle Ages, the status of women also declined in much of Christian Europe. In many ways this was directly related to Christian doctrine. St. Thomas Aquinas, ironically known within the Christian Church as the "angelic doctor" (Donahue, 1996), wrote that one should "only make use of a necessary object, woman, who is needed to preserve the species or to provide food and drink. . . . Woman was created to be man's [helper], but her unique role is in conception . . . since for all other purposes men would be better assisted by other men" (Thomas Aquinas as cited by Achterberg, 1990, p. 68). Centuries earlier, another Church leader, St. Jerome, frequently recognized for his support of matrons in their calling as nurses, remarked that "woman is the gate of the devil, the path of wickedness, the sting of the serpent, in a word a perilous object" (Heer, 1961, p. 322). These religious leaders were setting the stage for the persecution of women, which would last for hundreds of years and leave a persistent legacy of misogyny.

During the Middle Ages, religious and Christian Church–sanctioned secular nursing orders afforded the only legitimate avenue for women wishing to be nurses. The Church popularized the ideals of virginity, poverty, and a life of service. By the end of the thirteenth century, an estimated 200 000 women served as nurses within these orders (Achterberg, 1990). Caring for pilgrims in improvised infirmaries and clinics, women's nursing orders were particularly welcome during the Crusades. As was often the case, these orders were subordinate to the men's communities (Donahue, 1996). Nevertheless, some speculate that within the structure of the Church, these women exercised a degree of independence and autonomy. There is no doubt that they made a great contribution to the health care of the time.

During the Middle Ages, the Christian Church and the newly formed medical profession were actively engaged in the elimination of lay female healers. Women were excluded from newly formed degree-granting universities. Except for those devoting their lives to serving in religious nursing orders, women were not allowed by the Church to practise the healing arts. During a revival of learning in the thirteenth century, the Church imposed strict controls on the new profession of medicine and officially prohibited women from its practice (Achterberg, 1990, p. 15). Nevertheless, some women continued to secretly practise the healing arts, both within and outside the home. They used knowledge handed down for generations, intuitive knowledge, and empirical knowledge.

It was a popular religious view that women were essentially evil by nature. The pain of childbirth was believed to be punishment, and served the purpose of reminding women of their original sinful nature according to Christian doctrine. Those who dared provide pain relief to others during childbirth were severely punished (Achterberg, 1990). One can only speculate about the role of empathy in caring for labouring women during these difficult times. Later, the Original Sin of Eve would be used to justify torturing and murdering thousands of women during witch hunts.

Although the medical profession was officially sanctioned by the Christian Church, and male physicians were beginning to be trained in the university setting, there was scant scientific knowledge. Physicians relied solely on superstition (Ehrenreich & English, 1973). University-trained physicians used bloodletting, astrology, alchemy, and incantations. Their patients were almost exclusively wealthy. Physicians' treatments were usually ineffective, often dangerous, and inaccessible to the majority of the poor.

Much of the time, during and after the Crusades, people formed small communities around lords or "masters," who were often bishops or barons, usually with power related to land ownership or religion. In this feudal system, life for those who were lowest in the hierarchy was difficult. Peasants or serfs often worked on the land and, in exchange, were offered a safe haven by the lord. At the times of the Crusades, safety and defence were priorities for most. With the formation of any community, town, or small city, problems related to hygiene and sanitation are bound to occur. In the feudal system, peasants or serfs had serious problems related to poor sanitation and hygiene. Without antibiotics, the discovery of which would not occur until centuries later, most people died of infections, exposure, and diseases.

At this time, beliefs around the causes of illness and death were grounded in the concepts from the ancient Greek and Roman civilizations, and often tied to religious and spiritual beliefs. Concepts such as the four humours were popular notions of how the body worked. Directly related to the environment, the four humours existing in the human body were considered to be related to fire (yellow), earth (black bile), water (phlegm), and air (blood). Illness and death were thought to be related to an imbalance of humours or to "sins of the soul," and most treatments for ailments were related to creating balance in the humours through methods such as bloodletting, pilgrimages, and praying.

Peasant women were often the only healers for people who had no doctors and suffered bitterly from poverty and disease (Ehrenreich & English, 1973). These folk healers had extensive knowledge about cures that had been handed down for generations via oral tradition. They constantly improved their practice through empirical methods of observation, trial, and evaluation. While physicians continued to rely on superstition, these women developed an extensive understanding of bones and muscles, herbs, drugs, and midwifery (Barstow, 1994; Ehrenreich & English, 1973). Some authorities believed these peasant folk healers were actually practising some form of magic or witchcraft (Barstow, 1994). Others now speculate that women were honouring the old pagan religions, and worshiping the old gods who (to Church authorities) assumed the persona of the devil (Achterberg, 1990). It is likely that these women were simply assuming caring and curing roles in a manner that was consistent with prevailing folk belief. After all, almost everyone in medieval Europe believed in the reality of magic (Barstow, 1994). This atmosphere set the stage for Christian Church–sanctioned crimes against women in the form of the witch hunts.

In a sweep across Europe, the witch hunts lasted from the fourteenth to the seventeenth century. The atmosphere that led to the witch hunts was a critical mixture of war, disease, and poverty, combined with religious fervour, superstition, and political unrest. The witch trials were accomplished through an organized partnership among the Christian Church, state, and the emerging medical profession. Women, particularly women healers, represented a political, religious, and sexual threat to both Church and state, which were, during the middle ages, tightly bound together. An atmosphere of superstition and widespread belief in magic set the stage that would allow terrible crimes to be perpetrated against women (Achterberg, 1990; Barstow, 1994; Ehrenreich & English, 1973).

Armed with papal authorization to purge Germany of witches, Dominican inquisitors Kramer and Sprenger wrote *Malleus Maleficarum* (Barstow, 1994). In this witch hunters' manual, Kramer and Sprenger expressed virulent anti-feminine and anti-sexual opinions. They claimed that women are "liars, more superstitious than men, more impressionable, wicked minded, and in need of constant male supervision" (Barstow, 1994, p. 172). They wrote, "If a woman dare to cure without having studied she is a witch and must die" (Kramer & Springer as cited by Ehrenreich & English, 1973, p. 19); "No one does more harm to the Catholic Church than midwives" (p. 13). They also wrote, "When a woman thinks alone, she thinks evil. . . . Women are intellectually like children" (Barstow, 1994, p. 172). Kramer and Sprenger defined witchcraft as treason against God, and described it as female rebellion. According to Barstow, "the document reeks with fear and hatred of women, concluding with thanks to God 'who has so far preserved the male sex from so great a crime'" (1994, p. 62). The most authoritative document used by witch hunters, the *Malleus Maleficarum* was printed in four languages and at least twenty-nine editions between the years of 1486 and 1669 C.E.

What were the crimes of which the women were accused? Any woman who treated an illness, even if she applied a soothing salve to the diseased skin of her child, was likely to be accused of witchcraft. If the treatment failed, she was thought to have cursed the patient. If the treatment succeeded, she was believed to be in consort with the devil. Although women were permitted to practise midwifery (no one else wanted to do it), these women were in danger of being accused of witchcraft if anything went wrong with either mother or baby.

No one knows how many women were killed during the witch trials. When records were kept, they were abysmal. Often names were not used, and occasionally the verdict and sentence were not recorded. The most authoritative estimate of the number of executions is 200 000, although some estimates are as high as ten million. Women comprised 85 percent to 95 percent of those killed (Barstow, 1994). During the twelfth century in Russia, when looking for witches, authorities simply rounded up all the women in an area. Some small European towns were left with one woman or no women at all (Achterberg, 1990; Barstow, 1994; Ehrenreich & English, 1973).

It is difficult to comprehend the effect of the witch hunts on European society. Women had silently watched the public humiliation, torture, disfigurement, and death of other women. Barstow believes that this public acknowledgment of the evil nature of the female sex left all women humiliated and frightened. Because both the accused and those viewing the proceedings were powerless to prevent the torture and executions, the witch craze served to undermine women's belief in the ability and power of women. Indeed, this was likely the inference made by all of society. Achterberg writes, "women were never again given full citizenship in any country, nor was their role in the healing professions reinstated" (1990, p. 98). Even after the end of this terrible time, women were prohibited from independent healing professions by law in every country in Europe. This created a climate by which, under the protection and patronage of the ruling classes, males became the authoritative medical professionals (Ehrenreich & English, 1973). Although accounts of the witch hunts are absent in most popular nursing history texts, these events probably influenced the future of the profession more than any other single factor. As Ehrenreich and English write, "It was to become a theme of our history" (1973, p. 6).

The Renaissance and the Reformation

The sixteenth century heralded the beginning of two great movements: the Renaissance and the Reformation. Resulting from a revolutionary spirit and quest for knowledge, the Renaissance produced an intellectual rebirth that began the scientific era. The Reformation was a religious movement precipitated by the widespread abuses that had become a part of Christian Church life and doctrinal disagreement among religious leaders (Donahue, 1996).

The Renaissance gave birth to the scientific revolution and a new era in the healing arts. Beginning its gradual escape from the control of the Church, the scientific community made advances in mathematics and the sciences. René Descartes is credited with proposing a theory that quickly altered philosophic beliefs about the separation of mind and body. He proposed that the universe is a physical thing, and that everything in the universe is like a machine, which can be analyzed and understood. Descartes further theorized that the mind and body are separate entities (Durant, 1926), and that people are set against a world of objects that they must seek to master (McCarthy, 1990). Based on Descartes' work, **Cartesian philosophy** began to replace religious beliefs related to the physical and spiritual realms of humankind. As a direct result, a separation was created between the acts of caring and curing in the healing arts. The arrival of this philosophy, while elevating the sciences and making scientific inquiry possible, did not improve the status of nursing. Achterberg identifies this time as an important turning point. Regarding Cartesian philosophy, she says, "When spirit no longer is seen to abide in matter, the reverence for what is physical departs. Hence medicine no longer regarded itself as working in the sacred spaces where fellow humans find themselves in pain and peril, and where transcendence is most highly desired" (1990, p. 103). As Cartesian philosophy became popular, nurses' place in the health care system became limited to the "caring" realm. Caring was given lower priority than curing within the hierarchy of the healing arts. Some would argue that this legacy remains with nursing yet today.

In Canada, the earliest records of nursing begin in the seventeenth century, just after Jacques Cartier and Samuel Champlain's historic voyages to establish the settlements along the St. Lawrence River that would later become Canada, but which were then known as New France.

At the time of the establishing settlements, there were a number of prevailing systems of health care. Aboriginal persons living in the region had traditional healing methods, with remedies and treatments specific to their culture and beliefs. Other health care was provided by male priests who immigrated to New France and, while promoting Christianity, found themselves also caring for the ill and dying. While their main goal was promoting Christianity, they found that they needed help caring for the sick and sent pleas back to France for nurses to join the new settlements and help provide care, thus freeing the time and energies of the priests to carry out their missions.

The nursing traditions in Canada were by and large established with influence by France, not Britain. At that time, there were significant differences between the state of nursing as a profession or activity of women in Britain and France. In Britain, during the latter part of the Reformation when the struggle between the Catholic and Protestant groups were greatest, religious tensions between the Christian Church and the monarchy resulted in widespread rejection of the Catholic Church and subsequent release of nursing care from the nuns into the hands of incompetent staff. According to Donahue (1996), law and customs in Protestant countries discouraged the humane care of the "downtrodden and the weak" (p. 193). As religious orders were driven out of hospitals, conditions became deplorable and, in Britain, it was known as the "Dark Period of Nursing" (Donahue, 1996).

In Canada laywomen such as Marie Rollet Hébert came to assume nursing roles and be trained in providing care for the sick and dying. Her attitude towards Aboriginal persons and their practices established her as compassionate and open minded. She demonstrated respect for their belief and practices, and collaborated with them on providing health care, which was novel at the time. Instead of trying to change their beliefs or convince them to adopt different practices, she embraced the differences in beliefs and practices, and shared resources.

Jeanne Mance was another noteworthy woman in early nursing in Canada. One of the first female settlers, she was responsible for the first hospital establishment in the New World, what we now know as Hôtel-Dieu de Montréal, in 1645. Although like Marie Hébert, she was a laywoman, her hospital was staffed by nurses who belonged to the religious order Sisters of St. Joseph. She is seen as not only the founder of a hospital, but also one of the founders of the city of Montréal.

Later, into the modern era, women such as Marguerite D'Youville. Ethel Bedford Benwich, and Florence Nightingale all had important roles in the development of Canadian nursing.

THE MODERN ERA

Nursing as we known it today in North America began to emerge in the modern era. Known as the founder of modern nursing, Florence Nightingale (1820–1910) in her life and writing reflects the influence of the Renaissance and Reformation. Even though she was devoutly religious, Nightingale worked to free nursing from the bonds of the Christian Church, which she called "an over busy mother" (Roberts & Group, 1995). As a person, Nightingale remains an enigma. As a nurse, she remains a pioneer: researcher, leader and scholar. She saw nursing as a profession separate from the Church, yet she began her career as the result of a mystic experience (Simkin, 2001). According to Nightingale, God spoke to her four times, calling her into his service when she was sixteen years old (Selanders, 1998b). Her experience in the Crimean War was the direct result of her second revelation, which she termed a call from God (Showalter, 1981; Dossey, 2000). Although she was opposed to using church affiliation as a criterion for admission to nursing programs, her religious beliefs were evident in her practice and beliefs about nursing care. Nightingale's description of nursing as "caring for the mind and the body" was one of the first references to holistic nursing in the modern era.

Florence Nightingale became a model for all nurses. She was a nurse, statistician, sanitarian, social reformer, and scholar. She was politically astute, intelligent, and single minded. Contrary to accepted Victorian social order, Florence Nightingale addressed moral issues with courage and conviction. Additionally, she rebelled against the traditional expectations for women of that era: to become good wives and mothers. Her work was foundational in many ways. During the Crimean War, the rates of soldiers dying from poor living conditions and ailments related to sanitation and hygiene was incredibly high. Nightingale, on the front lines, recognized the importance of clean conditions in which to eat and provide nursing care, with separation between the clean and dirty areas of the soldiers' camps. What is basic knowledge to us today, when introduced and operationalized by Nightingale (her nurses went to work rearranging the camps and cleaning), remarkably decreased the mortality rate of soldiers on the front lines. Nightingale provided clear support and evidence of what eventually became known as the germ theory of disease. Having strong opinions on women's rights, she was not hesitant to challenge the established male hierarchy. Nightingale argued for the removal of restrictions that prevented women from having careers (Simkin, 2001). Her writings instructed nurses to "do the thing that is good, whether it is 'suitable for a woman' or not" (Nightingale, 1859, p. 76). Although some argue that Nightingale was not a feminist, her writings indicate that she felt women should have a more important place in the social structure. She wrote, "Passion, intellect, moral activity—these three have never been satisfied in woman. In this cold and oppressive conventional atmosphere, they cannot be satisfied" (Nightingale, 1852/1979, p. 29). It is certain that she did not ascribe to the popular Cartesian notion that women do not have minds and souls, and are put on the earth solely for man's purpose and pleasure (Roberts & Group, 1995).

Another of nursing's great modern leaders is Lavinia Lloyd Dock (1858–1956). Considered a radical feminist, Dock actively engaged in social protest, picketing, and parading for women's rights (Roberts & Group, 1995). She was concerned with the many problems plaguing nursing, warning that male dominance in the health field was the major problem confronting the nursing profession. Lavinia Dock's contemporaries ignored her concerns, and twentieth- and twenty-first-century nurses have found themselves fighting the same battles.

During this time, the force of nursing was moving through the country as settlement into the West increased. With the leadership of the Grey Nuns, missions were established throughout the West and nursing became a part of quality health care available to new settlers.

Ethel Fenwick, a British nurse, made a strong case that nurses should have their own professional organizations and that work needed to be done to increase standards for the educational preparation of nurses and to increase respect and legitimacy for the profession of nursing. Her work was fundamental in establishing what we now know as the International Council of Nurses (1899). Furthermore, she influenced the formation of nursing professional associations in both Canada and the United States.

In Canada, Mary Agnes Snively established the first national organization for nurses in 1907, known as the Canadian Society for Superintendents of Training Schools for Nurses. Snively was the first Ontario nurse to be trained in the Nightingale method of nursing. The following year, the Canadian National Association of Trained Nurses (CNATN) was established, again with Snively as president. Some years later, this organization, now with memberships from nursing schools (situated in hospitals) across the country, would become a formal part of the International Council of Nurses, further legitimizing the profession of nursing in Canada. The CNATN later became the Canadian Nurses Association (CNA). Snively was also superintendent of the Toronto General Hospital's School of Nursing and had significant influence on the standing of the profession in Canada, the improvement in hospital-based training of nurses, and the formation of leading nursing groups such as the CNA and professional organizations of nurses in Ontario.

Nursing further evolved as the identified needs and roles emerged. Public health nursing and military nursing were both important thrusts at this time, and significant leadership in both areas was seen in Canadian nursing. Nurses played important roles in both World wars. Nurses held ranks of officers, lost their lives, and tended to the wounded and dying in precarious and gravely dangerous situations. At this time, the image of nursing was described using words such as bravery, courage, loyalty, and dedication (Kalisch and Kalisch 1987). The evolving image of nurse from unskilled helper of the physician to independent and brave professional was an important step in improving the image of nursing in the public eye.

The mid-1900s heralded great advances for nurses. During these decades nurses moved into spheres of professional, social, and political responsibility. Although recurrent themes of paternalism and subjugation continued to affect the nursing profession, twentieth-century women became more politically active. The woman's movement encouraged political, social, and economic action to correct the wrongs suffered by women. Roberts and Group (1995) write that "Nurses' consciousness of their subordinated and oppressed group status became heightened, propelling some nurses to advocate radical role-breaking, risk-taking behaviors" (p. 187). The profession gained acceptance as a legitimate health care force.

After the World wars, the Canadian Red Cross Society provided grants and certification for nurses to become experts in public health nursing through university programs. Both the society and nurses alike recognized that the entrenchment of health care in the hospital system isolated many in communities and focused care on episodic, acute problems. Many persons, it was noted, suffered from chronic, manageable ailments and diseases, which could be better managed outside the hospital system by qualified caregivers, such as public health nurses. Additionally, there was recognition, at that time, of the need for strong well-established public health programs, health education, immunization, hygiene, and care for those living in poverty or without basic determinants of health. This trend is seen as one of the most important in health care today, articulated in documents such as the Lalonde Report (1975), the Epp Report (1986), and the Romanow Commission Report (2002). The most vocal and consistent supporters for strong and well-supported public health programs as well as the most prominent providers of public health today are still nurses. The establishment of the goal of "Health for All by the Year 2000" by the World Health Organization out of the Alma-Ata Declaration in 1978 is being embraced and acted upon by organizations such as the Canadian Nurses Association (2008). The CNA's vision for the future of nursing embraces the varied roles that nurses must play in order to provide holistic care to a diverse and changing Canadian population, ever mindful of the role of public health and the importance of the determinants of health for all Canadians (CNA, 2006). In *CNA's Preferred Future: Health For All,* the CNA states that,

> The need for equitable access has not changed, nor has it been met. And we are also facing new challenges on many fronts: shifting demographics, growing and unmet health needs, human resources shortages, as well as the globalization of economies and diseases. Other trends have created new opportunities through partnerships, research, innovation and evolving technology. The Canadian Nurses Association (CNA) accepts the challenge to re-frame and reinvigorate our approach to health care and human resources issues, from how nurses are educated and licensed to how their competencies are used to best advantage. Nursing education, job design and responsibilities must change as the country moves from the traditional model of treating illness to one that focuses on keeping people well, with both care and support for maintaining health delivered in the community. Making this model of health care a reality will require breaking down divisions within nursing as well as barriers between nursing and other professions. (CNA, 2008)

Many nurses have now claimed legitimate authority to provide independent skilled health care and assume institutional and political leadership positions. Perceiving a health care crisis of growing proportions, and recognizing a need for comprehensive, accessible, and sustainable health care, society challenged established institutions to foster greater use of nurses in expanded roles. Encouraged by a society in which health care has become a scarce resource, nurse practitioners, nurse midwives, and other advanced nurses have begun to assert themselves as independent professionals.

Entering the twenty-first century, nursing in Western culture has been shaped by spirituality and religion, ideas about gender roles, and cultural influences of the past. As a tapestry woven over time, nursing owns the heritage of those early times. Although many nurses have overcome social and institutional barriers to practise as full members of the profession, others continue to struggle within patriarchal, institutional hierarchy. Recognizing the legitimate need for both the caring and curing aspects of healing, nurses, committed to holistic practice, are charged with working together to improve their status and to ensure that the problems of the past are not repeated. Today's health care system is experiencing rapid change. Health care reform and proposed new models of health care delivery offer nurses opportunities and challenges. The position of the professional nurse within these systems is far from assured. Recalling lessons from the past, nurses remain acutely aware of threats to newly won professional recognition.

SUMMARY

Nursing is a profession that was created for the purpose of meeting specific perceived health needs. The profession is bound by the duty to competently meet the needs for which it was created. Individual nurses, therefore, have a duty to uphold the fiduciary commitment involved in being professionals.

In all cultures, the profession has been profoundly influenced by various aspects of gender roles, spirituality, and the dominant values and beliefs. Ideas and notions about health, illness, death, and the provision of care has always been influenced by prevailing ideas arising out of religion, scientific enquiry, philosophy, art, and literature. Sociological and anthropological approaches of examining the role of nursing in societies have uncovered ideas around the status of women and the valuing of feminized work that have had lasting effects on the legitimacy of nursing care and the status of nurses as autonomous professionals. In many cultures, women have been healers. Women's status in societies has directly determined the freedom they are given to become educated, to think and act independently, and to participate fully in the provision of skilled and unique health care. There were periods in history in which women were allowed freedom and responsibility, and there were dark periods in which women lived in subjugation. Even in the modern world, the notion of nursing as women's work persists, not only from a historical perspective but also in the kinds of challenges and unfortunate barriers that many males, seeking to enter nursing, encounter. Nursing today is at a crossroads, free of many of the restrictions and oppressions of the past, yet not fully franchised as a profession with power and authority.

Many religions have strong value-based statements about moral issues at the boundaries of life and death and, by virtue of this, have often had a profound influence on how many people, in the past and today, think about issues in health care. Throughout history, the strong relationship between religion and power has meant that the values of societies often were those espoused by the most powerful. Power gained through religion, historically, has often not been gained legitimately and often at the expense of others' well-being or values. Today, nursing and health care tend to be influenced by the state and not as much by the Church. In countries like Canada, in which there are many religions and belief systems, it is important to realize the historical influence of religion on nursing but to remember that in the modern world, there is not one set of overarching values and beliefs; instead, there is a legitimate and highly valued diversity of ideologies.

CHAPTER HIGHLIGHTS

- Throughout history, spiritual beliefs, religious practice, cultural norms, and political factors have influenced evolutionary changes in nursing. These factors continue to influence the practice of nursing today.
- Social need is the criterion for the existence of all professions.
- Moral reflection is required when desiring to meet the needs of others.

- The practice of nursing is focused on meeting the health care needs of others; therefore, the practice of nursing originates in moral thinking.
- Professions exist to meet the needs of society.
- Society grants professionals the exclusive right to practice within defined parameters.
- Professionals have a reciprocal duty to society to practise competently.
- Because nursing is primarily a profession of women, the social status of women affects the status of the profession.
- The status of the nursing profession determines members' ability to practise with freedom and responsibility.

DISCUSSION QUESTIONS AND ACTIVITIES

1. Talk with nurses and physicians. Ask their opinions about why some people choose to help others in need. In class, analyze and compare the responses.
2. Discuss the historical developments that caused the separation of the professions of medicine and nursing. How were the distinctions drawn as to the boundaries of the professions? How would you change the boundaries today?
3. Search the World Wide Web for information on Florence Nightingale. Pictures and a short history can be found at http://www.sparticus.schoolnet.co.uk/REnightingale.htm.
4. What is the relationship between the role of women in history and the status of nurses?
5. What is the relationship between the role of women today and the status of nurses?
6. Search out a few retired nurses. Ask them to describe the relationship between nurses and physicians in the mid-1900s. How was this related to the roles of women in society during the same time period?
7. Discuss the relationship between the role of nurses in the health care system today and their role in ethical decision making in the clinical setting.
8. Discuss the challenges that the profession of nursing faces related to attaining or maintaining an authoritative role in the health care system of the future.

REFERENCES

Achterberg, J. (1990). *Woman as healer*. Boston: Shambhala Publications.

American Nurses Association. (1980). *Nursing: A social policy statement*. Kansas City, MO: Author.

American Nurses Association. (1996). *Nursing's social policy statement*. Washington, DC: Author.

Barstow, A. L. (1994). *Witchcraze: A new history of the European witch hunts*. San Francisco: HarperCollins.

Canadian Nurses Association. (2006). *Towards 2020: Visions for nursing*. Ottawa: Author.

Canadian Nurses Association (2008). *CNA's preferred future: Health for all.* Ottawa: Canadian Nurses Association. Retrieved/from December 8, 2008 http://www.cna-aiic.ca/CNA/resources/webcastOct8/preferred_future/default_e.aspx.

Cartwright, F. F. (1972). *Disease and history.* New York: Dorset Press.

Dolan, J. A. (1973). *Nursing in society: A historical perspective* (13th ed.). Philadelphia: Saunders.

Dolan, J. A., Fitzpatrick, M. L., & Herrmann, E. K. (1983). *Nursing in society: A historical perspective* (15th ed.). Philadelphia: Saunders.

Donahue, M. P. (1996). *Nursing: The finest art.* St. Louis, MO: Mosby.

Dossey, B. M. (2000). *Florence Nightingale: Mystic, visionary, healer.* Springhouse, PA: Springhouse.

Dubois, A. E. (1921). *La Vénérable Mère d'Youville.* L'Oeuvre des Tracts: Montreal.

Durant, W. (1926). *The story of philosophy.* New York: Washington Square Press.

Ehrenreich, B., & English, D. (1973). *Witches, midwives, and nurses: A history of women healers.* New York: The Feminist Press.

Freire, P. (1993). *Pedogogy of the oppressed* (New rev. 20th Anniversary ed.). New York: Continuum.

Fulton, Y. (1997). Nurses' views on empowerment: A critical social theory perspective. *Journal of Advanced Nursing, 26,* 529–536.

Habermas, J. (1971). *Communication and the evolution of society.* Boston: Beacon Press.

Harden, J. (1996). Enlightenment, empowerment and emancipation: The case for critical pedagogy in nurse education. *Nurse Education Today, 16*(1), 32–37.

Hedin, B. A. (1986). A case study of oppressed group behavior in nurses. *Image: Journal of Nursing Scholarship, 18*(2), 53–57.

Heer, F. (1961). *The medieval world.* New York: New American Library.

Honderich, T., ed. (1995). *The Oxford companion to philosophy.* Oxford, England: Oxford University Press.

International Council of Nurses. (2006). *The ICN code of ethics for nursing.* Geneva: ICN.

Jameton, A. (1984). *Nursing practice: The ethical issues.* Englewood Cliffs, NJ: Prentice-Hall.

Kalisch, P., & Kalisch, B. (1987). *The changing image of the nurse.* Toronto: Addison-Wesley.

McCarthy, T. (1990). The critique of impure reason. *Political Theory, 18*(3), 437–469.

Nightingale, F. (1979). *Cassandra.* Old Westbury, NY: Feminist Press. (Original work published in 1852).

Nightingale, F. (1859). *Notes on nursing: What it is, and what it is not.* London: Harrison & Sons.

Plato. *Republic.*

Roberts, J. I., & Group, T. M. (1995). *Feminism and nursing: An historical perspective on power, status, and political activism in the nursing profession.* Westport, CT: Praeger.

Roberts, S. J. (1983). Oppressed group behavior: Implications for nursing. *Advances in Nursing Science, 5*(4), 21–30.

Selanders, L. C. (1998a). Florence Nightingale: The evolution and social impact of feminist values in nursing. *Journal of Holistic Nursing, 16*(2), 227–243.

Selanders, L. C. (1998b). The power of environmental adaptation: Florence Nightingale's original theory for nursing practice. *Journal of Holistic Nursing, 16*(2), 247–263.

Showalter, E. (1981). Florence Nightingale's feminist complaint: Women, religion, and suggestions for thought. *Journal of Women in Culture and Society, 6*, 395–412.

Simkin, J. *Florence Nightingale*. Retrieved January 14, 2001, from http://www.sparticus.schoolnet .co.uk/REnightingale.htm.

Stevens, P. E. (1989). A critical social reconceptualization environment in nursing: implications for methodology. *Advances in Nursing Science, 11*(4), 56–68.

Zolot, J. S., & Nelson-Hogan, D. (2000). News. *American Journal of Nursing, 100*(10), 32–37.

CHAPTER 2
Ethical Theory

OBJECTIVES

After completing this chapter, the reader should be able to:

1. Discuss the purpose of philosophy.
2. Define the terms "moral philosophy" and "ethics."
3. Discuss the importance of a systematic study of ethics to nursing.
4. Discuss the importance of ethical theory.
5. Describe utilitarianism.
6. Describe deontological ethics, defining the terms "categorical imperative" and "practical imperative."
7. Define the terms "virtue" and "virtue ethics."

INTRODUCTION

At its core, nursing deals with issues and situations that have elements of ethical or moral uncertainty. A growing dependence on technology and the resultant longer lifespans and higher health care costs, coupled with increasing professional autonomy, creates an atmosphere in which we are faced with problems of ever-increasing complexity. We need to be able to recognize situations with ethical and moral implications, and make coherent and logical ethical decisions based upon recognized ethical principles and theory. This text will prepare you to examine issues and in doing so, help you to come to logical, consistent, and thoughtful ethical decisions.

In order to be ethically aware professionals, nurses need to be able to recognize ethical issues and components of practice. This involves four key elements: having an awareness of our own beliefs and values; appreciating the diversity of views on ethical issues; recognizing that an issue is, in fact, an ethical dilemma; and, finally, having some sound basic knowledge of ethical theories and decision-making models.

Although being an ethically aware nurse entails being prepared to engage in ethical decision-making processes as part of a collaborative team, it also means that you must be prepared to examine your own values and beliefs. This can be a challenging and at times enlightening process. It may mean acknowledging that your values or beliefs are different from the institutions or agencies in which you work. It may also mean discovering that your values and beliefs are markedly different from your patients' or your co-workers' beliefs or cultural norms. Of course, this is a necessary and important part of evolving as an ethical professional—taking responsibility for your own beliefs while acknowledging and appreciating diversity. It does require moral courage and a willingness to be open to not only your own views but also others' views and the way in which you might be viewed by others for holding particular opinions or beliefs. It also requires an active avoidance of quick judgment of or assumptions about others. Finally, patience, sensitivity to others' concerns and priorities, and insightfulness are all key attributes of an ethically aware professional nurse, who makes dealing directly with ethical issues a priority in practice.

Ethical problems or dilemmas rarely have an easy answer and often require the most time, effort, and attention to try to sort out. By virtue of being ethical dilemmas, they could be resolved in a number of plausible ways that each might be pleasing to some stakeholders but problematic for others. In order to deal effectively with these types of dilemmas, first learn to recognize when something is in fact an ethical dilemma and not, for example, a purely professional or policy issue. Often ethical issues relate to professional demeanour, practice, or policy, but may not have a clear answer such as we might find in professional codes of ethics, institutional policies, or agency handbooks.

Having knowledge of ethical theories and ethical decision-making models, both of which are provided in this textbook, does not mean that you will find it easier to solve ethical dilemmas that may arise in your practice. However, this kind of knowledge can equip you in approaching an ethical problem in a way that everyone can understand and in which all stakeholders can participate. It may help you identify the most logical, fair, or rational decisions. Ethical theories can help you to understand a markedly different worldview than your own on a specific issue. Decision-making models may help you by taking you step by step through a difficult and complex issue. Furthermore, they may help you identify resources to help you, or alternative points of view that you may not have initially considered.

CASE PRESENTATION

Nursing Students Face an Ethical Dilemma

Santos and Lydia are two senior nursing students assigned to work in the intensive care unit with a critically ill patient. The patient, Mr. Dunn, is an eighty-seven-year-old retired ironworker. He lives alone in an old two-storey frame house. Mr. Dunn is diabetic. He is nearly blind and has moderately advanced prostate cancer and Alzheimer's disease. Mr. Dunn was admitted to the intensive care unit after he was discovered unconscious in his home by a neighbour. At that time he was ketoacidotic and had a very severe necrotic wound on his left leg. The surgeon attending Mr. Dunn is planning amputation of his left leg but has been unable to get consent from either Mr. Dunn or his next of kin, a niece who lives out of town.

Santos is proud of his efficiency as a nursing student. He makes rapid decisions. He insists that Mr. Dunn must have the amputation. He suggests to the physician that he have a substitute decision maker appointed for Mr. Dunn so that the surgery can proceed. The course is clear to him. Lydia, on the other hand, is not certain of the correct course of action. She talks to Mr. Dunn and his niece about his condition. She wonders if the amputation is the best solution to his problem. She thinks about his quality of life after the surgery. She worries about his ability to care for himself and about his state of mind should he be forced to live in a nursing home. She thinks about what she would want for her father if he were in the same situation. Lydia falls asleep at night pondering these thoughts. She does not know how to go about solving the problem. Santos is impatient with Lydia. He sees no benefit to the time and energy spent worrying about this problem when the solution is apparent to him.

In this example, we see nurses at two extremes. Santos makes quick decisions. In all likelihood he fails to recognize the ethical nature of the problem, the bearing the outcome may have on the people involved, or the conflicting possible solutions.

He has great pride in his ability to make decisions, and has confidence in the correctness of those decisions. Lydia, being more insightful and sensitive, recognizes intuitively that the problem presents no clear solution. She is troubled by the situation, but has no tools with which to deal with the predicament. One of the most important first steps to approaching an ethical dilemma is realizing that one exists. While Santos feels that there is a clear solution, he fails to recognize that there is more than one perspective in this situation, creating an ethical dilemma. By identifying that in fact there is no straightforward solution, Lydia has initiated the process of ethical decision making and deliberation. Each of these nurses will benefit from a study of nursing ethics.

? Think About It

Facing Ethical Dilemmas

- What alerts you to the presence of an ethical dilemma?
- How do you feel when confronted with difficult ethical decisions?
- What resources do you use to help you deal with ethical dilemmas?

Ethics and Nursing

Nursing is a profession that deals with the most personal and private aspects of people's lives. From the beginning of time, and by definition, nurses, whether called healers, caretakers, nurturers, or nurses, have cared for those in need in a very personal and intimate way. Nurses are often attentive to patients' needs over long periods of time. They may have made home visits and may know patients' families. They may have ongoing relationships with clients at clinics and community centres. They may care for patients at their bedside for hours and days on end. It is through the intimacy and trust inherent in the nurse–patient relationship that nurses become critical participants in the process of ethical decision making.

As participants in a dynamic profession, we are faced with ethical choices that affect the profession itself. For example, as the needs and demands of society change, boundaries of the domain of nursing contract and expand. This forces us to make decisions about such issues as the delegation of traditional nursing functions to non-nurse caregivers and the expanding boundaries of nursing. Because nursing is a regulated profession, we are obligated to review and discipline peers. This holds many ethical implications as we attempt to balance desires to protect the public, advance the profession, and maintain professional cohesiveness.

Nurses may also be called to take part in decision making on a broader scale. More than ever before, we are participating as members of policy-making bodies. Community, provincial, and national task forces; committees; and boards of advisors are just some of the health care decision-making groups in which nurses have become integral and respected members. It is imperative that nurses participating in decision making at this level be aware of the ethical implications of the decisions, particularly those dealing with the fair allocation of resources. These decisions affect both individuals and populations and, as such, compel those involved to cautiously deliberate every decision. A working knowledge of ethical theory enhances our abilities to deal with difficult ethical dilemmas by allowing us to appreciate diverse perspectives, explore rationale and interests that may be markedly different than ours, and understand our own approach to these kinds of complex issues. While knowledge of ethical theory does not guarantee that ethical decision making will necessarily be easier, it helps to ensure that an ethical dilemma does not become an ethical impasse.

PHILOSOPHY

Philosophy is the intense and critical examination of beliefs and assumptions. It is both natural and necessary to humanity. Philosophy gives coherence to the whole realm of thought and experience. It offers principles for deciding what actions and qualities are most worthwhile. Philosophy may also show inconsistency in meaning and context (Kneller, 1971). There are many philosophical schools of thought. Because of the nature of philosophy, it is impossible to verify philosophic beliefs or theories; nevertheless, the study of philosophy helps give order and coherence to beliefs and assumptions. It gives shape to what would otherwise be a random chaos of thoughts, beliefs, assumptions, values, and superstition.

Philosophers examine questions dealing with life's most important aspects. Typical questions include the following: What is the meaning of life? Is there a God? What is reality? What is the essence of knowledge? How can something be known? What is happiness? What is the ideal or virtuous human character? How can one understand human beliefs, values, and morals? Questions such as these have been asked by the most widely studied philosophers. Buddha asked, "How can one find the path that leads to the end of suffering?" Confucius asked, "What is the remedy for social disorder?" Socrates asked, "How should one live?" Through the centuries philosophy has concerned itself with topics that define the essence of human life. Martin Buber said, "With soaring power [man] reaches out beyond what is given him, flies beyond the horizon and the familiar stars, and grasps a totality" (1965, p. 61).

Ayn Rand, author and social philosopher, expressed her thoughts eloquently when she wrote the following:

> A philosophic system is an integrated view of existence. As a human being, you have no choice about the fact that you need a philosophy. Your only choice is whether you define your philosophy by a conscious, rational, disciplined process of thought and scrupulously logical deliberation—or let your subconscious accumulate a junk heap of unwarranted conclusions, false generalizations, . . . undefined

wishes, doubts and fears, thrown together by chance, but integrated
by your subconscious into a kind of mongrel philosophy and fused
into a single weight: self doubt, like a ball and chain in the place
where your mind's wings should have grown. (1982, p. 5)

Raphael (1994) describes philosophy as essentially divided into two branches: the
philosophy of knowledge and the philosophy of practice. The philosophy of knowledge is attentive to critical examination of assumptions about matters of fact and argument. Included in this branch are epistemology (the study of knowledge), metaphysics
(the study of ultimate reality), philosophy of science, philosophy of the mind, and
philosophical logic. Philosophy of practice, on the other hand, focuses on the critical
examination of assumptions about norms or values and includes ethics, social and
political philosophy, and philosophy of the law. It is philosophy of practice, particularly moral philosophy, that provides a groundwork for discussion of many of the troubling issues facing nurses.

Ethical theory provides a framework to guide cohesive and consistent ethical reasoning and decision making. This chapter is devoted to an examination of the two
ethical theories that have had the greatest influence on contemporary bioethics:
utilitarianism and deontology. A description of virtue or character ethics is also
included. There are many ethical theories, some more sound than others, and some
consisting of combinations of other theories. Theories related specifically to resource
allocation, such as libertarianism, are described in Chapter 15. Nurses who are interested in a more detailed examination of specific theories should read works by the
original theorists as well as analysis by contemporary writers.

MORALS/ETHICS

Ethics is concerned with the study of social morality and philosophical reflection on
its norms and practices. Moral issues are those that are essential, basic, or important,
and deal with important social values or norms, such as respect for life, freedom, and
love; issues that provoke the conscience or such feelings as guilt, shame, self-esteem,
courage, or hope; issues to which we respond with words like *ought, should, right,
wrong, good, bad*; and, issues that are uncommonly complicated, frustrating, unresolv-
able, or difficult in some indefinable way (Jameton, 1984, p. 4). Morality refers to traditions or beliefs about right and wrong conduct (Beauchamp & Walters, 1999). Morality is a social and cultural institution with a history and code of learnable rules. Morality
exists before we are taught its rules—we learn about them as we grow up
(Beauchamp, 2001). **Moral philosophy** is the philosophical discussion of what is considered good or bad, right or wrong, in terms of moral issues.

Ethics addresses the question, "What should I do in this situation?" Ethics offers a
formal process for applying moral philosophy. The study of ethics gives us a groundwork for making thoughtful and consistent decisions. These decisions may be based
upon morality or formal moral theory. In the end, though, ethics does not tell us what
we ought to do. We must decide that for ourselves.

Philosophical Basis for Ethical Theory

Unlike mathematics or other empirical sciences, there are no apparent absolute rules governing ethics. Mathematicians can say for certain that two plus two always equals four, regardless of the time factors, circumstances, feelings, or beliefs of those involved in the calculations. Ethical rules are less clear and difficult or impossible to prove. For example, while some people believe that killing for any reason is always wrong, others might argue that euthanasia can be beneficial either for the individual or the society, that abortion to save the life of the mother is permissible, or that killing during war is justified. There are reasonable arguments, based upon opposing viewpoints, that support any of these beliefs. How can rational people reach such different conclusions? The answer to this question may lie in the particular perspectives of the persons involved.

Ethical theories are derived from either of two basic schools of thought: naturalism or rationalism. An examination of these perspectives will help clarify the various theories.

Ask Yourself

What Is Your Personal Code of Ethics?

- Do you believe that there are some actions that are absolutely wrong in all circumstances? Why?
- Do you believe that you have an innate knowledge of right and wrong?
- How did you learn right and wrong? What was the influence of your parents? Society? Other forces?

Naturalism. **Naturalism** is a view of moral judgment that regards ethics as dependent upon human nature and psychology. Naturalism attributes differences in moral codes to social conditions, while suggesting that there is a basic congruence related to the possession, by nearly all people, of similar underlying psychological tendencies (Raphael, 1994). These similarities suggest that there is universality (or near-universality) in moral judgment. This viewpoint allows each group or person to make judgments based upon feelings about particular actions in particular situations. It further suggests that most people's judgments in similar circumstances will be much alike. Naturalism does not explain what others may consider to be aberrant, selfish, or cruel choices that are made by apparently rational people.

Naturalism holds that, collectively, all people have a tendency to make similar ethical decisions. Though there are many value differences among cultures, the variations are not as great as they may seem. Most people desire to be happy, to experience pleasure, and to avoid pain. There seems to be a natural tendency to sympathize with the wishes and feelings of others and, as a consequence, to approve of helping people in need. Raphael outlines similarities among cultures:

> All societies think that it is wrong to hurt members of their own group at least (or to kill them unless there are morally compelling reasons); that it is right to keep faith; that the needy should be helped; that people who deliberately flout the accepted rules should be punished. (1994, p. 16)

Raphael points to **sympathy** as a motivating factor in moral decision making. Sympathy is sharing, in imagination, of others' feelings. This entails imagining ourselves in the shoes of the other and consequently sharing their feelings. Sympathy involves such feelings as pleasure, the tendency have positive feelings about one who has pleased another, pain, and the tendency to feel hostile toward one who has caused pain to another. Sympathy, according to some, is a natural tendency and is the basis for moral reasoning.

Rationalism.   The opposing school of thought is **rationalism.** Rationalists argue that feelings or perceptions, though they may seem similar in many people, may not actually be similar. Rationalists believe there are absolute truths that are not dependent upon human nature. They argue that ethical values have an independent origin in the nature of the universe, and can be known to humans through the process of reasoning. Rationalists believe there are truths about the world that are necessary and universal, and that these truths are superior to the information that we receive from our senses (Raphael, 1994).

To rationalists, moral rules are necessarily true. Rationalists see the knowledge gained through the senses as only contingently true (Raphael, 1994). For example, the grass is perceived as green, but the colour may be different—or may be seen as different by some. One who feels bad when hearing of the misfortune of another may not feel the same way about all others. On the other hand, moral or ethical rules, originating from a higher source and being free of the variances in human nature, are always true. For example, rationalists argue that it is good to help those in need, and the truth of this maxim will not change based upon different circumstances or perceptions.

The differences in the two schools of thought revolve around the question of the origin of ethics. Is ethics a matter of feeling, or of reason? Are individuals free to make ethical choices based upon predictable human nature, or is the foundation of ethics based upon universal or theologic truth? The comparison between naturalism and rationalism is seen clearly in the study of ethical theories. We are challenged to consider these two viewpoints when reading ethical theory.

THEORIES OF ETHICS

Moral philosophy is the branch of philosophy that examines beliefs and assumptions about the nature of certain human values. Ethics is the practical application of moral philosophy; that is, given the moral context of good or bad, right or wrong, "What ought one to do in a given situation?" The philosopher reveals an integrated global vision in which elements, like pieces of a puzzle, have a logical fit. By developing theories of ethics, the philosopher hopes to explain values and behaviours related to cultural and moral norms. Each theory is based upon the particular viewpoint of the individual philosopher, and maintains, within itself, philosophical consistency. The discussion related to naturalism and rationalism explains, in part, one basic difference among moral philosophers. We chose utilitarianism and deontology for inclusion in this chapter because they are two of the major theories central to medical, nursing, and bioethics.

CASE PRESENTATION

Conflicting Duties

Hannah is the director of a visiting hospice outreach service for a large rural area. This week, she received notice that the funding to the hospice service from the federal and provincial governments was being drastically decreased. Without this funding, cuts must be made in the services provided to clients. When Hannah meets with the advisory board, they agree that one of two programs must be eliminated in order to cope with the decreased funding. One program is a common outreach program that provides assistance with activities of daily living for clients. This program helps a large number of clients, has been in place for many years and is consistently inexpensive to run. The other program is more innovative and costly, providing an opportunity for clients with highly complex and specific needs to get their nursing care at home, instead of visiting the local hospital on a regular basis, for specialized services. This program benefits a very few clients but does so in a significant way. While Hannah and the board recognize the importance of helping with complex, specific needs of the few, they are hesitant to advise eliminating a program that has been proven to help large numbers of clients.

Think About It

- What kinds of factors should Hannah and the board consider when making their decision? Why?
- What is the responsibility of the board to the large number of clients who would be denied assistance with daily living activities if the first program was eliminated?

- How would you decide what to do in this situation? What would you use to guide your decision making?

- As you continue to learn about the following ethical theories, return to thinking about this case and comment on what a utilitarian or a deontologist might do, and why?

Utilitarianism

Utilitarianism, sometimes called **consequentialism,** is a form of teleological theory. "Telos" comes from the Greek and literally means "end." Utilitarianism is the moral theory that holds that an action is judged as good or bad in relation to the consequence, outcome, or end result derived from it. Utilitarianism is an important ethical philosophy that has its basis in naturalism. According to the utilitarian school of thought, the right action is that which has greatest **utility** or usefulness. No action is, in itself, either good or bad. Utilitarians hold that the only factors that make actions good or bad are the outcomes, or end results, that are derived from them. Utilitarianism is, essentially, forward looking. In other words, a utilitarian is always looking into the future, assessing the potential outcomes and consequences of various courses of action and considering factors such as motivation, intention, or reasons behind action to be irrelevant in assessing the ethical soundness of a proposed action.

"Utilitarianism" is a broad term that relates to a number of important theories. One of the first utilitarians was the Roman philosopher Epicurus, whose teachings date to about 200–300 B.C.E. Epicurus believed that both good and evil lie in sensation, pleasure being good and pain being evil. He taught that pleasure can be gained by living a life of moderation, courage, and justice, and by cultivating friendship. Epicurus also believed that deities dwell apart from humans, and are not concerned with the state of human existence; therefore, humans control their own destinies (Honderich, 1995).

There was a rebirth of interest in utilitarian philosophy in the late eighteenth and early nineteenth centuries. Jeremy Bentham (1748–1832), a leading political philosopher, is considered to be the father of modern utilitarianism. According to Bentham's theory, actions can be considered to be right when they increase happiness and diminish misery, and can be considered to be wrong when they have the opposite effect. Following is Bentham's definition of the "principle of utility":

> By utility is meant that property in any object, whereby it tends to produce benefit, advantage, pleasure, good, or happiness . . . or . . . to prevent the happening of mischief, pain, evil, or unhappiness to the party whose interest is considered: if that party be the community in general, then the happiness of the community: if a particular individual, then the happiness of that individual. (Bentham, 1948, p. 2)

Bentham attempted to create a science derived from the principle of utility. He proposed that we should measure the product of an act in terms of the value of a proposed pleasure. Six criteria used to measure the pleasure included intensity, duration, certainty, propinquity (nearness in place or time), fecundity (the chance of it being followed by sensations of the same kind), and purity (the chance of it not being followed by sensations of the opposite kind). Bentham proposed that each criterion be given a value, and that the sum of the values related to the pleasure be weighed against a similar sum of values related to the pain that might result from any given act. The person should act in accordance with a mathematical formula, resolving ethical decisions based upon the sum total of the value of a given act.

Though many critics describe Bentham as having a hedonistic tendency (his theory is often referred to as hedonistic utilitarianism), it is clear from his writings that his interest extended far beyond physical pleasure. He wrote that *pleasure* is synonymous with many other terms such as *good, profit, advantage, benefit,* and so forth. In fact, his interest in the common good of the community refutes those who charge that his theory is hedonistic. He describes a type of justice in which action should have a tendency to augment the happiness of the community as a whole, rather than diminish it.

John Stuart Mill (1806–1873) was a leading nineteenth-century British moral philosopher. Like Bentham, Mill was a utilitarian. He described utilitarianism in terms of judging acts according to the end result. He wrote, "All action is for the sake of some end; and rules of action, it seems natural to suppose, must take their whole character and colour from the end to which they are subservient" (Mill, 1910, p. 2). The phrase *"the end justifies the means"* relates to Mill's theory. According to Mill, the only right actions are those that produce the greatest happiness. His "greatest happiness principle" holds that the right action in conduct is not the agent's own happiness, but the happiness of all concerned. He further believed that sacrifice is good only when it increases the total sum of happiness. For Mill, the object of virtue is the multiplication of happiness. He cautioned, however, that we must carefully attempt to avoid violating the rights of some people in the process of maximizing the happiness of others.

Mill defined his concepts in ways that make the meaning of this theory clearer. He described happiness as a state of pleasure that is not restricted to physical pleasure alone. In fact, Mill made a strong argument in favour of prioritizing pleasure, with intellectual pleasure having greater priority than physical or hedonistic pleasure. Further, Mill condemned those who chose sensual indulgences to the injury of health. He described the greatest sources of physical and mental suffering as "indigence, disease, and the unkindness, worthlessness, or premature loss, of objects of affection" (Mill, 1910, p. 14).

There are two basic types of utilitarianism. **Act utilitarianism** suggests that people choose actions that will, in any given circumstance, increase the overall good. **Rule utilitarianism,** on the other hand, suggests that people choose rules that, when followed consistently, will maximize the overall good.

Act utilitarianism. Act utilitarianism allows for different, sometimes opposing, action in different situations. For example, while act utilitarians probably believe that it is best to tell the truth (or keep promises, or avoid killing, and so on), they recognize that there are times when the overall consequences will be better for everyone concerned if this guideline is not followed, even if the rights of some individuals are violated (Beauchamp & Childress, 1994; Smart, 1997). Act utilitarians recognize that tenets should be used as rough guidelines rather than strict rules.

Rule utilitarianism. Rule utilitarianism, on the other hand, suggests that people should act according to rules that tend to maximize happiness and diminish unhappiness. Rule utilitarianism requires that people tell the truth (keep promises, avoid killing, and so on) in all circumstances, because the overall good is maximized by consistently following such rules. An example of rule utilitarian thinking regarding truth telling comes from the writing of Dr. Worthington Hooker, a prominent nineteenth century figure in medical ethics:

> The good, which may be done by deception in a few cases, is almost as nothing, compared with the evil which it does in many, when the prospect of its doing good was just as promising as it was in those in which it succeeded. And when we add to this the evil which would result from a general adoption of a system of deception, the importance of a strict adherence to the truth in our intercourse with the sick, even on the ground of expediency, becomes incalculably great. (Beauchamp & Childress, 1994, p. 51)

The argument of this rule utilitarian was that even though the patient's health is sometimes maximized through the use of deception, a widespread use of deception will eventually cause more harm than good. Thus, though rule utilitarians recognize that in some instances good might result from a particular act, in the end, the overall good is maximized by the following of strict rules in all situations.

In other words, in some cases, the rule utilitarian will act in a way that, for example, the act utilitarian would not approve as the good consequences of a particular act are not maximized. This is because the rule utilitarian seeks to follow the rule that will, overall, maximize good although, in some specific cases, it might well not lead to a decision that maximizes good.

Though utilitarianism is a widely accepted ethical theory, there are a few problems inherent in its use. Utilitarianism does not give sufficient thought to respect of persons. In fact, it is possible that harm can be done to minority groups or individuals in the name of overall good. It gives little recognition to the principle of autonomy, particularly when we consider utilitarian decision making relative to distributive justice. Critics argue that utilitarianism sacrifices rights of individuals in favour of the overall good.

Other limitations that are cited when referring to utilitarianism include the difficulty with defining what constitutes happiness or a "good" outcome. In a diverse world, there are many subjective and variable ideas about what defines a "good" consequence. When we consider the practical application of a utilitarian ethical theory, we also realize that we have a limited ability to accurately predict the future consequences of actions and that many times, there are unpredictable or unforeseeable factors that influence outcomes.

Many people criticize utilitarian approaches for aiming solely to optimize pleasure or happiness without considering that there may be other values that we should seek to optimize; there may be other values that are just as or more important than our own satisfaction or happiness.

Finally, utilitarianism provides no room for special relationships or interests. In evaluating what constitutes a "good" outcome, the interests of one person are considered as equal to any other person. This notion was revolutionary at its inception; a time of strong hierarchy, stringent notions of class and socioeconomic status, and feudal law. However, today, it is recognized that in some contexts and relationships, persons have and should be given special consideration or priority. Utilitarianism simply does not provide for this.

Even though there are problems inherent in utilitarianism, this ethical theory captures the imagination as an attractive moral philosophy. Its appeal lies in the simple precept of promoting happiness for as many people as possible. It is particularly useful as a method of deciding issues of distributive justice.

Ask Yourself

Is Utilitarianism Useful?

- What useful guidelines does utilitarianism provide in terms of distributing resources?
- To what degree is it permissible to sacrifice the rights of one to provide for the welfare of many?
- To what degree is it permissible to sacrifice the rights of many to provide for the welfare of one?
- Think about the strengths and weaknesses of utilitarianism in today's health care environments.

CASE PRESENTATION

Martin is a public health nurse in a large urban centre. This week there has been an outbreak of viral coughs, fever, and flu in the downtown community. Fearing a potential pandemic, public health has taken the extreme precaution of asking all health care professionals who work in acute care centres or in public health involved in direct client care to be quarantined when not at work. Martin is allowed to drive to work and home again but is prohibited to leave the house or have visitors at his home at all other times until the outbreak is controlled or the quarantine deemed no longer necessary. While an extreme precaution, Martin knows that these kinds of measures are necessary to prevent further spread of an unknown viral illness and adheres strictly to the guidelines for quarantine.

Leila is also a nurse in public health who is on home–work quarantine. While she also recognizes the importance of the quarantine, she is anxious to visit her mother, who lives a few kilometres from her house. She thinks to herself, "Well, no one will know and besides, who could it hurt? I'm only going to visit my mother for an hour and then I'll go straight home."

Think About It

- How is quarantine justified, from a utilitarian perspective?
- From a utilitarian perspective, is Leila's rationale for not following quarantine guidelines acceptable? Why or why not?
- How would you decide what to do in this situation? What ethical theories or principles would guide your actions?

Deontology

Deontological theories of ethics are based upon the rationalist view that the rightness or wrongness of an act depends upon the nature of the act, rather than its consequences. The term **deontology** is taken from the Greek word for "duty." Occasionally, deontology is called **formalism;** some writers refer to this type of ethical theory as **Kantianism.** Kantianism is based upon the writings of the German philosopher Immanuel Kant, who shaped many deontological formulations. For the purpose of this chapter, the terms *deontology* and *Kantian ethics* are used interchangeably.

Kant was born at Königsberg, Prussia, in 1724. After an uninspiring academic career, he surprised the world with his groundbreaking ethical theory. Late in his life, Kant published volumes of philosophical writings that shook the religious and political systems of his day, and continue to have strong influence on contemporary ethical philosophy. Kant contended that ethical rules are universal, and that humans can derive certain consistent principles to guide action. The awareness of these moral rules is the product of pure reason, rather than experience, as naturalists would maintain. Kant asserted that moral rules are absolute and apply to all people, for all times, in all situations. He believed that ethical rules could be known by rational humans. Knowledge of the right course of action in any given situation could be obtained by following a maxim that he called the **categorical imperative.** *Categorical* refers to moral rules that do not admit exceptions; imperative denotes a command that is derived from principle. Kant said there is only one categorical imperative:

> Act only according to that maxim by which you can at the same time will that it should become a universal law. (1959, p. 39)

In other words, when making a decision, one should imagine that, in all similiar cases, the same decision should be made. As an example, Kant related a moral problem in which a man needs money to feed his family. He knows that he will not be able to repay it, but knows that nothing will be lent to him if he does not promise to repay it at a certain time. In order to satisfy himself that the act of breaking the promise to repay the money is morally correct, the man asks himself the question, "Should every person always make promises which they know will not be fulfilled?" Through reasoning the man can see that this could not become a universal law, because no one would ever believe what has been promised. As a consequence, promise making would hold no meaning. Kant gave similar examples of situations related to suicide, squandering of talent, and helping others. Rather than compile a list of specific ethical rules, Kant proposed that each rational person should use the test of the categorical imperative to guide actions.

Following the categorical imperative, Kant also described the **practical imperative:**

> Act so that you treat humanity, whether in your own person or that of
> another, always as an end and never as a means only. (1959, p. 47)

To treat another person as a means according to Kant, is to use another person to fulfill your own needs or meet your own agenda. However, to treat a person as an end is to make their needs, agenda, or desires ends in themselves, and work toward them as you might work toward fulfilling your own needs or desires. Raphael (1994) makes the point that Kant's practical imperative automatically shows that domination of one person over another is morally wrong. Domination makes no allowance for the dominated person's power of decision making. He also notes that acting toward another as you would toward yourself mandates that, whenever possible, you must help people who need help. The practical imperative requires that we must fulfill certain duties owed to others, while keeping their needs foremost.

When the categorical imperative and the practical imperative are merged, there is a strong implication that each person is a member of a *realm of ends*—a politically organized society. Kant calls this "a systematic union of rational beings through common objective laws" (1959, p. 51). This requires that we should act as members of a community of equal and autonomous individuals, and that each member treat all others as moral beings. Each person should have regard for the desires of others, and allow them freedom of decision; in other words, respect their autonomous decisions. In Kantian theory, there is an inherent recognition that all people are equal and equally competent to make autonomous, universal decisions. According to Raphael (1994), "Kantian ethics is in fact an ethics of democracy. It requires liberty, equality, and fraternity" within a politically organized society (p. 57).

Deontology also implies that ethics are derived from fulfilling duties. When judging the ethical soundness of a proposed action, we are always "backward looking." In other words, one always must pay particular attention to the duties that lie behind our proposed actions, which motivate or drive us. An ethical person must act for the sake of duty or obligation. Kant believed that all *imperatives of duty* can be deduced from his categorical imperative (one should act as if one's actions could become universal law for all people) and must also comply with his practical imperative (treat all people as ends, none as means to an end). Deontology does not require that we ever look forward to the possible consequences or results of possible actions, merely to attend to the duties that underpin our actions, thereby making our actions ethically sound. He also believed that an action done from duty has its moral worth based upon reverence for the law and carrying out one's duty, rather than the results or outcomes of the act (Paton, 1961). Most professional codes of ethics are based upon Kantian principles. Nurses' codes of ethics stress the importance of fulfilling duties that are inherently owed to patients, and the importance of preserving the dignity and autonomy of each individual patient.

There are some acknowledged weaknesses with the practical application of deontological ethics. It has been noted to be exceptionless and rigid with no acknowledgment of special relationships and subsequent duties that result. Deontologists do not tell us how to decide between conflicting duties. Often, nurses find that they have clear, ethical duties that seem to present conflicts. How do we decide which duty has priority? Deontologists, such as Kant, offer little advice, noting only that a rational person will simply know his or her duties.

Finally, it does seem reasonable to assume that by failing to consider the possible consequences of given actions, we might create difficult, if not tragic or disastrous, situations.

Like utilitarianism, deontology is an attractive ethical theory. It is, in fact, a most popular foundation for many contemporary beliefs. It provides clear guidelines for judging the rightness or wrongness of action. It recognizes the dignity and autonomy of individuals, and allows all people equal consideration. It serves as a basis for much of the contemporary ethical thinking that guides health care delivery.

CASE PRESENTATION

Weighing Rights and Duties in Questions of Justice

Sumiko is the home health nurse for Mrs. B. Her patient is an eighty-nine-year-old widow who lives in the home that she and her husband shared until his death five years earlier. She suffers from severe rheumatoid arthritis and has a new colostomy. The colostomy was performed as a last resort for severe ulcerative colitis. Mrs. B. is unable to care for herself because of the advanced state of her arthritis. Her daughter, son-in-law, and two teenage grandchildren moved into her home to take care of her daily needs. After many months, the family feels that caring for the elderly woman has become an unbearable burden. They ask Sumiko to help arrange long-term care in a local nursing home. Mrs. B. wants to continue to live in her home.

❓ Think About It

Whose Rights Are More Important?

- Does Mrs. B. have the right to stay in her home, even if the entire family is made unhappy by her presence?

- According to deontology, what factors must the family consider in deciding?

- To whom does Sumiko owe a duty?

- To what degree should the rights of the other family members bear on the decision that Sumiko makes?

- Apply the categorical imperative to Sumiko's options.

- What would you do if you were Sumiko? On what basis would you make your decision?

Virtue Ethics

Virtue ethics, sometimes called **character ethics,** represents the idea that individuals' actions are based upon a certain degree of innate moral virtue. First noted in the writings of Homer, and subsequently in the works of Plato, Aristotle, and Socrates, the idea of cardinal virtues emerged: wisdom, courage, temperance, justice, generosity, faith, hope, and charity (Kitwood, 1990). Modern and contemporary writers also include such virtues as honesty, compassion, caring, conscientiousness, responsibility, integrity, discernment, trustworthiness, and prudence. Virtue ethics is reemerging as an important framework for examining ethical decision making and behaviour.

The concept of virtue ethics presents a challenge to deontological and utilitarian theories. These theories conceive of the demands of morality similarly; ethics provides guidelines to action that begins with the question, "What ought we to do?" (Beauchamp, 2001). In contrast, virtue ethics does not ask this question; instead, it posits that the basic function of morality is the moral character of persons and it shifts the focus from the action to the character of the actor. In doing so, it also moves away from the external to a greater involvement of self, persons, and relationships (Gardiner, 2003). Beauchamp (2001) suggests that virtues should not be thought of as moral requirements, because this confuses them with principles or rules. Rather, we could say that virtues are character traits that are socially valued. A *moral* virtue is a character trait that is morally valued, such as truthfulness, kindness, or honesty. A person with moral virtue has both consistent moral action and a morally appropriate desire.

The term "ethics" was derived from Aristotle's word *ethika*, which refers to matters having to do with character. Aristotle (384–332 B.C.E.) considered goodness of character to be produced by the practice of virtuous behaviour, rather than virtuous acts being the end result of a good character. According to Aristotle, virtues are tendencies to act, feel, and judge that are developed from a natural capacity by proper training and exercise. He believed that practice creates a habit of acting in a virtuous way, and that virtue can be learned and improved. Virtue, according to Aristotle, depends on "clear judgment, self-control, symmetry of desire, and artistry of means" (Durant, 1926, p. 75). He considered virtue to be the fruit of intelligent pursuit. "It is not the possession of the simple [person], nor the gift of innocent intent, but the achievement of experience in the fully developed [person]" (Durant, p. 75). He considered excellence to be won by training and habituation, and believed that virtuous character is created by repeatedly acting in a virtuous manner. Aristotle's traits of a virtuous character provided three criteria:

1. Virtuous acts must be chosen for their own sake.

2. Choice must proceed from a firm and unchangeable character.

3. Virtue is a disposition to choose the mean.

The *golden mean* of virtuous behaviour, for Aristotle, meant practising moderation: avoiding both excess and deficiency. Aristotle did not list a number of moral principles. For him, the basic moral question is not "what should one do" but rather "what should one be" (Mayo, 1958).

Phillipa Foot adds another perspective to Aristotle's concept of a virtuous person. Foot proposes that virtue lies not only in engaging in virtuous acts, but also in will. She defines will as "that which is wished for as well as what is sought." According to Foot, a positive or moral will is sometimes the necessary ingredient in success. She says,

> sometimes one man succeeds where another fails not because there is some specific difference in their previous conduct but rather because his heart lies in a different place; and the disposition of the heart is part of virtue. What this suggests is that a man's virtue may be judged by his innermost desires as well as by his intentions and this fits with our idea that a virtue such as generosity lies as much in someone's attitudes as in his actions. (1997, p. 330)

According to Foot, virtue is not like a skill or an art. It cannot merely be a practised and perfected act: it must actually engage the will. In other words, an act, though apparently kind or generous, for example, cannot be considered to be virtuous if the intention is not good. Although Aristotle's idea of virtue is one of hope (everyone has the capacity to learn virtuous action), Foot makes the road to virtuous character less easily travelled.

Focal Virtues. In the discussion of virtue as related to biomedical ethics, Beauchamp and Childress define character as being "comprised of a set of stable traits that affect a person's judgment and action" (2001, p. 30). Like Aristotle, these authors suggest that although people have different character traits, all have the capacity to learn or cultivate those that are important to morality. Beauchamp and Childress propose that there are five focal virtues that are more pivotal than others in characterizing a virtuous person: compassion, discernment, trustworthiness, integrity, and conscientiousness.

Compassion. **Compassion** is the ability to imagine oneself in the situation of another. Beauchamp and Childress (2001) define the term in the following manner: "The virtue of compassion is a trait combining an attitude of active regard for another's welfare with an imaginative awareness and emotional response of deep sympathy, tenderness, and discomfort at the other person's misfortune or suffering" p. 32 (2001). This virtue embodies internalizing of the golden rule. Compassion is so important that many times the patient's need for a compassionate and caring presence outweighs the need for technical care. We must be careful, however, that compassion does not impede our ability to make objective decisions.

Discernment. The virtue of **discernment** is related to the classical concept of wisdom. "The virtue of discernment brings sensitive insight, acute judgment, and understanding to action. Discernment involves the ability to make judgments and reach decisions without being underly influenced by extraneous considerations, fears, personal attachments and the like." (Beauchamp and Childress, 2001, p. 34). Discernment gives an insight into appropriate actions in given situations. It requires sensitivity and attention attuned to the demands of a particular context. For example, a discerning nurse will recognize when a patient needs comfort and reassurance rather than privacy. Discernment requires that we continually strive to recognize and understand important nuances in human behaviour.

Trustworthiness. **Trustworthiness** is another focal virtue for nurses. "Trust is a confident belief is and reliance upon the moral character and competence of another person. Trust entails a confidence that another will act with the right motives and in accordance with appropriate moral norms." (Beauchamp and Childress, 2001, p. 34). Trustworthiness is measured by others' recognition of the nurse's consistency and predictability in following moral norms. In practical terms, trustworthiness is accounted for in the reputation we have among coworkers. This virtue is important for us in relationships with patients, physicians, and other nurses.

Integrity. **Integrity** is perhaps the cardinal virtue. **Moral integrity**, according to Beauchamp and Childress (2001), means "soundness, reliability, wholeness and integration of moral character." (p. 36). Integrity refers to two parts of a person. First, it refers to the integration of all parts of a person, which can include aspects such as values and beliefs along with emotions, wishes, and actions. Secondly, it encompasses the moral trait of being steadfast to one's values and beliefs and standing up for them, even when faced with adversity. It also refers to our continuing to follow moral norms over time. A person with integrity has a consistency of convictions, actions, and emotions and is trustworthy. Integrity is compromised when the nurse acts consistently or in a way that is not supported by professed moral beliefs. Deficiencies in moral integrity may include hypocrisy, insincerity, and bad faith.

Conscientiousness. A person acts in a conscientious way, according to Beauchamp and Childress (2001), if he or she consistently, with explicitly good intentions tries to do what is right, after putting an effort into determining what constitutes the "right" choice of action. Conscientiousness involves significant effort and strong intentions to do what is right.

While there are many different writings on virtues, there is no set list of virtues. Ancient writings tended to consider virtues as existing on a spectrum, from excess to deficiency. For example, when considering truthfulness as a virtue, the deficient extreme is deception while the excessive extreme is forthrightness. Similarly, in considering the virtue of compassion, the deficient extreme is disinterest while the excessive extreme would be entanglement. If we examine conscientiousness, the deficient extreme might be carelessness contrasted with the excessive extreme of obsession. Finally, when thinking about the virtue of integrity, we can identify that the deficient extreme would be corruption while the excessive extreme is self-righteousness (Gardiner, 2003). Considering the virtues as existing along a spectrum demonstrates that one can have "too much" of what might be considered a good virtue, and that in turn, this excess might be equally problematic as a deficiency.

Virtue Ethics in Nursing.   How does the concept of virtue or character ethics fit with nursing as a principled profession? It is likely that principled behaviour, while not the sole domain of a good moral character, is more likely to occur in the presence of one. Certainly Florence Nightingale thought virtue was an important trait of the good nurse. Traditionally recited by graduating nurses, the Nightingale Pledge implies virtue of character as nurses promise purity, faith, loyalty, devotion, trustworthiness, and temperance. It is reasonable to say, according to the Pledge, that good character is the cornerstone of good nursing, and that the nurse with virtue will act according to principle. If Aristotle was correct in his belief that virtue can be practised and learned, then we can learn, through practice, those acts which, by their doing, create a virtuous person.

Virtue theory is not without its limitations. One assumption is that there are shared virtues or a kind of metanarrative about what constitutes virtue. While many people may agree that compassion or truthfulness is a virtue, this view may be neither universal nor shared. Additionally, virtue theory assumes that all agents share a goal of becoming more virtuous as they grow and evolve. This, in turn, leads to the assumption that all people share this goal and aim of becoming as virtuous as possible. Moreover, if virtuousness does in fact, then, exist in degrees, how do we approach those with "evolving" virtuousness?

One critically important feature of virtue theory is that it shifts the locus of ethical decision making from outside the person, driven by ethical principles or theories, to the actual person, and her views, attributes, and inner motivations. This may be a more realistic view of how people make difficult ethical decisions on one hand. On the other hand, to expect everyone to be virtuous decision makers fails to acknowledge the fact that when motivations and emotions play a part in judgment, we may not succeed at putting those emotions aside and acting in the most virtuous way. However, it is a strength of virtue ethics theory, that it recognizes that good decision making may in fact be strengthened by habit and that virtue and virtuous character traits may be developed over time.

Feminist and Relational Ethics

Typically, traditional ethical theories have focused on abstract approaches (couched in philosophical theories) to complex ethical issues. In the past decades, feminist perspectives on ethics and bioethical issues have challenged these traditional approaches to solving moral dilemmas, which often aim to uncover the rational, just, and fair course of action or solution. Relational ethics approaches emphasize, as feminist ethics does, the importance of the relationships between the "players" in ethical dilemmas.

Much of the potential problem-solving methods and plausible outcomes to moral dilemmas from traditional perspectives, such as utilitarianism or deontology, tend to focus on justice and the rights of persons, and not attend to issues of power or the nature of relationships. Feminist ethics theorists posit that ethical dilemmas, especially in social constructs such as health care, are often laden with issues of power and an imbalance of power. Along with those using relational ethics, they ask that when considering an ethical issue, one attends to the relationships between the persons involved, the power differentials, and the perception of hierarchy, marginalization, or oppression of persons involved (Keatings and Smith, 2000; Sherwin, 1992).

❓ Think About It

Consider the case of an illiterate woman, Grace, without legal status who is new to Canada, faced with a complex health system that is difficult to access and navigate, who has a sick child. She knows that there is a local medical clinic near to the shelter where she is currently living but has no idea if they will see her as she has no identification and no money. She has a small network of persons who help her out, and they have identified that her child is very ill and should see a doctor immediately. They cannot reach the physician who comes to the shelter once weekly in time for her child to be seen today.

Consider that she is a refugee from a country where she has endured civil unrest and, along with other women in her family, has been physically beaten and oppressed with a threat of rape or further violence if she remained in her country of origin. This is not an unrealistic case. When faced with barriers to accessing care for her child—that include her own gender perhaps; her lack of understanding of English and inability to read or understand in a predominantly English-speaking system; her illegal status; her fear of being uncovered as a person without legal status; and her feeling that she would take significant personal risks to access care for her child—all these things make her vulnerable.

Add to that the oppression and violence she endured in her home country—and her resultant fear of males in authority positions. The relationships she has experienced and those that she might experience as part of her health care experience are clearly all important to sort through when considering her case from a perspective of feminist ethics.

- What kinds of issues make Grace *most* vulnerable, in your opinion?
- Grace does not have provincial coverage for health care as she is not a citizen nor a landed immigrant or permanent resident. Her lack of legal

status is not her fault, as she has immigrated here to escape torture and possibly death for her and her children. Do you think it is fair that she, technically, cannot access adequate health care? What would a feminist ethicist say?

- If you were a nurse who first encountered Grace in a local medical clinic, how would you go about making her comfortable and addressing her needs? What are the priorities?

That ethical approaches such as utilitarianism or deontology do not allow for considerations of important contextual issues, like past experiences, relationships, and vulnerability, is clear in the case above. The traditional theories fail to acknowledge or address issues of vulnerability, the nature of special relationships (e.g., mother and child, adult child and elderly parent) and caring roles and duties, often traditionally taken on by women in society and unrecognized as unique and important in history. Often classified as systematic and based on primarily male-biased perspectives, these traditional ethical theories are seen as limited in their usefulness for approaching the kinds of complex, contextual, relational and sometimes engendered health care dilemmas that arise in the modern world.

CASE PRESENTATION

Mr. Wey is an eighty-three-year-old retired bus driver who is being seen in the respirology clinic today as he has had some unusual shortness of breath over the past few weeks, accompanied by transient pain and discomfort. He is accompanied by his wife and two sons. His daughter-in-law, Mary, is a physician in the radiology department and has been in and out during Mr. Wey's day of testing.

When the tests are completed and Mr. Wey is getting changed down the hall, the family, along with Mr. Wey's daughter-in-law, approaches the doctor and asks him what, if anything, was found. The doctor is a colleague of Mary's and looks concerned. He discloses that they have found Mr. Wey has a significantly large growth in his lungs and it is likely cancerous. He wants to schedule more tests, a biopsy, and likely surgery as soon as possible.

Mr. Wey's wife and one son insist that the doctor not tell Mr. Wey his diagnosis now. They inform him that they have a family trip planned, on a cruise ship and then at a resort in the southern United States. The trip will take about a month and a half. Mrs. Wey tells the doctor that they have been saving for this trip for two years. They will finally be able to see their eldest son again, who has been overseas and estranged from them for over ten years, and meet their only grandchildren for the first time.

Mary also adds that Mr. Wey has a history of depression and alcohol abuse, which has been very hard on the family and especially their eldest son, who left home because of the strained relationship with his father. She agrees that it might be a good idea to not tell him at this time, to let him enjoy his family trip and then, upon his return, inform him and begin treatment.

Before Mr. Wey returns, the family and his physician quickly agree not to tell him until after his trip. They feel that by allowing him to enjoy his trip, they are acting in his best interests. His youngest son, however, feels that this is not the right thing to do and voices his discomfort over this hasty decision.

Think About It

- What would a deontologist do, and why?
- What would a utilitarian recommend, and why?
- What virtues should the family and physician exercise in making a decision?
- What ethical principles are most important to consider in this situation?
- If you were the physician, would you tell Mr. Wey of his diagnosis? How would you justify your decision?
- Think about Mr. Wey's perspective. How might he feel, in either case, if he is told right now or after his trip?
- Why might Mr. Wey's youngest son be uncomfortable with the option of not telling his father about his diagnosis?

SUMMARY

Ethical theory helps us understand the origin and process of ethical and moral thinking and behaviour. Two important theories are particularly important to nursing ethics. The ethical theory of utilitarianism was developed in part by Jeremy Bentham, and later refined by John Stuart Mill. Utilitarianism suggests that ethical decisions should be made in regard to the outcome or end result. Accordingly, no action in itself is inherently right or wrong. This theory also provides for the greatest good for the greatest number. Utilitarianism is particularly useful in situations of distributive justice but tends to ignore the rights of the minority or the individual.

Deontology, or Kantian ethics, was initially developed by Immanuel Kant. This theory, through the use of the categorical imperative, assists one in making ethical decisions. The categorical imperative demands that the agent ask the question, Can this action be a law for all people in all circumstances? Additionally, the theory presents the practical imperative, which requires that we treat all individuals as if they were ends only, rather than means. Kantian ethics provides clear guidelines for making ethical decisions, but does not provide for making decisions when there are conflicting duties or obligations.

Virtue, or character, ethics, as described by Aristotle, describes each person as capable of practising and learning virtue through repetition of virtuous acts. Thus, the virtuous person is one in whom virtue is habituated. Virtue ethics complements other ethical theories, and can be used to nurture or predict character in individuals. Ethical theories can help us understand ethical decision-making models, and assist in developing a cohesive and logical system for making individual decisions.

CHAPTER HIGHLIGHTS

- Philosophy is the intense and critical examination of beliefs and assumptions.
- Moral philosophy is the philosophical discussion of what is considered to be good or bad, right or wrong.
- Ethics is a formal process for making logical and consistent decisions, based upon moral philosophy.
- As the morally central health care profession, nursing requires astuteness of moral and ethical issues.
- Ethical theories explain values and behaviour related to cultural and moral norms.
- Utilitarianism holds that right action is that which has the greatest utility or usefulness, and no action is in itself either good or bad.
- Deontology is based upon the rationalist view that the rightness or wrongness of an act depends upon the nature of the act, rather than the consequences that occur as a result of it.
- Kantianism is a particular deontological theory developed by Immanuel Kant.
- The categorical imperative is the Kantian maxim requiring that no action can be judged as right which cannot reasonably become a law by which every person should always abide.
- The practical imperative is the Kantian maxim requiring that one treats others always as ends and never as a means.
- Virtue ethics, usually attributed to Aristotle, represents the idea that individuals' actions are based upon innate moral virtue.

DISCUSSION QUESTIONS AND ACTIVITIES

1. Describe the differences in beliefs about the origin of ethical rules.

2. Describe a hypothetical situation in which an ethical dilemma exists, and discuss solutions to the dilemma in terms of act utilitarianism and rule utilitarianism.

3. Identify specific health care funding policies, and discuss them in terms of utilitarian theory.

4. Identify different ethical codes, including professional codes, that are based upon Kantian or deontological ethics.

5. Describe a real or hypothetical situation in which there is an ethical dilemma. Relate a solution to the dilemma, using the rule of the categorical imperative.

6. List and describe the virtues that you feel are important for nurses.

7. Consider the following situation: Two nursing students are discovered to have cheated on several assignments. After being questioned by the instructor, both students deny having cheated, even though the evidence is irrefutable. Discuss these students in terms of virtue ethics and Kantian ethics. Do these students have integrity? Do these students have the character to become good nurses? How would you apply the categorical imperative?

REFERENCES

Beauchamp, T. L. (2001). *Philosophical ethics* (3rd ed.). Boston: McGraw Hill.

Beauchamp, T., & Childress, J. (2001). *Principles of biomedical ethics* (5th ed.). New York: Oxford University Press.

Beauchamp, T. L., & Walters, L. (1999). *Contemporary issues in bioethics*. Belmont, CA: Wadsworth.

Bentham, J. (1948). *An introduction to the principles of moral legislation*. New York: Hafner Press.

Buber, M. (1965). *The knowledge of man: A philosophy of the interhuman*. New York: Harper & Row.

Durant, W. (1926). *The story of philosophy*. New York: Washington Square Press.

Foot, P. (1997). Virtues and vices. In C. Sommers & F. Sommers, eds., *Vice and virtue in everyday life: Introductory readings in ethics* (4th ed., pp. 328–343). Fort Worth, TX: Harcourt Brace College. (Reprinted from P. Foot, *Virtues and vices*, Berkeley, CA: University of California Press)

Gardiner, P. (2003). A virtue ethics approach to moral dilemmas in medicine. *Journal of Medical Ethics, 29*, 297–302.

Hesse, H. (1971). *Siddhartha*. New York: Bantam.

Honderich, T., ed. (1995). *The Oxford companion to philosophy*. New York: Oxford University Press.

Jameton, A. (1984). *Nursing practice: The ethical issues*. Englewood Cliffs, NJ: Prentice-Hall.

Kant, I. (1959). *Foundations of the metaphysics of morals* (L. W. Beck, trans.). Indianapolis: Bobbs-Merrill.

Keatings, M., & Smith, O. B. (2000). Ethical and legal issues in Canadian Nursing. (2nd ed.) Toronto: Saunders.

Kitwood, T. (1990). *Concern for others. A new psychology of conscience and morality*. New York: Routledge.

Kneller, G. F. (1971). *Introduction to the philosophy of education*. (2nd ed.). New York: John Wiley & Sons.

Mayo, B. (1958). *Ethics and the moral life*. London: MacMillan.

Mill, J. S. (1910). *Utilitarianism*. London: Dent & Sons.

Paton, H. J., trans. & ed. (1961). *The moral law*. London: Hutchinson & Co.

Rand, A. (1982). *Philosophy: Who needs it?* New York: Bobbs-Merrill.

Random House, et al. (1987). *The Random House Dictionary of the English Language* (2nd ed., unabridged). New York: Random House.

Raphael, D. D. (1994). *Moral philosophy* (2nd ed.). New York: Oxford University Press.

Sherwin, S. (1992). *No longer patient.* Philadelphia: Temple University Press.

Smart, J. J. C. (1997). Utilitarianism. In C. Sommers & F. Sommers, eds., *Vice and virtue in everyday life: Introductory readings in ethics* (4th ed., pp. 110–123). Fort Worth, TX: Harcourt Brace College. (Reprinted from J. J. C. Smart & B. Williams, eds., *Utilitarianism: For and against,* New York: Oxford University Press)

Thomas, J. (1998). Ethical frameworks for decision making. In Thomas, J. & Waluchow, W. (Eds.) Well and Good: Case Studies in Biomedical Ethics. Peterborough, Ontario: Broadview Press, 1–55.

CHAPTER 3
Ethical Principles

OBJECTIVES

After completing this chapter, the reader should be able to:

1. Discuss the principle of autonomy in terms of patients' rights, informed consent, parentalism, and noncompliance.
2. Discuss the principle of beneficence as it relates to nursing practice.
3. Define the principle of nonmaleficence, and weigh actions in terms of harm and benefit.
4. Relate the principle of veracity to nursing practice.
5. Examine the principle of confidentiality in nursing practice, recognizing legal implications and reasonable limits to confidentiality.
6. Discuss the principle of justice as it relates to the delivery of health care goods and services.

7. Relate the principle of fidelity to nursing's promise to society.

8. Discuss situations in which there is a conflict between two or more ethical principles.

INTRODUCTION

Ethical issues are commonly examined in terms of a number of **ethical principles**. Ethical principles are basic and obvious moral truths that guide deliberation and action. Major ethical theories utilize many of the same principles, though either the emphasis or meaning may be somewhat different in each. For example, autonomy is a dominant principle in deontological theory but is less important in utilitarian theory. It is vital for nurses to understand ethical principles and be adept at applying them in a meaningful and consistent manner. (See Figure 3–1.) It is the authors' contention that consistent adherence to principle is an important basis for ethical practice in nursing. This chapter examines the following ethical principles: autonomy, beneficence, nonmaleficence, veracity, confidentiality, justice, and fidelity.

Figure 3–1 **Principles of Ethics**

Autonomy
Beneficence
Nonmaleficence
Veracity
Confidentiality
Justice
Fidelity

Respect for Persons

All of the principles discussed in this chapter presuppose that nurses have respect for the value and uniqueness of persons. Occasionally viewed as an ethical principle in its own right, **respect for persons** implies that one considers others to be worthy of high regard. Certainly, genuine regard and respect for others serves as the cornerstone of any caring profession. Discussion of the ethical principles in this chapter is based upon the belief that we value the principle of respect for persons.

AUTONOMY

The word **autonomy** literally means self-governing. Autonomy is a word that is frequently used, yet poorly understood. We are told to respect the autonomy of patients, but are given little guidance in understanding the meaning of this abstract concept. The term is more frequently used as a contrast to undesirable states such as dependency, coercion, paternalism, thoughtlessness, and habit (Jameton, 1984). We are expected to understand the concept and be advocates to ensure the maintenance of autonomy for all patients.

Aveyard (2000) suggests that the ambiguous use of the term *autonomy* should be replaced by a concept with a specific meaning and working definition. The term *autonomy* denotes having the freedom to make choices about issues that affect one's life. Autonomy is closely linked to the notion of respect for persons, and is an important principle in cultures where all individuals are considered to be unique and valuable members of society. In cultures that do not regard all members as being of equal worth or that respect social structure above individual rights, autonomy is less important. Autonomy implies that each person has the freedom to make decisions about personal goals. It is a state in which each of us is free to choose and implement our own decisions, free from lies, restraint, or coercion (Edge & Groves, 1994, p. 31). In societies where slavery exists, where women are expected to be subservient to men, where there is a lack of respect for cultures, races or religious identities, or where children are exploited, the notion of autonomy is meaningless. Autonomy cannot thrive in a climate that does not allow for either the independent planning of personal goals or the privilege of examining and choosing options to meet goals.

Implied in the concept of autonomy are four basic elements. First, the autonomous person is respected. It is logical that those choosing the nursing profession would inherently value and respect the unique humanness of others. This element is essential to assuring autonomy. Second, the autonomous person must be able to determine personal goals. These goals may be explicit and of a global nature, or may be less well defined. For example, the patient with an ankle injury may have a goal to return to athletic play within two weeks of the injury, or may simply wish to be pain free. In each case the patient develops personally chosen goals that are consistent with a particular lifestyle. In keeping with the notion of choice as an expression of one's lifestyle, values, and beliefs is the notion of autonomy as authentic articulation. When considering the choices made by persons who are ill, in pain, or frightened, one must try to ensure that their choice reflects who they are, in a broader way and that the choice they might make today would be the same or a similar choice they might make on any other day, when pain free, well, and less scared or burdened (Yeo and Moorhouse, 2002). Third, the autonomous person has the capacity to decide on a plan of action. The person must be able to understand the meaning of the choice to be made and deliberate on the various options, while understanding the implications of possible outcomes. Imagine, for example, ordering from a restaurant menu written in a language you do not understand. You have the freedom and responsibility to make a choice, but cannot make a meaningful choice without an understanding of the various foods offered. Additionally, a person must be able to demonstrate a kind of moral reflection, not just the practical ability to understand the differences between the choices. In other words, persons must be able to reflect upon the values and beliefs that they hold when weighing options and making decisions. This also implies that one has adopted these values and beliefs in a meaningful way and not simply through a process lacking in critical contemplation or conscious choice (Yeo and Moorhouse, 2002). When we believe that a patient is not able to comprehend the meaning of choices, goals, or outcomes, we say that the person is incompetent to make decisions, or lacks decision-making capacity. There are certain groups of patients that are generally thought of as unable to make informed choices. Children, fetuses, and those with some kinds of developmental disabilities may be among these groups. Fourth, the autonomous person has the freedom to act upon the choices. In situations where persons are capable of formulating goals, understanding various options, and making decisions, yet are not free to implement their plans, autonomy is either limited or absent. Autonomy may be limited in situations where the means to accomplish autonomously devised plans do not exist. An example is seen in the case of a person living in a remote region of Ontario, who does not have the same access to timely, inclusive care as the person living in downtown Ottawa or Toronto. In order to assure autonomy, each of the four elements must be present to a reasonable degree.

A number of intrinsic factors may threaten patient autonomy. The patient's role is often a dependent one. The patient seeks health care assistance because of a real or perceived need and, as a result, can be thought of as being dependent upon the health care provider. The role of the health care professional, on the other hand, is one of power. This power is based upon knowledge and authority and is inherent in the role. This complementary relationship, while a necessary one, can potentially, lead to violations of patient autonomy.

Ask Yourself

Is the Patient Role a Dependent One?

- Describe a time when you or a family member experienced the role of hospitalized patient.
- How did you or your family member feel when interacting with members of the health care team who were dressed, while you or your family member were in pajamas or a hospital gown or, worse yet, naked?
- Describe the degree to which you or your family member were able to maintain dignity and autonomy.

Health care professionals are often insensitive to the way in which the health care industry systematically dehumanizes and erodes the autonomy of clients. Patients are forced to comply with rules that require them to be and act dependent often without consideration of individual, religious, or cultural differences, beliefs, and practices. Immediately upon admission to a hospital, patients are disrobed, asked questions about personal and private matters, forced to relinquish money and belongings, and expected to remain in a bed, emphasizing the dependency of the patient role. Patients are placed in rooms with doors that are seldom closed and asked to wear pajamas. Workers, who are strangers to patients, freely enter and leave the patients' rooms, making privacy impossible. Regardless of patients' personal habits or knowledge of their own health care, they are forced to bathe at certain times, eat at certain times, take medications at certain times, and are often prohibited from practising self-care measures that may have been their habits for many years. Patients are expected to follow each plan that is made. Otherwise, they may be labelled difficult or *noncompliant*. While there is strong emphasis on the importance of autonomy, health care professionals are often guilty of creating a climate of dependency for patients—of coercing otherwise autonomous, intelligent, and independent adults essentially into a very dependent role. Moreover, often patients lose their sense of self as they are acclimatized to a standard routine and care plan. While individualized and holistic care should always be the goal of nursing care, often time and resource constraints prohibit the extra efforts and time it takes to consistently deliver individualized care.

Recognizing Violations of Patient Autonomy

Often, nurses and other health care workers fail to recognize subtle violations of patient autonomy. This especially occurs when nurses perceive choices to be self-evident. At least four factors are related to this failure. First, nurses may falsely assume that patients have the same values and goals as themselves. This state of mind compels some nurses to believe that the only reasonable course of action is the one that is consistent with their own values. This leads to faulty conclusions. For example, if an elderly person chooses to stay in her own home, even though to others she seems to be incapable of caring for herself, the choice might be viewed as unreasonable and might become grounds to believe the patient incompetent to make decisions. In other words, "If you don't make the choices that seem correct to me, you must be incompetent to make decisions." In truth, the elderly person may recognize that life is drawing to a close and may want to remain in familiar surroundings, maintain dignity, remain independent, and prevent needless depletion of her life savings. The decision is based upon her thoughtful consideration of the consequences of staying home versus the consequences of living in a long-term care facility. There are some who would insist that she should be allowed to stay at home, even if she places herself at considerable danger, as long as she does not jeopardize the autonomy of others.

CASE PRESENTATION

Noncompliance Versus Autonomy

Cora is a forty-five-year-old woman who looks years older than her stated age. She has very limited monthly income. Cora smokes two and one-half packs of cigarettes per day. She has severe COPD with constant dyspnea and frequent exacerbations. The nurse who sees her at a local clinic is interested in at least preventing further problems, and speaks to Cora often about the importance of quitting smoking. The situation becomes very frustrating for all involved when Cora returns repeatedly for increasingly severe problems, having failed to quit smoking. Cora, becomes labelled by the health care team as noncompliant. During a particularly severe exacerbation, the nurse says to Cora, "You know you are committing suicide by continuing to smoke." Cora's reply is, "You don't understand. I live alone. I have no money, no friends, no family, and will never be able to work. I know the damage I'm doing, but smoking is the only pleasure I have in life." (Nathaniel, 2000)

Think About It

Do Nurses Coerce Patients?

- In attempting to persuade Cora to stop smoking, to what degree is the nurse disallowing Cora's right to autonomy?

- Does Cora have the right to choose to continue smoking?

- If rights and responsibilities are correlative, how should the clinic respond to Cora's continuing to smoke? Would you suggest that the clinic continue to serve Cora, even though she is not following the plan of care? How might Cora be better included in creating a collaborative care plan?

- To what degree is coercion employed in situations such as Cora's? Is coercion ever an appropriate strategy?

- What would you do?

The second cause of failure to recognize subtle violations of patient autonomy lies in our failure to recognize that individuals' thought processes are different. Discounting a particular decision as incorrect may not take into consideration the fact that people process information in different ways. For example, there are those whose thought processes are very logical and methodical; others think in ways that are creative and free flowing. It is particularly important to recognize these types of differences when several people are working together to come to a common decision. What is obvious to one will not be obvious to all—not necessarily because of a difference in values, knowledge base, or intellect, but because of different backgrounds and styles of thinking (Harrison & Bramson, 1982). This is an important consideration when collaborating with patients, families, and other professionals.

The third cause of failure to recognize subtle violations of patient autonomy lies in our assumptions about patients' knowledge base. It is easy for us to forget that we have gained a specialized body of knowledge through our programs of basic nursing education and extensive work experience. Knowledge about such things as basic anatomy and physiology, disease processes, and the mechanism of action of drugs, and so forth is so ingrained in our minds that it is easy to presume everyone has at least some of the same type of knowledge. We often assume patients have more knowledge than is reasonable for them to have. Consequently, we may discount or criticize patients' decisions, even though flaws lie in the patients' level of knowledge, rather than the appropriateness of decisions. Recall that an understanding of the choices, outcomes, and implications are inherently necessary for autonomous decision making. The nurse must accurately assess the patient's level of understanding in order to assure autonomy.

The fourth cause of our failure to recognize subtle violations of patient autonomy lies in the unfortunate fact that in some instances the "work" of nursing becomes the major focus. This produces a climate of industrious habit. As we go about our work—doing procedures, giving medications, writing care plans, and trying to keep up a frantic pace—attentiveness to assuring patient autonomy is sometimes neglected.

In today's climate of advanced technology, fiscal uncertainty, staffing reductions, and bottom-line management, we should guard against focusing on work rather than caring.

Autonomy for patients is more frequently discussed in terms of larger issues, such as informed consent, paternalism, compliance, and self-determination. Let us review this principle as related to these and other recurrent themes.

Barriers to Autonomy

Autonomy exists within the confines and constructs of the world around us. As we have noted, it is often difficult for patients to express autonomous choices in different kinds of health care settings. However there are also social, political, and relational contexts that may affect one's ability to express an autonomous choice. Many of us have had our autonomy restricted at one time. Think about how that felt. For many people who are poor, institutionalized, or marginalized, they feel this way on an ongoing basis, as their autonomy is constrained by their position in the world. Their social status, position, relationships, perceptions, visible, or invisible attributes may make them unable to exercise their autonomy. As nurses, we must always be keenly aware of broader social, political, or relational constraints on persons that might affect them and their ability to be free and autonomous decision makers for themselves.

Informed Consent

Informed consent relates to a process by which patients are informed of the possible outcomes, alternatives, and risks of treatments, and are required to give their consent freely. The notion of informed consent is embedded in the principle of autonomy. The same barriers and facilitating factor relevant to autonomy apply to the informed consent process. It assures the legal protection of a patient's right to personal autonomy in regard to specific treatments and procedures. The concept of informed consent is one that has come to mean that patients are given the opportunity to autonomously choose a course of action in regard to plans for medical care. This is usually discussed in relation to surgery and complex medical procedures. Informed consent will be discussed in more depth in Chapter 11.

Paternalism/Parentalism

Paternalism is a gender-biased term that literally means acting in a *fatherly* manner. The traditional view of paternal actions includes such role behaviours as leadership, benevolent decision making, protection, and discipline. As commonly used in nursing, the term *paternalism* carries negative connotations, particularly related to implied dominant male versus submissive female roles.

In the health care arena, the concept of parentalism translates to professionals who restrict others' autonomy, usually to protect that person from perceived or anticipated harm or with a goal of acting in a person's best interests. Parentalism may be appropriate when a patient is judged to be incompetent or to have diminished decision-making capacity. As advocates, we choose to do for the patient that which it is reasonable to believe the patient would choose for him- or herself, if that were possible. We can consider parentalism a form of advocacy when we combine genuine concern for the patient with a well-founded belief that the patient is unable to make autonomous decisions. However, this combined concern can be misguided if it is used to coerce, control, or extent influence over persons, or if the person's best interests are not carefully and thoroughly articulated.

The risk of harm is not enough by itself to judge a person incompetent. Virginia Henderson, the well-known nursing leader and author, recounts her experience as a hospitalized patient:

> I was in the room with another patient, and I couldn't stand being in bed any longer, and I would sit in a chair. This nurse came in and saw me sitting in the chair, and she said "Ms. Henderson if you keep doing that, we are going to have to tie you down" . . . I thought, You just try it. . . . (Goldsmith, 1992, p. 4)

Even though Ms. Henderson was ninety-four years old at the time of her hospitalization, she was certainly competent to make decisions for herself. Patients who are competent must be allowed to act autonomously—even if the choices can be predicted to cause them harm or render them incompetent (Quinn & Smith, 1987). One exception that can be made is that even competent persons cannot be allowed to act in a way that would cause harm to others.

The term *paternalism* generally evokes negative sentiments among nurses and other health care professionals. This is due in part to a recognition that in the past patients' autonomy was frequently violated in the name of beneficence. Professionals sometimes make the dangerous assumption that they are uniquely qualified to make health care decisions by virtue of their professional knowledge and, further, that professional knowledge is the only knowledge needed to make decisions for patients. "Health care professionals often [believe they] understand better than patients do the full clinical implications of health risks, for they have seen the clinical results of its total actual results" (Quinn & Smith, 1987, p. 37). This kind of thinking allows us to ignore multiple contextual factors that might be unrelated to physical outcomes, yet affect the whole person. These factors include, among others, economic considerations, lifestyle, values, role, culture, and spiritual beliefs. In making decisions, all possible factors must be taken into consideration. This dictates that the patient must be autonomously engaged in the decision-making process and considered as an individual with unique beliefs, values, and lifestyle choices. In today's health care environments, it is widely accepted that patients are "experts" on themselves and only they can provide the important contextual information that is necessary for autonomous decision-making processes.

It is interesting to compare discussion of the concept of paternalism in the nursing and medical literature. Nursing literature generally describes paternalism in a negative way. Nurses often think of paternalism as behaviour that precludes autonomy. Medical literature, on the other hand, traditionally discusses paternalism as a benevolent quality. The following passage illustrates this point:

> In its strong version, the principle of paternalism justifies restricting someone's autonomy if by doing so we can benefit her. In such a case, our concern is not only with preventing the person from

harming herself, but also with promoting her good in a positive way. The principle might be appealed to even in cases in which our actions go against the other's known wishes. (Munson, 1992, p. 43)

The differences between the nursing and medical community in relation to beliefs about paternalism probably relate to historical, cultural, and gender factors. Now, in medicine, just as in nursing, the beliefs and practices around the person as autonomous have evolved markedly and paternalistic approaches to medical care are becoming a trend of the past. Interdisciplinary discussion is needed in order to reach a consensus about the appropriateness of paternalism in health care decision making.

Ask Yourself

Who Should Make Decisions?

- How do you feel when someone else makes a decision about you without your input?
- Since nurses and doctors may know more about the science of health care, is it ever appropriate for them to make decisions about the health care regimen without participation of the patient?

Noncompliance

The term **noncompliance** is generally thought of as denoting an unwillingness of the patient to participate in health care activities. This commonly entails lack of participation in a regimen that has been planned by the health care professional but must be carried out by the patient. Examples of such activities include taking medication as scheduled, maintaining a therapeutic or weight loss diet, exercising regularly, and quitting smoking. Use of the term *noncompliance* is just as likely to represent failure of the nurse as that of the patient. Discussion about noncompliance and care of the noncompliant patient centres around two basic factors. First, the autonomous participation of the patient in the health care plan is essential to success. When patients are fully aware of the choices in health care therapies and the consequences of nontreatment and are encouraged to make health care decisions, they are more likely to assume ownership of them and, as a result, to participate in care. Often nurses formulate plans of care that are consistent with a scientific base of knowledge but seem unreasonable to the patient, or fail to recognize diverse or unique needs or qualities of individuals. The nurse is amiss if she does not do her best to ensure that the patient is not an autonomous participant in the formulation of the plan. Second, nurses and other health care professionals must assess patients' abilities to follow plans of care. Patients may be unable to adhere to plans of care for a variety of reasons including lack of resources, lack of knowledge, lack of support from family members, psychological factors, and cultural beliefs that are not consistent with the proposed plan of care. Many times, patients are unable to participate in plans of care as they have not been included in the crucial planning processes and, therefore, their needs are not reflected in the proposed plans. An example of patients' inability to comply with a plan of care is seen every day in physicians' offices and emergency departments. Often patients are given prescriptions for medications that are prohibitively expensive. Many patients do not have private insurance or workplace plans to cover the costs of medication. These costs are not covered by the *Canada Health Act*, and are paid by individuals or private insurers. When they return with the same symptoms, not having taken the prescribed medication, they are invariably labelled as noncompliant. The problem is not one of compliance, but rather health care professionals' negligence in assessing patients' ability to follow a plan of care.

What are we to do when patients are well informed and apparently able to follow plans of care, yet do not? One hears stories of physicians who refuse to continue to care for patients who do not comply with instructions—smoking cessation, for example. In a climate of limited resources, this is a question worthy of contemplation. Codes of ethics for nurses universally support respect for individuals and individual choice, and are not restricted by considerations of social or economic status (ANA, 2001; ICN, 2006; Canadian Nurses Association, 2008). Further, the nurse must not be affected by patients' individual differences in background, customs, attitudes, and beliefs. Because health care practices are an integral part of patients' backgrounds, customs, and beliefs, refusal to participate in a plan of care, regardless of the outcome, is the prerogative of the patient, and must not affect the care given by the nurse. Ultimately, choices about health care practices belong to patients. If allowed to choose, patients should not be labelled in a negative way for choices with which nurses do not agree. It is not appropriate for professionals who express the belief that all competent patients have the right to autonomous choice to make value judgments about the choices made, and subsequently label patients as noncompliant (Nathaniel, 2000).

BENEFICENCE

The principle of **beneficence** is one that requires nurses to act in ways that benefit patients. There is no controversy as to whether nurses are obligated to act beneficently—beneficent acts are morally and legally demanded by our professional role (Beauchamp & Walters, 2001). The objective of beneficence provides nursing's context and justification. It lays the groundwork for the trust that society places in the nursing profession, and the trust that individuals place in particular nurses or health care agencies. Perhaps this principle seems straightforward, but it is actually very complex. As we think about beneficence certain questions arise: How do we define beneficence—what is *good*? Should we determine what is good by subjective, or by objective, means? Furthermore, is it possible to have an objective definition of the notion of good? When people disagree about what is good, whose opinion counts? Is beneficence an absolute obligation and, if so, how far does our obligation extend? Does the trend toward patient autonomy outweigh obligations of beneficence? As Veatch (2000) asks, "Is the goal really to promote the total well-being of the patient? Or is the goal to promote only the *medical* well-being of the patient?" (p. 41) We must keep these questions in mind as we practise.

The ethical principle of beneficence has three major components. (See Figure 3–2.) It maintains, first, that we ought to do or promote good (Beauchamp & Childress, 2001). Even with the recognition that *good* might be defined in a number of ways, it seems safe to assume that the intention of nurses in general is to do good. Questions arise when, in particular situations, those involved cannot decide what is *good*. For example, consider the case of a patient who is in the process of a lingering, painful, terminal illness. There are those who believe that life is sacred and should be preserved at all costs. Others believe that death is preferable to a life of pain and dependence. The definition of *good* in any particular case will determine, at least in part, the action that is to be taken.

Figure 3–2 **Beneficence**

> Do or Promote Good
> Prevent Harm
> Remove Evil or Harm

CASE PRESENTATION

Making a Difficult Decision

Anthony is 23 years old and has been in a vegetative state for over three years. At the age of 19, he and his friends were diving off a rugged cliff face on a graduation trip in Costa Rica. When he dove, he struck a rock. It was hours until he received medical attention and he has never regained consciousness since that day.

He is in a long-term rehabilitation centre and has had numerous severe complications, including infections, respiratory illnesses, and serious pressure sores, despite constant nursing care. In the past few months, he has had more serious respiratory infections and may require ventilation if these episodes continue. The nurses have mentioned to the physician that they recommend Anthony have a "Do not resuscitate" order on his chart, in case of a respiratory or cardiac arrest.

His mother and father visit daily, and the strain is beginning to show. They also note that Anthony appears to be deteriorating. They have been told, from the beginning, that there is no chance of recovery and that the remainder of his life would be spent in a vegetative and unresponsive state.

His parents feel that, with the increased respiratory infections, he may be suffering. They call for a health care team meeting. His mother agrees with the nurses and does not wish him to be placed on a ventilator and that he not be resuscitated in the case of a respiratory or cardiac arrest. She tells the health care team that would be more "merciful" to her son and that he would have wanted this. On the other hand, Anthony's father disagrees and insists that his son have all measures taken in case of any serious adverse event. He tells the team that he is a "good Catholic" and believes that by not doing all that could be done, he would be allowing his son to be "murdered." He also believes that it is in his son's best interests to be kept alive, "in case something new comes along and he can be helped. After all," his father continues, "he is still so young and has so much promise. He loved life and would want me to fight for him."

❓ Think About It

- In this case, what does each person or group of persons (his mother, his father, the nurses) consider to be in Anthony's best interests and why?
- How could Anthony's best interests be determined, if at all?

The principle of beneficence also maintains that we ought to prevent evil or harm (Beauchamp & Childress, 2001). In fact, some believe that doing no harm, and preventing or removing harm, is more imperative than doing good. All codes of nursing ethics require us to prevent or remove harm. For example, the International Council of Nurses (ICN) *Code of Ethics for Nurses* (2006) says, "The nurse takes appropriate action to safeguard individuals, families and communities when their health is endangered by a co-worker or any other person" (p. 3). Similarly, the Canadian Nurses Association *Code of Ethics for Registered Nurses* (2008), states:

> "Nurses question and intervene to address unsafe, non-compassionate, unethical or incompetent practice or conditions that interfere with their ability to provide safe, compassionate, competent and ethical care to those to whom they are providing care, and they support those who do the same. Nurses are attentive to signs that a colleague is unable, for whatever reason, to perform his or her duties. In such a case, nurses will take the necessary steps to protect the safety of persons receiving care." (CNA, 2008, p. 41)

Appendix D of the 2008 revision of the Canadian Nurses Association *Code of Ethics* outlines practical suggestions for the application of the *Code of Ethics* in minimizing the possibilities of potential harm to others, in various, specific circumstances.

Appendix D
Applying the Code in Selected Circumstances

Responding Ethically to Incompetent, Noncompassionate, Unsafe, or Unethical Care

- Maintain a high level of confidentiality about the situation and actions at all times.
- Review all information available about the current situation.
- Separate personal from professional issues. Concentrate on the situation at hand.

- Where appropriate and feasible, seek information directly from the colleague(s) whose behaviour or practice has raised concerns.

- Pay attention to the moral distress nurses are experiencing in trying to find an ethical course of action. Consider the risks of not taking action to persons receiving care, colleagues, self, and the organization, and reflect on the potential harms and breaches in trust that could result if no action is taken. Nurses need to consider as well the consequences that may occur for them and for others in taking various courses of action.

- If possible, speak with an impartial and trusted colleague outside of the situation who can preserve appropriate confidential information and help validate or rule out the conclusions being drawn.

- Seek information from relevant authorities (e.g., supervisor or manager) on expected roles and responsibilities for all of the parties who share responsibility for maintaining safe, competent, compassionate and ethical care.

- Consult, as appropriate, with colleagues, other members of the team, professional nursing associations or colleges or others who are able to assist in addressing and resolving the problem.

- Advise the appropriate parties regarding unresolved concerns and, when feasible, inform the colleague(s) in question of the reasons for your action. Know what immediate help is available to colleague(s) and be ready to help the colleague(s) find these resources.

(CNA, 2008, p. 41)

Ethical Considerations in Addressing Expectations That Are in Conflict with One's Conscience

- The nurse who decides not to take part in providing care on the grounds of moral objection communicates his or her desires in appropriate ways.

- Whenever possible such refusal is made known in advance and in time for alternative arrangements to be made for persons receiving care.

- Moral objections by the nurse are motivated by moral concerns and an informed, reflective choice and are not based upon prejudice, fear or convenience.

- When a moral objection is made, the nurse provides for the safety of the person receiving care until there is assurance that other sources of nursing care are available.

- Employers and co-workers are responsible for ensuring that nurses and other co-workers who declare a conflict of conscience receive fair treatment and do not experience discrimination (RCNA, 2000, p. 2).

- Nurses need to be aware that declaring a conflict of conscience may not protect them against formal or informal penalty.

(CNA, 2008, p. 45)

Ethical Considerations for Nurses in a Natural or Human-Made Disaster, Communicable Disease Outbreak, or Pandemic

A. In anticipation of the need for nursing care in a disaster or disease outbreak, nurses:

- work together with others in positions of leadership to develop emergency response practice guidelines, using available resources and guidelines from governments, professional associations and regulatory bodies;
- learn about and provide input into the guidelines the region, province or country has established regarding which persons are to receive priority in care (e.g., priority based on greatest need, priority based on probability of a good outcome and so on);
- learn how support will be provided for those providing care and carrying the physical and moral burden of care;
- request and receive regular updates about appropriate safety measures nurses might take to protect and prevent themselves from becoming victim to a disaster or disease;
- assist in developing a fair way to settle conflicts or disputes regarding work exemptions or exemptions from the prophylaxis or vaccination of staff; and
- help develop ways that appeals or complaints can be handled.

B. When in the midst of a disaster or disease outbreak, nurses have an ethical obligation to:

- refer to regulations and guidelines provided by government, regulatory bodies, employers and professional associations;
- help make the fairest decisions possible about the allocation of resources;
- help set priorities in as transparent a manner as possible;
- provide safe, compassionate, competent and ethical care (in disasters, as much as circumstances permit);
- help determine if, when and how nurses may have to decline or withdraw from care; and
- advocate for the least restrictive measures possible when a person's individual rights must be restricted.

(CNA, 2008, pp. 48–49)

Ethical Considerations in Relationships with Nursing Students

- All teacher–student interactions are to be in keeping with ethical nursing practice.
- All nurses and nursing students treat each other with respect and honesty.
- All nurses endeavour to provide nursing students with appropriate guidance for the development of nursing competence.
- The primary responsibility for the care of the person remains that of the primary nurse to whom the person has been assigned.

- Nursing students ensure that persons receiving care are informed of their student status. The person's right to refuse care or assistance provided by a student is to be treated with respect.
- Nursing students are expected to meet the standards of care for their level of learning. They advise their faculty clinical instructor and their clinical unit nurse supervisors if they do not believe they are able to meet this expectation.
- If nursing students experience difficulties with disrespectful actions from nurse(s) in practice that they are not able to overcome through conversation with the nurse(s) involved, they discuss these incidents with their faculty clinical instructor and, failing helpful outcomes from that discussion within an appropriate period, they enlist the assistance of the appropriate nursing education administrator in their nursing program.

(CNA, 2008, p. 50)

Acting Ethically in Situations That Involve Job Action

- Each nurse is accountable for decisions made about her or his practice at all times in all circumstances, including during a legal or an illegal strike (Nurses Association of New Brunswick [NANB], 2004).
- Individual nurses and groups of nurses safeguard persons receiving care when planning and implementing any job action.
- Individuals and groups of nurses participating in job action, or affected by job action, share the ethical commitment to the safety of persons in their care. Their particular responsibilities may lead them to express this commitment in different but equally appropriate ways.
- Persons whose safety requires ongoing or emergency nursing care are entitled to have those needs satisfied throughout any job action.
- During job action, if nurses have any concern about their ability to maintain practice and ethical standards or their ability to ensure the safety of persons in their care, they are responsible for communicating this concern in accordance with identified lines of accountability so that corrective action can be taken as quickly as possible (NANB, 2004).

(CNA, 2008, p. 51)

NONMALEFICENCE

The principle of **nonmaleficence** is related to beneficence. This principle requires us to act in such a manner as to avoid causing harm to patients. Included in this principle are deliberate harm, risk of harm, and inadvertent harm that occurs during the performance of beneficial acts. Most ethicists today tend toward the Hippocratic tradition that states, first do no harm (the principle of nonmaleficence), placing this principle above all others. It is obvious that we must not commit acts that cause deliberate harm. This principle prohibits, for example, experimental research that assumes negative outcomes for the participants, and the performance of unnecessary procedures for economic gain or solely as a learning experience. Nonmaleficence also means avoiding harm as a consequence of doing good. In such cases, the harm must be weighed against the expected benefit. For example, sticking a child with a needle for the purpose of causing pain is always bad—there is no benefit. Giving an immunization, on the other hand, while causing similar pain, results in the benefit of protecting the child from serious disease. Arguably, the harm caused by the pain of the injection is easily outweighed by the benefit of the vaccine. In day-to-day practice, we encounter many situations in which the distinction is less clear, either because the harm caused may appear to be equal to the benefit gained, because the outcome of a particular therapy cannot be assured or accurately predicted, or as a result of conflicting beliefs and values. For example, consider analgesia for patients with painful terminal illness. Narcotic analgesia may be the only type of medication that will relieve very severe pain. This medication, however, may result in dependence and can hasten death when given in amounts required to relieve pain. Cammon and Hackshaw (2000) offer another common example. Orders for patients to have nothing by mouth before procedures and tests are common practice, unquestioned by most nurses. The authors cite examples in which elderly patients were denied food for up to six days as tests and procedures were completed. The consequences of starvation in the elderly are unquestionable, yet the practice of following NPO orders for long periods of time is seldom questioned. As nurses, we must be alert to situations such as these in which harm may outweigh benefit, taking into account our own values and those of patients.

CASE PRESENTATION

Beneficence Versus Nonmaleficence

A middle-aged nurse recounts an incident that she believes relates to the principle of nonmaleficence. As a senior nursing student she was responsible for the care of a man who had a shotgun wound to his abdomen. Surgery had been performed, and the surgeon was unable to adequately repair the damage. The man was not expected to survive the day. He was, however, awake and strong, though somewhat confused. He had a fever of 107° Fahrenheit. He was receiving intravenous fluids and had continuous nasogastric suction. The man begged for cold water to drink. The physician ordered nothing by mouth in the belief that electrolytes would be lost through the nasogastric suction if water were introduced into the stomach. The student had been taught to follow the physician's orders. She repeatedly denied the man water to drink. She worked diligently—giving iced alcohol baths, taking vital signs, monitoring the intravenous fluids, and being industrious. He begged for water. She followed orders perfectly. After six terrible hours she turned to find the man quickly drinking the water from one of his ice bags. She left the room, stood in the hallway, and cried. She felt she had failed to do her job. As a result of the gunshot wound, the man died the next morning. Today her view of the situation is different.

Think About It

Weighing Harm Against Benefit

- Was this patient harmed? Discuss your answer.
- What was the benefit of the nothing by mouth order?
- Discuss whether the harm of thirst or the benefit of maintaining nothing by mouth should take precedence.
- What other ethical principles are relevant?
- Why did the student experience such extreme distress?
- Why do you think that the nurse's view of the situation is different today?

This case illustrates the difficulty encountered when attempting to *honour* the principles of beneficence and nonmaleficence.

VERACITY

The term **veracity** relates to the practice of telling the truth. Truthfulness is widely accepted as a universal virtue. Most of us were taught as children to always tell the truth. Philosophers, in general, favour openness and honesty. The philosophers most frequently cited in nursing literature, Immanuel Kant and John Stuart Mill, agree in *favour* of truth telling. Nursing literature promotes honesty as a virtue and truth telling as an important function of nurses. However, there are some differences in perspective among health care professionals. Bioethicists disagree on the absolute necessity of truth telling in all instances, but in most cases, it is agreed that truth telling is better than deception (Hébert, Hoffmaster, and Glass, 2008).

Ask Yourself

Is Truth Telling Always Beneficent?

- A patient's family member asked you to lie to the patient about the seriousness of their diagnosis or prognosis, in order to "protect the patient." How would you feel? What would you do?

- A fellow nurse discloses to you, over lunch, that she mistakenly gave an incorrect dosage of medication to a patient earlier that day. She adds that the patient hasn't experienced any adverse effects due to the lower dose and that he is unaware of the mistake. She asks you to keep it a secret. What would you do? Is the patient owed the truth, despite the lack of serious adverse effects? Why or why not?

- One of your patients is being seen by a new clinical clerk from another medical service, who is very busy and overwhelmed with referrals. The patient asks the clerk about the results of the tests that were done two days ago, stating that she is very anxious and worried about the possible results. The clerk tells the patient "not to worry" and that the results aren't in yet, but they'll probably be just fine. When you read the chart, you see that in fact the results are there, and they indicate a serious condition and need for further surgery and treatment. When you confront the clerk about what he told the patient, he tells you, "She isn't my primary patient. I need to leave it up to her attending physician to give her that news. I just don't have the time or the knowledge of her case to tell her all that." What could the clerk have done instead? What would you do now?

- You are a registered nurse in a public health clinic in an underserved area of the city. You see many patients with a variety of social and economic challenges, every day. One of your regular patients, a young single mother with three children, comes in to see you today, in obvious distress. She has run out of her medication as she found someone on the street to sell it to, in order to make some extra money to buy food, as the food banks are tightening up their allowances for families. She begs you to provide her with more medication as she now requires it. You know that you can dispense more medication to her but you need to have the approval of the nurse practitioner to do so. You also know that the nurse practitioner will not approve dispensing medication if she knows that the patient sold it on the street. You decide that you will tell her that the patient simply lost the medication and now requires extra. Are health care professionals owed the same right to truth telling and veracity as patients? Who might be harmed as a result of not telling the truth in this case?

We can support nurses' practice of telling the truth in many ways. Truth telling engenders respect, open communication, trust, and shared responsibility. It is promoted in all professional codes of nursing ethics. Truth telling advances and ensures the genuineness and trust between patient and the health care professional, and establishes an environment of authenticity and openness.

A very general interpretation of the ideas of the contemporary philosopher Martin Buber (1965) suggests that true communication between people can take place only when there are no barriers between them. Lying or deception creates a barrier between people and prohibits both meaningful communication and the building of relationships. Recognizing that communication is the cornerstone of the nurse–patient relationship, an argument can be made that nurses must be truthful in order to communicate effectively with patients.

Violating the principle of veracity shows lack of respect. Telling lies, or avoiding disclosure, implies that the specific function of the nurse or other person involved assumes prominence over the patient or, at the very least, the autonomy of the patient.

Jameton (1984) suggests that manipulating information for the purpose of controlling others is like using coercion to control them. In essence this keeps them from participating in decisions on an equal basis. Used to benefit the patient, it is paternalism; used against the patient, it is fraud (Myers, 2000).

Jameton (1984) also suggests that deceiving others may constitute an unnecessary assumption of responsibility. When unfortunate consequences occur, the one responsible for the deception can also be assumed to be responsible for consequences. It is often impossible to foresee all potential future negative consequences of deception. When bad consequences occur after we have reported the truth, we can attribute responsibility to unfortunate circumstances.

Truth telling enables trust. We can make the argument that truth telling is imperative in assuring that patients continue to trust nurses and other health care professionals. It is by virtue of the trust in these relationships that patients are willing to suspend some measure of autonomy and seek help in meeting health care needs. Without this trust the nurse–patient relationship would be destroyed.

Veracity is described as a key element in the professional–patient relationships (Beauchamp & Childress, 2001; Hébert, Hoffmaster, and Glass, 2008). The American Medical Association notes that physicians must be honest in all dealings with patients (American Medical Association, 2001). While many documents mention truth telling as an ethical attribute and obligation, veracity as a separate notion is rarely addressed and not mentioned in the Codes of Ethics of either the Canadian Nurses Association Code or the Canadian Medical Association. Veracity compels health care professionals to provide "comprehensive, accurate, and objective transmission of information, as well as to the way the professional fosters the patient's or subject's understanding" (Beauchamp and Childress, 2001, p. 284)

As with other principles, there is a some discrepancy between nursing and medical literature in regard to veracity. Recognizing that health care is an interdisciplinary effort, and that disclosure of information to patients involves both nurses and physicians, along with other members of the health care team, it is important for us to understand differing perspectives on the notion of veracity. It is also imperative to note two important considerations in this discussion. First, this discussion does not further a claim that "all physicians" believe that the truth should be withheld in specific circumstances nor does it further a mistaken belief that all nurses believe in veracity in all circumstances. This would be an error, based on an inaccurate assumption and a furthering of stereotypes about groups of health care professionals and the differences between these groups. Second, the perspectives and views on veracity in the medical, nursing, and bioethics literature and in practice are always changing, responsive to other trends in medical care, legal, and ethical obligations, as well as the specific contexts or situations.

Some medical literature makes the claim that patients do not want bad news, and that truthful information has the potential to harm them. Lipkin (1991) argues that physicians should sometimes deceive their patients or withhold information from them. It is his view that patients do not have sufficient information about how their bodies function to interpret medical information accurately, and sometimes do not want to know the truth about their illness. Joseph Ellin (1991) discusses special considerations that have been posed by the medical profession in relation to truth telling. He suggests that it does not seem beneficent to adopt an ethic of absolute veracity in which it is an obligation to cause avoidable anguish to someone who is already ill, especially when hope and positive outlook may promote healing and help prolong life. He writes, "One could hope to avoid this dilemma by holding that the duty of veracity, though not absolute, is to be given very great weight, and may be overridden only in the gravest cases . . ." (p. 82). Ellin draws a distinction between lying and deception: lying is the purposeful telling of untruths, whereas deception is usually accomplished through nondisclosure. He argues that there is an absolute duty to avoid lying to patients; however, there is no duty not to deceive. Examples he gives include withholding information about a poor prognosis or giving placebo medication. Consider the following situation: A mother of four is admitted to the emergency department after an automobile accident in which two of her children are killed. Recognizing that she is in very serious condition, according to Ellin, it would be appropriate to avoid telling her of the death of her children at this point in time. If, however, she asks about their condition, she must be told the truth.

Ask Yourself

Is the Truth Sometimes Harmful?

- Do you think it is acceptable to deceive a patient in order to prevent unnecessary suffering?
- How would you feel if you were a patient and the health care team and your family conspired to deceive you—if, for example, you were ill and you had a bleak prognosis?

Bok (1991) examines the practice of physicians deceiving patients in the name of beneficence. She writes that lying to patients has historically been seen as an excusable act. "Some would argue that doctors, and only doctors, should be granted the right to manipulate the truth in ways so undesirable for politicians, lawyers, and others" (p. 75). In fact, truth telling has never been a principle that was given consideration in the medical literature. Veracity is absent from virtually all oaths, codes, and prayers. Even the Hippocratic Oath makes no mention of truthfulness. The 1847 version of the American Medical Association Code of Ethics endorses some forms of deception by stating that the physician has a sacred duty to avoid "all things which have a tendency to discourage the patient and to depress his spirits" (Bok, 1994, p. 1683).

Nursing and medicine view veracity from two different perspectives. It is clear that physicians have traditionally seen disclosure or nondisclosure to be a facet of care within their control that can have implications for patient welfare and have exercised veracity in ways which were felt to be in the best interests of their patients. To withhold bad news is often considered a beneficent act if disclosure of the information is predicted to harm the patient. Nursing, on the other hand, upholds veracity as supporting individual rights, respect for persons, and the principle of autonomy. Recognition of the viewpoint of others is imperative for professionals who must collaborate. Chapter 4 discusses methods of making decisions about ethical problems when there are differences of perspective among those involved.

CONFIDENTIALITY

Confidentiality is the ethical principle that requires nondisclosure of private or secret information with which one is entrusted. Support for this principle is found in codes and oaths of nursing and medicine dating back many centuries. Nursing codes of ethics require that we maintain confidentiality of patient information. According to the ICN *Code of Ethics for Nurses* (2006), "The nurse holds in confidence personal information and uses judgement in sharing this information." Similarly, the ANA *Code of Ethics for Nurses* (2001) and the Canadian Nurses Association *Code of Ethics for Registered Nurses* (2008) direct nurses to maintain confidentiality. Confidentiality is the only facet of patient care mentioned in the Nightingale Pledge, recited for decades by graduating nurses: "I will do all in my power to elevate the standard of my profession and will hold in confidence all personal matters committed to my keeping and all family affairs coming to my knowledge in the practice of my profession." The Hippocratic Oath is also very clear: "Whatever, in connection with my professional practice, or not in connection with it, I see or hear, in the life of men, which ought not to be spoken of abroad, I will not divulge, as reckoning that all such should be kept secret." Though there are compelling arguments in favour of maintaining confidentiality, there is disagreement about the absolute requirement of confidentiality in all situations.

The ability to maintain privacy in one's life is an expression of autonomy. The capacity to choose what others know about us, particularly intimate personal details, is important, because it enables us to maintain dignity and preserve a measure of control over our own lives. Markus and Lockwood discuss the importance of privacy:

> Privacy is thus a value closely related to, and perhaps ultimately grounded on, the value of personal autonomy. To take this value of privacy seriously is to subscribe to a number of familiar precepts. It means that we should be reluctant to pry, that we should respect personal confidences, and that when we enter into relationships with others that render us privy to sensitive or intimate personal information, we should be [careful] about passing this information on, even in the absence of any specific request not to do so. (1991, p. 349)

Thus, maintaining confidentiality of patients is an expression of respect of persons and, in many ways, is essential to the nurse–patient relationship. Consider the following case presentation.

CASE PRESENTATION

Making the Best Choice

Lora is a seventeen-year-old high school student. She comes to the local family planning clinic requesting birth control pills. In the process of completing the initial physical examination, the nurse practitioner finds evidence of physical abuse, including a recent traumatic perforated ear drum. Lora hesitantly and tearfully admits that her biological father slapped her across her left ear prior to her coming to the clinic. She reports that she recently moved into his home after living most of her life with her mother and stepfather. She reports that her stepfather was sexually abusive to her and that she wishes to remain with her biological father. She says that she can tolerate her father hitting her occasionally, and she does not want to get him in trouble or be forced to move back to her stepfather's home. The law requires that the nurse report any suspicion of child abuse to adhere to mandatory reporting laws. However, the CNA *Code of Ethics* requires the nurse to maintain confidentiality.

Think About It

To Tell or Not to Tell

- What are the principles involved?
- Does the nurse's obligation to report the incident of child abuse supersede the obligation to maintain confidentiality—particularly considering that the patient requested confidentiality? What if Lora was fourteen years old?
- What are the options for the nurse?
- What are the possible outcomes of the different options?
- Does Lora's autonomy outweigh the nurse's responsibility to report the abusive situation?
- Review the legal obligation in Canada to report cases of suspected child abuse. What other kinds of situations require mandatory reporting?

There are at least two basic ethical arguments in favour of maintaining confidentiality. The first of these is the individual's right to control personal information and protect privacy. The second argument is one of utility.

This right to privacy flows from autonomy and respect for persons. On one level, patients have the right to expect that personal and private information will not be shared unnecessarily among health care providers. Patient information is not an appropriate topic for elevator or dinner conversation. It is most likely that violations of this nature were what authors had in mind when writing early creeds and oaths that promise confidentiality. Nurses and other professionals often casually discuss private patient matters. On another level, nurses must keep in mind the number of people who have legitimate access to patient records. In a hospital situation, patient charts are accessible to many personnel. Nurses, physicians, dieticians, respiratory therapists, utilization review staff, financial officers, students, secretaries, physical therapists, and others have legitimate reason to view patient records. Information of a sensitive and private nature that the patient intends for the nurse alone can become widely known in a large health care facility. Care must be taken in choosing information to be recorded in patients' charts. Special care must be taken to avoid inadvertent breaches of confidentiality (Erlen, 1998) including those involved with electronic records (Muldoon, 1996). It is important for nurses to be aware of the many threats to patient confidentiality.

Confidentiality is particularly important when revelation of intimate and sensitive information has the potential to harm the patient. Harm can take various forms such as embarrassment, ridicule, discrimination, deprivation of rights, physical or emotional harm, marginalization, and loss of roles or relationships. Consider the plight of many persons with AIDS whose diagnoses have become public knowledge without their consent. Confidentiality is particularly important when dealing with vulnerable populations (Winston, 1988).

The second argument is one of utility. If patients suspect that health care providers reveal sensitive and personal information indiscriminately, they may be reluctant to seek care. Government policy makers recognize this problem. In Canada, significant privacy legislation exists at both the federal and provincial levels to protect the confidentiality of personal information for Canadians. At a federal level, Canada has two privacy laws. The *Privacy Act*, first enacted in 1983, outlines the obligations of federal government agencies and institutions to respect the privacy rights of citizens by treating the collection and disclosure of personal information with great care. It also clearly states that individuals have the right to access their own information, about themselves, without interference or constraints (Office of the Privacy Commissioner of Canada, 2004). Second, the *Personal Information Protection and Electronics Document Act*, also known by the acronym PIPEDA (2000) sets out rules for how personal information should be sought and managed by private-sector organizations and in commercial activities (Kardash & Penta, 2005). Each province, in turn, has individual legislation and acts governing the management of personal and health information. For example, Alberta has the following legislation and acts pertaining to personal and health information: The *Freedom of Information and Protection of Privacy Act*; the *Health Information Act*, which took effect in 2001; and the *Personal Information Protection Act* (PIPA) which came into force January 1, 2004. Ontario has the *Freedom of Information and Protection of Privacy Act* and the *Personal Health Information Protection Act*, which came into effect in 2004.

Each province has its own privacy commissioner to oversee relevant legislation and the challenges that arise with complex legislation and rules governing the collection, use, storage, and dissemination of personal identifiable information, which includes health information, across a variety of contexts, including education and health care. The Privacy Commissioner of Canada has a website that describes the kinds of oversight the federal government and each province has, in regards to private information of Canadian citizens (http://www.privcom.gc.ca/resource/prov/index_e.asp). Because of the intimate and private nature of reproductive health issues, confidentiality of those seeking family planning services, for example, is mandated. Those caring for patients with AIDS also recognize the need to maintain confidentiality. According to Winston (1988), many who work with AIDS patients find such arguments particularly compelling, believing that disclosure of patients' antibody status or a diagnosis of AIDS would have a "chilling effect," discouraging those in high-risk groups from seeking care. There are other diagnoses, such as mental illness, alcoholism, and drug addiction that, if revealed without the permission of the person involved, could lead to public scorn, and subsequently discourage others from seeking care. In Canada, the issue of mandatory reporting of gunshot wounds is an example of a debate in which those opposed fear that victims of gunshot wounds will not seek medical treatment for fear of criminal charges or police involvement.

CASE PRESENTATION

Francis is a new graduate nurse, working in a busy downtown hospital. Today, he has a quick lunch by himself. He hasn't had time yet to make good friends and finds himself very busy, as a fresh graduate on a new unit. A group of more senior nurses from the unit are having lunch at an adjoining table, close by. Francis and his colleague hear them discussing a particularly challenging patient quite loudly, disclosing details about the patient and his wife and joking. He recognizes that it was a very difficult morning and that his fellow nurses are "letting off steam." He also notes that at nearby tables, there are patients, families, and staff from other units, who can easily hear the conversation.

The group of nurses catch Francis's eye and motion, in a friendly way, for him to come over and join them. This is the first time that they have extended this kind of friendly invitation to him and he is eager to join them. However he is very uncomfortable with discussing patients in a crowded cafeteria. He also thinks that he should mention something to them about not talking about patients in public places, but he is afraid that they will then not allow him to be part of the group.

Think About It

- What should Francis do, and why?
- Have you ever been in a similar situation? How did you feel? What did you do?
- What ethical principles are important to consider, in this case?
- What might a utilitarian or a deontologist advise Francis to do, and why?

Limits of Confidentiality

Should the principle of confidentiality be honoured in all instances? There are arguments that favour questioning the absolute obligation of confidentiality in certain situations. These arguments include theories related to the principles of harm and vulnerability (Winston, 1988). The harm principle can be applied when the nurse or other professional recognizes that maintaining confidentiality will result in preventable wrongful harm to innocent others. Mandatory testing of pregnant women for HIV and syphilis, for example, is intended to prevent the spread of a serious communicable disease to the fetus. In this instance, society chooses to override the privacy of the individual to protect the health of the innocent. Though directing nurses to maintain confidentiality and advocate for continuous policy development and safeguards for protection of privacy, the CNA *Code of Ethics* (2008) notes that there are situations in which the obligation of confidentiality is not absolute. The *Code of Ethics* states that if disclosure of information without a person's authorization is necessary or legally required, it must be carried out with great care, by disclosing the minimum amount of information to the fewest number of persons in order to meet requirements. Additionally, the persons in their care must always be told that their information is being disclosed to others as well as informed about the rationale for doing so. Finally, the *Code of Ethics* compels nurses, when disclosing health information without a person's consent, to do so in ways that do not further marginalize or stigmatize that person, their family, or community, by virtue of having that information known to others.

In rare instances, case law supports the harm principle. In July of 1976, the California Supreme Court ruled that a psychologist, Dr. Lawrence Moore, and his superior, Dr. Harvey Powelson, and the agency for which they worked were liable in the wrongful death of Tatiana Tarsoff. Prosenjit Poddar killed Tatiana Tarsoff in October of 1969. According to Tatiana's parents, two months earlier Poddar confided his intention to kill Tatiana to his psychologist, Dr. Moore. Though Dr. Moore initially tried to have his patient involuntarily committed, Dr. Powelson intervened and allowed Poddar to return home. Neither Tatiana nor her parents were informed of the patient's threats. The court found that the defendants were responsible for the wrongful death of Tatiana because they knew in advance of the patient's intentions. The obligation to protect the innocent third party superseded the obligation to maintain confidentiality. According to the majority opinion in this case, the duty to warn arises from a special relation between the patient and the psychologist that imposes a duty to control the patient's conduct (Tobriner, 1991).

Foreseeability is an important consideration in situations in which confidentiality conflicts with the duty to warn. The nurse or other health care professional should be able to reasonably foresee harm or injury to an innocent other in order to violate the principle of confidentiality in favour of a duty to warn. This consideration precludes blanket disclosure of private information that might predict harm to others. The Tarasoff case exemplifies reasonable application of the harm principle. Subsequent court cases support the decision in the Tarasoff case. Courts have found that privacy is not absolute and is subordinate to the state's fundamental right to enact laws that promote public health.

The harm principle is strengthened when one considers the vulnerability of the innocent (Haggarty, 2000). The duty to protect others from harm is stronger when the third party is dependent on others or is in some way especially vulnerable. This duty is called the vulnerability principle. Vulnerability implies risk or susceptibility to harm when vulnerable individuals have a relative inability to protect themselves (Winston, 1988). For example, nurses have a legal and absolute duty to report child abuse. Because children are dependent and vulnerable, they are at greater risk of harm. Coupling the harm principle with the vulnerability principle produces a rather strong argument for abandoning the principle of confidentiality in certain instances.

❓ Think About It

Can Nurses Violate Confidentiality?

- How do you think confidentiality and the harm and vulnerability principles can be reconciled?

- How would you feel if a relative contracted a sexually transmitted infection from a source who public health officials knew was infected, and had reason to believe would infect your relative, but neglected to warn?

- How would you feel if you were HIV infected and your health care provider violated your right to confidentiality?

Actions that are considered ethical are not always found to be legal. Though there is an ethical basis for subsuming the principle of confidentiality in special circumstances, and there is some legal precedent for doing so, there is legal risk to disclosing sensitive information. There is dynamic tension between the patient's right to confidentiality and the duty to warn others. Nurses need to recognize that careful consideration of the ethical implications of actions will not always be supported in bureaucratic and legal systems.

JUSTICE

Justice is the ethical principle that relates to fair, equitable, and appropriate treatment in light of what is due or owed to persons, recognizing that giving to some will deny receipt to others who might otherwise have received these things. Within the context of health care ethics, the relevant application of the principle focuses on distribution of goods and services. This application is called **distributive justice**. Unfortunately, there is a finite supply of goods and services, and it is impossible for all people to have everything they might want or need. One of the primary purposes of governing systems is to formulate and enforce policies that deal with fair and equitable distribution of scarce resources.

Decisions about distributive justice are made on a variety of levels. The federal and provincial governments are responsible for deciding policy about broad public health access issues, such as establishment of new programs or hospitals. These decisions are made at a "macro" level. Hospitals and other organizations formulate policy on an institutional or "meso" level and deal with issues such as how decisions will be made concerning who will occupy intensive care beds and how patients will be triaged in emergency rooms. Nurses and other health care providers frequently make decisions of distributive justice on an individual basis or, literally at the bedside. For example, having assessed the needs of patients, nurses decide how best to allocate their time (a scarce resource) between their assignments of patients, all with varied needs and levels of required care.

There are three basic areas of health care that are relevant to questions of distributive justice. First, what percentage of our resources is it reasonable to spend on health care? Second, recognizing that health care resources are limited, which aspects of health care should receive the most resources? Third, which patients should have access to the limited health care staff, equipment, and so forth? (Jameton, 1984).

In making decisions of distributive justice, one must ask the question, "Who is entitled to these goods or services?" Philosophers have suggested a number of different ways to choose among people. Figure 3–3 lists some of the ways that people have historically made these types of decisions.

Figure 3–3 **Distributive Justice**

> To each equally
> To each according to need
> To each according to merit
> To each according to social contribution
> To each according to the person's rights
> To each according to individual effort
> To each as you would be done by
> To each according to the greatest good to the greatest number

There are those who believe that all should receive equally regardless of need. On the surface, nationalized health care systems would seem to meet this criterion, since all citizens are eligible for the same services. However, because some citizens would necessarily require more health care services than others, nationalized systems also are required to meet the criterion of need. Countries with different health care systems do this in different ways. In Canada, the allocation of health care resources, through what is known as universal health care, is based upon an egalitarian model—one in which everyone receives an equal share of available resources. The values underlying this approach include equal access to health care and the preservation of basic human rights through health care, social democracy, and social justice and humanitarianism. These values are closely related to our identity as Canadians and many persons feel that they should be upheld and protected closely (Romanow, 2002). With the development of the first universal social health care program in post–Second World War Canada, the health care system has continued toward addressing the varied health needs of the constituents and supporting the poor, elderly, and disabled through complex social systems. Dramatic cuts in health care funding in the 1980s had dramatic effects on social programs, such as health care, education, and social support; however the values underlying the system, even one constrained by financial limitations and sustainability concerns, remain constant.

As health needs differ between persons, some citizens necessarily "use" more resources while others "use" less. However, the notion that a universal system is there, if we require it, is a fundamental value inherent in the Canadian system.

The principles of the *Canada Health Act* outline the values and practical application and administration of them within the Canadian health care system.

PRINCIPLES OF THE *CANADA HEALTH ACT*
The Criteria

1. **Public Administration:** Health care insurance plans are to be administered and operated on a non-profit basis by a public authority, responsible to the provincial/territorial governments and subject to audits of their accounts and financial transactions.

2. **Comprehensiveness:** The health insurance plans of the provinces and territories must insure all insured health services, which include hospital, physician care, surgical-dental care and, where permitted, services rendered by other health care practitioners, such as nurse practitioners.

3. **Universality:** One hundred percent of the insured residents of a province or territory must be entitled to the insured health services provided by the plans on uniform terms and conditions.

4. **Portability:** Residents moving from one province or territory to another must continue to be covered for insured health care services by the "home" province during any minimum waiting period, not to exceed three months, imposed by the new province of residence. After the waiting period, the new province or territory of residence assumes health care coverage.

   Residents temporarily absent from their home provinces or territories, or from the country, must also continue to be covered for insured health care services. This allows individuals to travel or be absent, within prescribed limits, from their home provinces or territories but still retain their health insurance coverage.

   The portability criterion does not entitle a person to seek services in another province, territory or country, but is more intended to entitle one to receive necessary services in relation to an urgent or emergent need when absent on a temporary basis, such as on business or vacation.

   If insured persons are temporarily absent in another province or territory, insured services are to be paid at the host province's rate. If insured persons are temporarily out of the country, insured services are to be paid at the home province's rate.

   In some cases, coverage may be extended for elective (non-emergency) service in another province or territory, or out of the country. Prior approval by one's health insurance plan may also be required.

5. **Accessibility:** The health insurance plans of the provinces and territories must provide:

   Reasonable access to insured health care services on uniform terms and conditions, unprecluded, unimpeded, either directly or indirectly, by charges (user charges or extra-billing) or other means (age, health status or financial circumstances); reasonable access in terms of physical availability of medically necessary services has been interpreted under the *Canada Health Act* using the "where and as available" rule. Thus, residents of a province or territory are entitled to have access to insured health care services at the setting "where" the services are provided and "as" the services are available in that setting.

The German philosopher, Friedrich Nietzsche, had a different perspective to the egalitarian model outlined above. He believed that there are superior individuals, and that society's goal should be to enhance these "supermen." For Nietzsche, the choice of distribution was a clear one—to each according to his present or future social contribution (Durant, 1926). To each according to that person's rights indicates a libertarian viewpoint, and to each as you would be done by is a reflection of the golden rule. The idea that each should receive according to effort is a common belief in our culture and indicates the traditional "work ethic." Entitlement programs in the United States generally award benefits based upon a combination of need and the greatest good that can be accomplished for the greatest number of people. In other words, the American system is often viewed as a libertarian system. Chapter 15 discusses the application of the principle of distributive justice in greater detail.

FIDELITY

The ethical principle of **fidelity** is often related to the concept of faithfulness and the practice of keeping promises. Society has granted nurses the right to practise nursing through the processes of licensure and registration (*Regulated Health Professions Act*, 1991). The process of licensure is one that ensures no other group can practise within the domain of nursing as defined by society and the profession or practise using the label of "registered nurse." Thus, to accept licensure and become legitimate members of the profession mandates that nurses uphold the responsibilities inherent in the contract with society and inherent as members of a regulated profession. Members are called to be faithful to the society that grants the right to practice—to keep the promise of upholding the profession's code of ethics, to practice within the established scope of practice and definition of nursing, to remain competent in practice, to abide by the policies of employing institutions, and to keep promises to individual patients. To *be* a nurse is to *make these promises*. In fulfilling this contract with society, nurses are responsible to faithfully and consistently adhere to these basic principles.

On another level, the principle of fidelity relates to loyalty within the nurse–patient relationship. It gives rise to an independent duty to keep promises or contracts (Veatch, 2000) and is a basic premise of the nurse–patient relationship. Problems sometimes arise when there is a conflict between promises that have been made and the potential consequences of those promises in cases in which carrying them out will cause harm in other ways. Though fidelity is the cornerstone of a trusting nurse–patient relationship, most ethicists think there are no absolute, exceptionless duties to keep promises—that, in every case, harmful consequences of the promised action should be weighed against the benefits of keeping the promise.

SUMMARY

As we participate in meeting the health care needs of society, we must be constantly aware of ethical implications inherent in many situations. Each nurse must develop a philosophically consistent framework from which to base contemplation, decision, and action. It is this framework that gives shape to our concept of various ethical principles. The principles discussed in this chapter presuppose nurses' innate respect of persons. Ethical principles include autonomy, beneficence, nonmaleficence, veracity, confidentiality, justice, and fidelity.

CHAPTER HIGHLIGHTS

- All ethical principles are embedded in a respect for persons.
- Autonomy denotes having the freedom to make choices about issues that affect one's life.
- Various intrinsic and extrinsic factors may threaten patient autonomy.
- The principle of beneficence maintains that one ought to do or promote good, prevent evil or harm, and remove evil or harm.
- The principle of nonmaleficence requires one to avoid causing harm, including deliberate harm, risk of harm, and harm that occurs during the performance of beneficial acts.
- The principle of veracity relates to the universal virtue of truth telling.
- Confidentiality is the ethical principle that requires nondisclosure of private or secret information with which one is entrusted.
- Justice is the ethical principle that relates to fair, equitable, and appropriate treatment in light of what is due or owed to persons, recognizing that giving to some will deny receipt to others who might otherwise have received these things.
- Fidelity is the ethical principle that relates to faithfulness and promise keeping.

DISCUSSION QUESTIONS AND ACTIVITIES

1. Find the CNA *Code of Ethics for Nurses* on the CNA website. Read the code and discuss how the various statements relate to the principles discussed in this chapter.

2. Read the following hypothetical situation and answer the questions that follow:
An elderly gentleman presents himself to the emergency department of a small community hospital. The patient has contractures and paralysis of his left hand; he apparently has complete expressive and at least partial receptive aphasia. Upon questioning, the man takes off his right shoe and points to his right great toe and grimaces, apparently indicating a problem in that area. The nurse is unable to gather any further information from him because of his difficulty in communicating. In attempting to help him, she asks if he has a neighbour or friend accompanying him. He shakes his head, indicating that he is alone.

Curious, the nurse asks him how he came to the hospital. The patient smiles and proudly produces a driver's licence from his shirt pocket. Subsequently, the nurse leaves the room and returns a few minutes later to find that the patient left the hospital, having received no care. The nurse suspects that because of his current physical condition the man is unsafe to drive a motor vehicle.

- What are the ethical implications in this situation?
- What ethical principles are involved?
- Should the nurse pursue avenues to locate the patient and ensure that he is not endangering himself or others by driving? Would this be a breach of confidentiality? Autonomy?
- How does the nurse express fidelity in this situation?
- What is the beneficent action?

3. Describe situations you have witnessed in which decisions were made for patients in a paternalistic manner. Discuss your perception of the appropriateness of paternalism in given situations.

4. Read the following hypothetical case and answer the questions that follow:

Martha is a seventy-five-year-old woman who has terminal cancer of the bladder. During the course of her therapy, she sustains third-degree radiation burns to her lower abdomen and pelvic area. Her wounds are extensive and deep, involving her abdominal wall, bladder, and vagina. The physician orders frequent medicinal douches and wound irrigations. These treatments are very painful, and the patient wants the treatments discontinued but is too timid to actually refuse them. The physician will not change the order.

- Discuss the situation in terms of beneficence and nonmaleficence.
- How does this patient express her autonomy?
- What is the nurse's responsibility in assisting the patient to maintain autonomy?
- How does the nurse deal with conflicting loyalties and principles?

5. Do you think health care professionals should disclose information to patients related, for example, to a poor prognosis, even though the information may cause distress? Discuss your views in depth.

6. Jameton (1984) says that for nurses to be less than competent is unethical. Discuss this statement in terms of fidelity.

7. Read the following hypothetical case and answer the questions that follow:

Nels Gruder is a forty-year-old disabled truck driver. He was injured several years ago in a trucking accident. He subsequently has had back surgery but continues to have severe pain. He has been seen by every local neurosurgeon and, for one reason or another, is not pleased with the care he has gotten. Because of the seriousness of his initial injuries, there is little doubt that Mr. Gruder has chronic back pain. Even though the local emergency room policy of not prescribing narcotic analgesics for chronic pain is clearly stated on signs in the waiting area, Mr. Gruder comes there frequently complaining of severe back pain. He reports a history of gastric ulcers and allergy to nonsteroidal anti-inflammatory drugs (NSAIDs). The nurse practitioner who sees Mr. Gruder is faced with a man who is in obvious pain. She wishes to help him relieve the pain he is experiencing. At the same time she realizes that narcotic analgesia is not appropriate for this type of problem, and is unable to prescribe NSAIDs because of his reports of gastric ulcers and allergy. He says he has tried exercises and a local pain clinic, neither of which was effective. He is aware of the emergency room policy regarding narcotic analgesics for chronic pain, but he comes there in desperation. He insists that his pain is relieved only by narcotic analgesia.

- What ethical principles are involved?
- Does the benefit of pain relief outweigh the harm potentially caused by long-term narcotic analgesic use for this patient?
- Should Mr. Gruder's perceived need for narcotic pain medications be honoured even though the nurse practitioner feels he has a problem with drug dependence?
- How does the nurse do what she thinks is right and yet respect Mr. Gruder's autonomy?
- Is it important whether or not the nurse's actions please the patient?

REFERENCES

American Hospital Association. (1975). *Statement on a patient's bill of rights*. Chicago: Author.

American Medical Association. (2001). *Code of medical ethics. Principles of medical ethics*. Chicago: AMA.

American Nurses Association. (1995). *Nursing's social policy statement*. Washington: Author.

American Nurses Association. (2001). *Code of ethics for nurses*. Washington, DC: Author.

Aveyard, H. (2000). Is there a concept of autonomy that can usefully inform nursing practice? *Journal of Advanced Nursing, 32*(2), 352–358.

Beauchamp, T., & Childress, J. (2001). *Principles of biomedical ethics* (5th ed.). New York: Oxford University Press.

Beauchamp, T. L., & Walters, L. (2001). *Contemporary issues in bioethics*. Belmont, CA: Wadsworth.

Bok, S. (1991). Lies to the sick and dying. In T. A. Mappes & J. S. Zembaty, eds. *Biomedical ethics* (pp. 74–81). New York: McGraw-Hill.

Bok, S. (1994). Truth telling. In W. Reich, ed., *Encyclopedia of bioethics* (pp. 1682–1686). New York: Macmillan.

Buber, M. (1965). *The knowledge of man: A philosophy of the interhuman*. New York: Harper & Row.

Cammon, S. A., & Hackshaw, H. S. (2000). Are we starving our patients? *American Journal of Nursing, 100*(5), 43–46.

Canadian Nurses Association. (2008). *Code of ethics for registered nurses*. Author.

Durant, W. (1926). *The story of philosophy*. New York: Washington Square Press.

Edge, R. S., & Groves, J. R. (1994). *The ethics of health care: A guide for practice.* Albany, NY: Delmar.

Ellin, J. S. (1991). Lying and deception: The solution to a dilemma in medical ethics. In T. A. Mappes & J. S. Zembaty, eds., *Biomedical ethics* (pp. 81–87). New York: McGraw-Hill.

Erlen, J. A. (1998). The inadvertent breach of confidentiality. *Orthopedic Nursing, 17*(2), 47–50.

Goldsmith, J., ed. (1992). Virginia Henderson, RN: Humanitarian and scholar. *Reflections, 18*(1), 4–5.

Haggarty, L. A. (2000). Informed consent and the limit of confidentiality. *Western Journal of Nursing Research, 22*(4), 508–514.

Harrison, A. F., & Bramson, R. M. (1982). *Styles of thinking.* New York: Doubleday.

Hébert, P. C., Hoffmaster, B., & Glass, K. C. (2008). *Truth telling.* In P. Singer & A. M. Viens, eds., *The Cambridge textbook of bioethics.* Cambridge, England: Cambridge University Press.

International Council of Nurses (2006). *The ICN code of ethics for nurses.* International Council of Nurses, Geneva Switzerland. Retrieved January 23, 2001, from the World Wide Web: http://icn .ch/indes.html/

Jameton, A. (1984). *Nursing practice: The ethical issues.* Englewood Cliffs, NJ: Prentice-Hall.

Kardash, A., & Penta, A., eds. (2005). *A compendium of Canadian legislation respecting the protection of personal information in health research.* Ottawa: Canadian Institutes of Health Research.

Lipkin, M. (1991). On lying to patients. In T. A. Mappes & J. S. Zembaty, eds., *Biomedical ethics* (pp. 72–73). New York: McGraw-Hill.

Markus, A., & Lockwood, M. (1991). Is it permissible to edit medical records? *British Medical Journal, 303,* 349–351.

Muldoon, J. D. (1996). Confidentiality, privacy and restriction for computer-based patient records. *Hospital Topics, 74*(3), 32–37.

Munson, R. (1992). Major moral principles. In *Intervention and reflection: Basic issues in medical ethics* (4th ed., pp. 31–45). Belmont, CA: Wadsworth.

Myers, M. T., Jr. (2000). Lying for patients may be a violation of federal law. *Archives of Internal Medicine, 160*(4), 2223–2224.

Nathaniel, A. (2000). An examination of ethical principles as they relate to noncompliance. Continuing education case study. Sigma Theta Tau International Honor Society of Nursing. Retrieved January 13, 2001, from the World Wide Web: http://www.nursingsociety.org/

Quinn, C. A., & Smith, M. D. (1987). *The professional commitment: Issues and ethics in nursing.* Philadelphia: Saunders.

Romanow, R. (2002). *Building on values: The future of health care in Canada. Commission on the future of health care in Canada. Final report.* Canada.

Tobriner, M. O. (1991). Majority opinion in *Tarsoff v. Regents of the University of California.* In T. A. Mappes & J. S. Zembaty, eds., *Biomedical ethics* (pp. 165–169). New York: McGraw-Hill.

Veatch, R. (2000). *The basics of bioethics.* Upper Saddle River, NJ: Prentice Hall.

Winston, M. E. (1988). AIDS, confidentiality, and the right to know. *Public Affairs Quarterly, 2,* 91–104.

Yeo, M., & Moorhouse, A. (2002). *Concepts and cases in nursing ethics* (2nd ed.). Peterborough, ON: Broadview Press.

PART II

DEVELOPING PRINCIPLED BEHAVIOUR

Recognizing that values and beliefs are culturally relative, Part II describes theories related to moral development and values clarification. This section examines the process of ethical decision making and its application to clinical situations. Because personal values and moral development influence perceptions and decisions, readers are encouraged to become aware of their own values and to examine personal levels of moral development in light of the different theories presented in Part I. Benefiting from this knowledge, readers can begin to be more sensitive to the perspectives, decision-making abilities, and tendencies of other people and to acknowledge the influence of their own values and moral development on various decision-making processes.

CHAPTER 4

Values Clarification

OBJECTIVES

After completing this chapter, the reader should be able to:

1. Define and differentiate personal values, societal values, professional values, organizational values, and moral values.
2. Discuss how values are acquired.
3. Discuss self-awareness as a tool for ethical practice.
4. Explain the place of values clarification in nursing.
5. Explain the valuing process.
6. Describe values conflict and its implications for nursing care.
7. Consider the interaction between personal and institutional values.
8. Discuss the importance of attending to both personal values and patient values.

INTRODUCTION

Principled behaviour flows from personal values that guide and inform our responses, behaviours, and decisions in all areas of our life. Ethical decision making requires self-awareness and knowledge of ethical theories and principles. Such awareness of self includes knowing what we value or consider important. The branch of philosophy that studies the nature and types of values is called **axiology**, a word that comes from the Greek for *worth* or *worthy*. Axiology includes the study of values in art, known as aesthetics; in human relations and conduct, known as ethics; and in relation to beliefs regarding relationship with the Divine, known as religion. This chapter discusses the importance of being aware of personal values and how these values influence the way we relate to self and others within personal and professional arenas.

WHAT ARE VALUES?

Values are ideals, beliefs, customs, modes of conduct, qualities, or goals that are highly prized or preferred by individuals, groups, or society. Omery (1989) notes that the fundamental nature of values includes a pattern of a "subjective, strongly motivational preference or disposition toward a person, object, or idea that is more likely to be manifest in an affective situation . . . and [is] more likely to be mobilized by the individual in a hierarchical order" (p. 500). Values, which are learned in both conscious and unconscious ways, become part of a person's makeup and provide guidance as we set priorities. When we are faced with choices, our preferences and their hierarchy becomes evident. For example, if we value truth telling in all types of situations without exception, others may see us as overly forthright or direct. What we value becomes apparent in how we conduct ourselves on a daily basis. When a friend asks how her new haircut looks, if we indeed value truth telling, we may well choose to tell her that the cut does not suit her. These kinds of decisions and how we enact our values, on a daily basis, shape who we are as moral persons and how those in our world perceive us. Our values influence choices and behaviour whether or not we are conscious that the values are guiding the choices. Values provide direction and meaning to life and a frame of reference for integrating, explaining, and evaluating new experiences, thoughts, and relationships. Values may be expressed overtly, as espoused behaviours or verbalized standards, or may manifest in an indirect way through verbal and nonverbal behaviour.

Moral Values

As discussed in Chapter 2, individual cognitive evaluation of right and wrong, good, and bad, is reflective of **moral thought.** Flowing from this, preferences or dispositions reflective of right or wrong in human behaviour are considered **moral values** (Omery, 1989). Moral values constitute a special case of values because the particular circumstances that call them forth deal with ethical issues or dilemmas. These kinds of values are what we refer to, implicitly, when we are deciding, "What is the right thing to do?" We are often faced with moral or ethical dilemmas that challenge our beliefs or force us to articulate our values in an explicit way, through our actions or decisions. These kinds of ethical dilemmas may be encountered in a professional context or in our personal lives as we interact and form relationships with others. Moral values help us to decide what we "ought" to do or should do, according to our deeply held beliefs and priorities. These kinds of values are acquired over a lifetime, may be dynamic and iterative, and are influenced by any number of contexts or factors, such as our family, culture, spirituality, education, friendships, philosophical orientation, workplace, or profession, to name a few. These values may be acquired within contexts and social constructs such as the family, through our religious, educational or philosophical orientation, or through our profession.

ACQUIRING VALUES

Personal ethical behaviour flows from values held by an individual that develop over time. Cultural, ethnic, familial, environmental, educational, and other experiences of living help to shape our values. We begin to learn and incorporate values into our beings at an early age and continue the process throughout our lives. As noted previously, values are acquired in both conscious and unconscious ways. Values may be learned in a conscious way through instruction by parents, teachers, mentors, religious leaders and educators, and professional or social group leaders. Many values are formally adopted by groups and are written in professional codes of ethics, religious doctrines, societal laws, and statements of an organization's philosophy. Socialization and role modelling, other ways values are acquired, lead to more subconscious learning. Some values stay with us for much of our lives, and others may change or be altered in response to our own development and experiences. "The most important step in values formation is one's freedom to choose those values that are most cherished and to relinquish those that have little meaning" (Seroka, 1994, p. 11). The process of value formation, as Seroka calls it, and the choosing or rejecting of values, might also be referred to as the development of one's moral autonomy.

As children, we often adopt the values and beliefs of our parents. We are told what school we will attend, what religion we are affiliated with, and, in our interactions with those all around us, we encounter our culture, environment, and socioeconomic status relative to others. In one sense, we simply assume the values and beliefs of those with the most influence over us. Adolescents often identify more strongly with friends and peer groups, social networks, and both school and extracurricular activities. Through exploration of the world around them in a more independent way, adolescents may find that they are questioning the values of their parents, religion, culture, or environment in which they are growing up. This is often referred to as a kind of "teenage rebellion" and it is an important step in the development of our moral autonomy.

Later in youth, as we take on new roles away from home, as college or university students, as workers, new professionals or careerists, we are compelled to, again, explore new sets of values, beliefs, and priorities and find a way in which these new values can be incorporated or overlapped onto our existing set of values and beliefs.

As we develop new relationships with people outside our immediate families, who may be from diverse cultures, environments, or religions than our own, we also may reflect upon our own values, and, as Seroka notes, discover which of our held values are especially important, while renouncing those without meaning. In addition to these processes, we may also adopt or assume new values or change our values based on our experiences, relationships, and environments.

While many of us have "core" values that we find are relatively unchanging over time, they may be adaptable as we learn new perspectives or worldviews. Additionally, we may find a new perspective that better helps us to articulate our long-held values in a novel way. For example, consider Beatrice, a young nursing student who was raised by parents who identified themselves as agnostic and who instead focused their moral teaching toward Beatrice on doing good for others in all aspects of one's life and rejecting money or possessions as motivation for action or success. After travelling to do missionary work in Nepal, Beatrice found herself drawn to Buddhism. She identified strongly with the messages and philosophical stance of Buddhists and decided to embrace Buddhism in her own life. While she did not change her own values, she found that her identification with Buddhism allowed her a means by which to articulate the values that were instilled from her parents, in a unique and meaningful way.

Because values become a part of who we are, they often enter into decision making in less than conscious ways. We constantly make judgments that reflect our values, though not always realizing that we have a given set of values or that these values are affecting our decisions (Davis, Aroskar, Liaschenko, & Drought, 1997; Engebretson & Headley, 2000; Simon, Howe, & Kirschenbaum, 1995). Becoming more aware of one's values is an important preliminary and ongoing step in being able to make clear and thoughtful decisions. Reflecting upon one's own values in a conscious way, and being able to help others to articulate their values clearly, are particularly important in the area of ethical decision making.

Ask Yourself

How Have Your Values Developed?

Think of three ideals or beliefs that you prize in your personal life. For example, you may value a clean house and orderly life or you may instead place a lower value on keeping your house clean and tidy, and instead focus on valuing quality time with your children each day. As another example, you may find that you place a high value on being married while others may feel that it is not necessary to be married to have a long-term, meaningful relationship. Finally, you may set priorities in your working life to work fewer hours and spend more time relaxing and with your family, but have less disposable income while others may value working harder and longer hours in order to provide their family with more disposable income and time away on luxurious vacations.

When you think of what you value, your ideal or belief, try to think back to how that belief or value came into your awareness. Reflect upon how it evolved

(Continued)

to become something that you identify as important or a priority. Try to trace each belief or ideal back to the earliest time in your life when you were aware of its importance or presence.

- When and how did you learn to view each belief or ideal as important?
- How have they changed or evolved over time?
- Where do you find your support for them?
- How prevalent do you think these beliefs or ideals are among other people?
- What do you think of people who hold different beliefs or ideals?
- Think of a time in your life when one of these beliefs or ideals has been challenged. How did you feel? How did you react?

SELF-AWARENESS

Ethical relationships with others begin with self-knowledge and the willingness to express that awareness to others honestly and appropriately. Self-knowledge is an ongoing, evolving process that requires us to make a commitment to know the truth about ourselves. This is not an easy commitment to make. We must remember that what we believe to be the truth is always coloured by our perceptions, and surrounding contextual factors, and can change over a time (Covey, 1990). Keep in mind that most situations are not black or white. All sides are present in each situation. Like the aperture of a camera, what we see in any situation depends upon where we are standing and the angle from which we are looking. From this perspective, there can be many views of a situation, depending upon how many people are picturing it. Understanding the truth of a situation is usually more accurate if people appreciate that there can be different views, and openly share these perspectives (Banonis, 1997). While sharing diverse perspectives is key to any kind of exercise in which we identify or explore values, we must keep in mind the importance of remaining open to multiple perspectives. While we can never "walk in the shoes" of another person, truly, we can, however, remain open to how others' realities, experiences, cultures, spirituality, and environments have shaped their perspective. We also need to attend to and actively understand the reasons and rationales others have for decisions they make and priorities they set, especially if they are different from what our own decisions or actions might have been in a similar situation. The ability to be open to multiple perspectives, to try to understand the reasons others have for their decisions or actions, is an important part of becoming an ethically aware person. In a professional context, developing this ability is essential to interacting with and providing holistic and client-centred care to a diverse population of persons.

The term **values clarification** refers to the process of becoming more conscious of and articulating what we value or consider worthy. It is an ongoing process that is grounded in our capacity for reflective, intelligent, self-directed behaviour (Gaydos,

2000; Keegan, 2000). By focusing time, energy, and attention to reflecting on our values, we shed light on our personal perspective and discover our own answers to many concerns and questions. Developing insight into our values improves our ability to make value decisions. No one set of values is appropriate for everyone; we must appreciate that values clarification may lead to different insights for different people (Engebretson & Headley, 2000; Gaydos, 2000). Engaging in values clarification promotes a closer fit between our words and actions, enabling us to more clearly "walk our talk," thus enhancing personal integrity. As noted in Chapter 3, **integrity** refers to adherence to moral norms that is sustained over time. Moral integrity could also be called authenticity. Authenticity, in terms of moral development, refers to the attribute of maintaining and articulating consistent fundamental values and beliefs, over time. As we noted above, sometimes our values and beliefs may change or iterate, as we age, as well as question, and learn new perspectives. However, for many persons, our very fundamental "core" beliefs persist over time, despite being exposed to many different influences. These might include fundamental beliefs such as believing that hurting others is wrong, that truth telling is preferred over deception, or that those who are vulnerable or dependent on our care must be protected from harm. Being authentic, or maintaining moral integrity, signifies that we hold such beliefs or values in a way that is consistent and unwavering. Note, however, that this does not imply that, as persons with strong moral integrity, we automatically reject others who hold markedly different beliefs. Instead, we must be as steadfast in exploring, understanding, and appreciating the values of others as we are in holding onto our own. Trustworthiness and a consistency of convictions, actions, and emotions is implicit in integrity. It is only to the extent that we appreciate our own values that we can begin to understand the values of another.

Since values include dimensions of knowing and of feeling, the process of becoming more clear about what we consider to be overarching values needs to address both the cognitive and the affective domains. Through analyzing our behaviour and becoming more in touch with our feelings, we learn to discern which choices are rational, thoughtful, and dynamic, and which are the result of preconditioning (Seroka, 1994). Assessment of personal values requires a readiness and willingness to take an honest look at our ideals and behaviours; at our words, actions, and motivation; and at the congruencies and incongruencies among them. Moving toward the point of choosing our own values, rather than merely acting out prior programming, is a goal of the process and part of our ongoing development of our moral autonomy.

Enhancing Self-Awareness

Self-awareness is the ultimate tool for living a personally ethical life. Values clarification and **self-awareness** go hand in hand. The first and most important step in awareness of the self is the conscious intention to be aware. Being conscious of our thoughts, feelings, physical and emotional responses, and insights in various situations can promote appreciation of our values. Conversely, by identifying and analyzing personal values, we become more self-aware (Burkhardt & Nagai-Jacobson, 2002; Rew, 1996; 2000). We can enhance insight by developing the ability to step back and see what is going on in any situation, and being aware of ourself and our reactions in the present moment. Self-awareness can begin with as simple an act as tuning in to our breathing, noting its rate, rhythm, depth, and other characteristics without any effort to change it. Self-awareness is a way of becoming conscious of an act that usually occurs quite unconsciously. Another way to become more aware is to pay attention to how we are feeling physically and emotionally in any given situation—to name the feelings without judging them. We might ask, "What do I think I am reacting to here, and can I identify where that reaction comes from?" or "Why am I uncomfortable with this person's choice or decision?" For example, when you see a beautiful sunset, you might note a feeling of peace, exhilaration, or relaxation, and realize you are responding to beauty, with an ensuing memory that your mother was always one to be observant of beauty in her world. You thus recognize that you learned this value, at least in part, from your mother. Introspection, observation, reflection, meditation, journalling, art, writing, therapy, reading, discussion groups, and feedback assist us in expanding self-awareness.

Individual reflection and discussion with another person or in small groups help us to become more aware of and to analyze our values. Group discussion enables us to react and to hear the reactions of others. Such processes may lead us to see more clearly those values we have accepted because of programming, and to articulate better those values we have chosen. These processes may also lead us to modify our perspective based on the insights of others. Active listening and reflection upon the diverse views and beliefs of others is an important part of these processes. Alongside listening and reflecting, self-awareness requires that we maintain on openness to the views of others, as we reflect upon our own. Other tools that open our perspective include taking the other side of a debate, interviewing people with differing opinions, walking in another's shoes and defending his or her position, and asking for feedback on your positions. Another way to look at values is to ask general questions like "If I knew I would die in six weeks, what would I be doing today?" or "If I had to leave my house and could take only three things with me, what would they be?" or "Where would I like to be five/ten/twenty years from now?"

Simon and colleagues (1995) suggest that the valuing process includes three areas:

Prizing and cherishing one's beliefs and behaviours, which includes knowing what one does and does not support and communicating this to others;
Choosing one's beliefs and behaviours by evaluating values received from others, which includes examining alternatives and their consequences then deciding what is one's own;
Acting on these beliefs with a consistent pattern that reinforces actions supportive of the values.

The intent of values clarification is to help us become more aware of our own values and the valuing process in our lives; it does not aim to impose or instill particular values in our lives.

Journalling.   Kolkmeier (1995) describes **journals** as "records that are kept on a periodic or regular basis and contain factual material and subjective interpretations of events, thoughts, feelings, and plans" (p. 336). For many people, keeping a diary or journal of experiences and personal reactions to situations is a useful tool in developing awareness. A number of books such as those by Progoff (1992), Adams (1990), Kahn (1996), and Baldwin (1991) are available to guide someone new to journalling. Figure 4–1 offers guidelines that may help students utilize the journalling process to gain insight into personal values. The following are a few general considerations that may enhance the ability to gain insight through journalling. When writing in a journal, let your thoughts flow as freely as possible without censoring or judging what you are writing. Allow yourself time and privacy when you are journalling, and keep the journal in a place where you feel comfortable that you control who has access to it. Commit to journalling on a regular basis. Recognize that journalling is a personal process, so go with your style. If a format such as that suggested in Figure 4–1 helps you, go for it! If not, write as the thoughts flow from you.

Figure 4–1 **Journalling for Values Awareness**

- Describe a situation in your personal or professional experience in which you felt uncomfortable or felt that your beliefs or values were being challenged, or in which you felt your values were different from others involved.
- As you record the situation, include how you felt physically and emotionally at the time you experienced the situation.
- Write down your feelings as you remember the situation. Are your reactions now any different from when you were actually in this situation?
- What personal values do you identify in the situation? Try to remember where and from whom you learned these values. Do you completely agree with the values, or is there anything about them that you question?
- What values do you think were being expressed by others involved? How are they similar or different from your values?
- What do you think you reacted to in the situation?
- Can you remember having similar reactions in other situations? If yes, how were the situations similar or different?
- How do you feel about your response to the situation? Is there anything you would change if you could repeat the scene? Rewrite the scene with the changes or alternative endings.
- What do you need to do to reinforce behaviours, ideals, beliefs, or qualities that you have identified as personal values in this situation? When and how can you do this?

VALUES IN PROFESSIONAL SITUATIONS

Values clarification is important to nurses in several ways. To know and appreciate our own value system provides a basis for understanding how and why we react and respond in decision-making situations. Knowing our own values enables us to acknowledge similarities and differences in values when interacting with others, which ultimately promotes more effective communication and care. Commitment to developing more awareness of personal values enables us to be more effective in facilitating the process with others. In the professional realm, these others may be colleagues, patients, families, or institutions.

Values Conflict. When personal values are at odds with those of patients, colleagues, or the institution, internal or interpersonal conflict may result. This can subsequently affect patient care and can have serious personal and professional implications for the nurse. Dealing in an effective way with **values conflict** requires conscious awareness of our own values, as well as awareness of the perceived values of the others involved. Such awareness enables the nurse to be more alert to situations in which the behaviours of others are judged according to his or her own values, or in which personal values are being imposed upon another. When differences in values are identified, the nurse can choose to respond to the other's viewpoint, in a way that seeks understanding and common ground, rather than reacting in a "knee-jerk" fashion. In this way the integrity of the caring relationship can be maintained.

The following case presentation provides an example of values conflict. As you read the case, think about the values that are evident in the situation. Put yourself in the position of each of the participants and ask yourself what you might do if you were in their shoes.

CASE PRESENTATION

A Conflict of Values

Nine-year-old Benton is a patient on the pediatric unit with a diagnosis of terminal stage Ewing's sarcoma. He has three sisters, aged seven, six, and three, who are currently being cared for by a grandmother. His father is self-employed and works long hours. His mother has never worked outside the home. Both parents have high school educations, and their primary activities outside the family are church related. They belong to a small nondenominational rural church and state that they hold fast to what is taught in the Bible and put their faith in the word of God.

Prior to his illness, Benton, a healthy child, had been brought to the clinic only for acute health concerns. Shortly after entering second grade two years ago, he began limping. The family attributed the limp to a playground injury. When he continued to complain of pain and the limp persisted after three months, his mother took him to a local health clinic. Above-the-knee amputation followed diagnosis, but metastasis was evident in nine months. Chemotherapy has been only palliative.

The physician has discussed Benton's poor prognosis with the parents, recommending comfort care. The parents say they want everything possible to be done for him, and the father conducts nightly prayer sessions at Benton's bedside, affirming that God is healing Benton. Although Benton has asked whether he is going to die, his father refuses to allow staff to speak with him regarding fears or concerns about his condition. When asked what Benton has been told, the father responds, "He knows God is trying us and we must have faith." The mother, who appears less confident of a healing, is there twenty-four hours a day. She supervises Benton's care relentlessly, at times irritating staff with questions and demands. She keeps a notebook record of her son's care, including medication, times of care, intake and output, and personal assessments. Although Benton used to talk to staff, he now appears frightened and remains quiet, sleeping off and on.

Think About It

Dealing with Values Conflict

Respond to these questions from the vantage point of the nurse in the situation:

- What is your first personal reaction to this situation? Identify your values relative to the situation.
- What do you perceive to be the values of the others involved?
- Identify value incongruencies that might lead to conflict. Give specific examples of how such a conflict can potentially affect patient care.
- Describe specific nursing interventions aimed at managing the conflict in a professional manner, and give examples of how nursing codes would guide such actions.
- Describe your own strengths and limitations as you consider dealing with this situation.

Impact of Institutional Values

Nurses need to be conscious of both the spoken and unspoken values in their work settings. Values of individual institutions and organized health care systems that are explicitly communicated through philosophy and policy documents, such as mission or vision statements, are called **overt values**. Values may also be implicit in expectations that are not in writing. Implicit or **covert values** are often identified only through participation in or controversies within the setting (Omery, 1989). When seeking employment, nurses should identify congruencies or incongruencies between personal values and those of the institution, because accepting employment implies committing to the value system of the organization. Consider, for example, Leila, who has worked for many years at a small but busy downtown hospital that provides care for HIV and AIDS patients and is especially sensitive to the community of gay and transgendered individuals who live locally. Many of the staff there are members of the community and identify with the unique needs and concerns of their clients. Clients, in turn, feel supported and treated in a holistic and meaningful way. A decision by the provincial government has resulted in an amalgamation between Leila's small hospital and a larger hospital, located on the other side of town. Traditionally, the larger hospital has been affiliated with the Catholic Church but now, as the merger approaches, it has publicly acknowledged that the amalgamated hospital structure will be one that embraces diversity and provides holistic, client-centred care for all persons. While Leila is appreciative of this public acknowledgement, she is worried that there may well be difficulties in merging the collective but diverse values of the two groups of staff members. She has heard from some friends who work there that some of the staff members at the larger hospital are not in favour of the merger and do not wish to provide care to HIV positive or AIDS patients who are gay or transgendered. She worries that her clients may not be treated in a way that is respectful or inclusive, and that they may feel further marginalized, despite what the public announcements have portrayed.

Schoof notes that what one believes and how one thinks about a job or institution is important, and has a direct impact on job performance. Such internal belief systems tend to shape a person's thinking and direct him or her to do what he or she thinks is right, regardless of the employer's philosophy. Schoof suggests that it is better to identify what is valued by the employer, that is, where he or she stands and pays attention to and rewards, and then to decide if one can work in that environment. As an example, he indicates that there are three primary ways to approach patient care: focus on meeting patient needs (intrinsic care), focus on doing all the tasks (extrinsic care), and focus on following the rules (systemic care) (personal communication, February 12, 1996). If there is a conflict between our values regarding patient care and the values of the institution, physician, and family we may experience moral distress. **Moral distress** is the reaction to a situation in which there are moral problems that seem to have clear solutions, yet we are unable to follow our moral beliefs because of external restraints. Jameton notes that moral distress is "knowing the morally right course of action to take" (Jameton, 1984, p. 542), but being prevented from taking it, due to institutional conflicts, structures, or constraints (Jameton, 1984). This distress is often evidenced in anger, dissatisfaction, frustration, and poor performance in the work setting. We will be discussing moral distress in greater detail in Chapter Six, as we examine models of ethical decision making.

Ask Yourself

How Should Values Influence Job Selection?

Maria, a recently divorced mother of three, desperately needs to return to work, but nursing jobs in her area are scarce. There is one opening at a women's health clinic that performs abortions. The job, which has excellent salary and benefits, including on-site child care, looks great to Maria, except that abortions are contrary to her personal and religious beliefs. A friend who works at the clinic said that, unless they are short staffed, Maria would not have to assist with abortions if she had objections.

- What dilemmas are evident in this situation?
- What are the value incongruencies?
- What are your values related to this situation?
- What factors should Maria consider in deciding whether to take the job?

Gingerich and Ondeck (1993) describe one process for defining and making organizational values more explicit. This process includes determining what is valued by staff, board members, management, and health care professionals regarding the elements of the organization's philosophy, and identifying specific expectations for each group. Exercises focused on self-awareness, clinical priorities, and opinions about value-laden issues are conducted within each of the groups to develop awareness of and consensus around the values. This allows all involved to have an investment in the value system.

The Hartman Value Profile is another approach to looking at values within an organization (Hartman, 1967; Edwards & Davis, 1991; H. Schoof, personal communication, 1996). The process involves having the institution select a number of employees representing two groups within the organization: those considered to be the *shining stars*, and those considered least satisfactory. Those identified complete the profile, which is a forced ranking, from best to worst or most despicable, of eighteen items relating to how persons perceive the world around them and eighteen items related to how they perceive their inner selves. Patterns are identified by analyzing the participants' responses utilizing a computerized mathematical system that identifies how each item compares with the others that are ranked. The resulting information provides a profile of the underlying values within the organization. Decision makers can use this information to examine how prevailing belief systems are influencing performance, and to seek potential employees whose values are most consistent with those of the organization.

CASE PRESENTATION

Differences in Personal and Organizational Values

Joan has been the nurse manager of her unit for the past ten years and is highly regarded by the hospital's administration. For the past several months, however, she has been feeling more frustrated and less satisfied with her work because of staffing cuts and other institutional decisions. Attending to patient needs has always been the most rewarding part of her job. However, many of the institutional decisions, in Joan's opinion, have negatively affected patient care. Recently she feels that she has been forced to overlook these needs and attend more to the needs of the organization. She considers leaving, but she has seniority, good benefits, and two children to support. She is also aware that her distress at work is affecting her family, because she carries a lot of the frustration home with her.

Think About It

How Values Affect Choices

- Identify values evident in this situation. Which of these reflect your personal values?
- What conflicts might arise from these values?
- What do you think Joan should do?
- If you were in Joan's position, what beliefs, ideals, or goals would guide you in making a decision to stay or leave? Identify potential consequences of each choice.

Clarifying Values with Patients

Values of both nurses and patients influence patient care situations. Since patients are the recipients and consumers of health care, it is good to know what they expect or value. Patient and provider perceptions of what constitutes quality care can be quite different. Great discrepancies in these perceptions may lead to patient dissatisfaction. This can have a variety of consequences, including affecting a patient's attitude and decisions regarding following recommendations for care and treatment (which may affect recovery), marring the reputation of the health care agency or institution or potentiating poor relationships between patients and providers. Allanach and Golden (1988) describe the process of a service audit aimed at identifying patient expectations and clarifying their opinions about the level of service. Nursing care behaviours identified as valued by patients in this study relate to the amount of care and time spent with patients and to the technical quality of nursing care. Consider the potential conflict of values when patients expect nurses to spend time with them and the institution puts more emphasis on getting the tasks done.

Ask Yourself

What Would You Do?

- You are busy and two call lights go on at the same time. What factors enter into deciding which one you respond to first?
- Consider that in the above situation one patient is in serious condition and has been verbally abusive to staff, while the other is not quite as serious and is someone you really enjoy being with. Whom would you respond to first and why?

- Your patients let you know how much they appreciate the extra care and time you give them compared to the other nurses. At the same time, your evaluation is coming up and your supervisor has indicated that you need to be more efficient with your time. What would you do in this situation and why?

When working with patients regarding health care decisions, nurses need to be aware of personal values and patients' values pertaining to health. When the health values of the nurse and those of the patient are different, the patient may become labelled as "difficult," uncooperative, self-destructive, noncompliant, ignorant, or unwilling to take responsibility for her or his own health. Part of being an ethical practitioner involves the ability to see the world from others' perspectives and to realize that they are just as valid as our own, although they may be markedly different. Cultural differences in values, beliefs, and choices should be viewed as opportunities for learning and expanding our understanding of the world around us, without assuming that our perspective is the "right one." Instead, these differences are often seen as variances from a cultural "norm" and efforts are put less into understanding the divergent views of others, and more into trying to change these views to more closely resemble our own. This is a dangerous stance to take and one that is ethically problematic, at the very least. In today's world, **globalization** and the multicultural nature of most societies compel us to attend to, engage with, and be respectful of the varied views, values, and choices of others.

Pender (1987; 1996) discusses the role of values in health promotion. She notes that knowing personal values is important, as is the need to avoid imposing our values on patients. Consider, for example, the client at a youth outreach centre, an impoverished young woman living on the street, with few supports and almost no financial arrangements. She admits to drug use, cigarette smoking, and alcohol abuse. She also discloses to you that she has had sex with men for money, drugs, and alcohol. While she admits it is dangerous, she uses condoms and ensures that she always works with another friend, in order to be safe. She tells you that she likes "partying," doing drugs and drinking, and while living on the street would not be a choice for many, for her it represents an escape from a home life that was, according to her, highly abusive and much more oppressive and dangerous. If priorities on her care plan include improved nutrition, stopping sexual activity for money, smoking cessation, drug rehabilitation and cessation, and alcohol abstinence, while well intentioned, these goals may simply demonstrate nursing values being imposed on the client. Instead, exploring the client's wishes, reasons for seeking care, and ways to advocate, support her, and help ensure her safety in her chosen lifestyle, at this time, would be a more meaningful and worthwhile health promotion activity.

With self-awareness the nurse can be more effective in helping patients to identify their own values. Assisting patients to clearly articulate their values is important because a lack of clarity about values may result in inconsistency, confusion, misunderstanding, and inadequate decision making. It can also lead to feelings of being influenced or coerced, for patients who do not have an opportunity to clearly articulate their values, choices, and rationales. The ability to make informed choices, including the process of informed consent, is enhanced by having clarity about our values. "Assisting clients to clarify values; understand the personal and social consequences of acting on current values; achieve greater consistency among values, attitudes, and behaviours; and plan health-related experiences that may result in self-initiated changes in value hierarchies" are key nursing actions (Pender, 1987, p. 161).

Many instruments and processes are available to facilitate exploring values in general and health values in particular. One example is a process that asks people to rank a list of ten health values from most important to least important. The list includes a comfortable life, an exciting life, a sense of accomplishment, freedom, happiness, health, inner harmony, pleasure, self-respect, and social recognition (Pender, 1987, p. 165). Pender notes that if health appears within the top four on the list, the person places a high value on health. However, definitions of health will vary, since each person defines health according to personal beliefs and values.

Another approach to analyzing health values described by Doyle (1994) asks people to identify from a list of ten health-related behaviours what they do and why they do it. Behaviours include activities such as exercising a minimum of three times per week, talking to a close friend or relative about worries, and having sex without using a condom. Doyle notes that the response to why a behaviour is practised provides insight into values surrounding the behaviour, such as choosing not to exercise in order to have more time, or choosing to exercise because it helps in weight control.

SUMMARY

This chapter has discussed the importance of self-awareness regarding values and the valuing process. Values are learned and change in response to life situations as a person develops. The process of values clarification enables persons to begin to identify and choose their own values rather than merely act out of prior programming. The interaction between personal values and those of patients and organizations can affect job satisfaction and patient care. The reader is encouraged to explore various processes that facilitate values clarification, both those presented in this chapter and those found in other resources.

CHAPTER HIGHLIGHTS

- Values are highly prized ideals, behaviours, beliefs, or qualities that are shaped by culture, ethnicity, family, environment, and education, and are acquired in both conscious and unconscious ways.
- The process of incorporating values begins at an early age and continues throughout life. Some values remain consistent while others change in response to growth and life experiences.

- Awareness of personal values undergirds the ability to make clear and thoughtful decisions, and enables us to acknowledge similarities and differences in values when interacting with others, thus promoting more effective communication, care, and facilitation of values clarification with others.

- Values clarification is not intended to instill values; rather, the aim is to facilitate awareness of personal values and the valuing process in order to move toward the point of choosing our own values rather than merely reacting from prior programming.

- The valuing process includes prizing and cherishing, choosing, and acting on beliefs and behaviours.

- Dealing effectively with values conflict requires attention to personal values, the perceived values of others, and the ability to recognize both overt and covert expression of values in a situation.

- Congruence between personal values and those of an institution is an important consideration for a nurse seeking employment.

- Assisting patients to articulate their values and beliefs, an important part of nursing care, may help prevent deleterious consequences related to not addressing differences in values between patients and providers.

DISCUSSION QUESTIONS AND ACTIVITIES

1. A non-nursing classmate asks you what studying values has to do with nursing. How would you respond? Incorporate your understanding of the nature of values and how they become part of us into your response.

2. What values guide your personal life? How did you learn these values? Select something that you consider important in professional nursing practice and trace how you learned this value.

3. Discuss why values clarification is important both personally and professionally.

4. Identify the overt values of your health care agency and identify overt and covert values of nurses and others within the agency. Explain the importance of knowing about both.

5. Describe a situation in which you experienced someone (it could be you) reacting from values that were not conscious at the time. How did this affect the interaction?

6. Determine the health values of three patients or people you do not know well and discuss why nurses need to be attentive to what patients value.

7. Describe a situation in which you experienced values conflict and how you dealt with the conflict.

8. Find current examples of public or professional figures whose personal values seem at odds with their professional or public trust. Discuss your reaction to the discrepancy in values that you identify and the interplay between personal values and professional integrity.

REFERENCES

Adams, K. (1990). *Journal to the self: Two paths to personal growth*. New York: Warner Books.

Allanach, E. J., & Golden, B. M. (1988). Patients' expectations and values clarification: A service audit. *Nursing Administration Quarterly, 12,* 17–22.

Baldwin, C. (1991). *Life's companion: Journal writing as a spiritual quest*. New York: Bantam Books.

Banonis, B. C. (1997). *Principled behavior applied to everyday life*. Charleston, WV: Unpublished manuscript.

Burkhardt, M. A., & Nagai-Jacobson, M. G. (2002). *Spirituality and healing*. Albany, NY: Delmar Publishers.

Chinn, P. L. (1995). *Peace and power: Building communities for the future* (4th ed.). New York: National League of Nursing Press.

Covey, S. R. (1990). *The seven habits of highly effective people*. New York: Simon & Schuster.

Davis, A. J., Aroskar, M. A., Liaschenko, J., & Drought, T. S. (1997). *Ethical dilemmas and nursing practice* (4th ed). Norwalk, CT: Appleton & Lange.

Doyle, E. I. (1994). Recognizing the value-health behavior connection: "What I do and why I do it." *Journal of Health Education, 25,* 116–118.

Edwards, R. B., & Davis, J. W. (1991). *Forms of value and valuation*. Lanham, MD: University Press of America.

Engebretson, J. C., & Headley, J. A. (2000). Cultural diversity and care. In B. M. Dossey, L. Keegan, & C. E. Guzzetta, eds., *Holistic nursing: A handbook for practice* (3rd ed., pp. 283–310). Gaithersburg, MD: Aspen Publishers.

Gaydos, H. L. B. (2000). The art of holistic nursing and the human health experience. In B. M. Dossey, L. Keegan, & C. E. Guzzetta, eds., *Holistic nursing: A handbook for practice* (3rd ed., pp. 51–66). Gaithersburg, MD: Aspen Publishers.

Gingerich, B. S., & Ondeck, D. A. (1993). Values incorporation throughout the organization. *Caring Magazine, 12,* 18–23.

Hartman, R. S. (1967). *The structure of value*. Carbondale, IL: Southern Illinois University Press.

Jameton, A. (1984). *Nursing practice: The ethical issues*. New Jersey: Prentice-Hall.

Kahn, S. (1996). *The nurse's meditative journal*. Albany, NY: Delmar Publishers.

Keegan, L. (2000). Holistic ethics. In B. M. Dossey, L. Keegan, & C. E. Guzzetta, eds., *Holistic nursing: A handbook for practice* (3rd ed., pp. 159–170). Gaithersburg, MD: Aspen Publishers.

Kolkmeier, L. G. (1995). Self-reflection: Consulting the truth within. In B. M. Dossey, L. Keegan, C. E. Guzzetta, & L. G. Kolkmeier, eds., *Holistic nursing: A handbook for practice* (2nd ed.). Gaithersburg, MD: Aspen.

Omery, A. (1989). Values, moral reasoning, and ethics. *Nursing Clinics of North America, 24,* 499–507.

Pender, N. J. (1987). *Health promotion in nursing practice* (2nd ed.). Norwalk, CT: Appleton & Lange.

Pender, N. J. (1996). *Health promotion in nursing practice* (3rd ed.). Norwalk, CT: Appleton & Lange.

Progoff, I. (1992). *At a journal workshop*. New York: Tarcher.

Rew, L. (1996). *Awareness in healing*. Albany, NY: Delmar Publishers.

Rew, L. (2000). Self-reflection: Consulting the truth within. In B. M. Dossey, L. Keegan, & C. E. Guzzetta, eds., *Holistic nursing: A handbook for practice* (3rd ed., pp. 407–424). Gaithersburg, MD: Aspen Publishers.

Seroka, A. M. (1994). Values clarification and ethical decision making. *Seminars for Nurse Managers, 2,* 8–15.

Simon, S. B., Howe, L. W., & Kirschenbaum, H. (1995). *Values clarification: A handbook of practical strategies for teachers and students*. New York: Hart.

CHAPTER 5
Values Development

OBJECTIVES

After completing this chapter, the reader should be able to:

1. Discuss influences of culture on values development.

2. Contrast theoretical approaches to moral development.

3. Describe and differentiate the ethic of care and the ethic of justice.

4. Evaluate the personal phase of moral development.

5. Discuss gender bias and cultural bias regarding theories of moral development.

INTRODUCTION

Nurses frequently encounter situations that present ethical dilemmas. In some situations the "right" choice seems quite evident, while in other circumstances a considerable lack of clarity about what is "right" may exist. How do we come to know what is right or how to respond in a principled way in a given situation? This chapter reviews factors that influence values formation, theoretical perspectives related to stages of values development, and considerations for nursing regarding moral development.

TRANSCULTURAL CONSIDERATIONS IN VALUES DEVELOPMENT

Human values development, often referred to as **moral development,** is a product of the sociocultural environment in which we live and develop. We learn what is considered right and wrong within the culture in formal ways such as by precept and admonition, through informal processes such as role modelling, and by technical learning in a teacher to student process (Hall, 1973). Norms for etiquette and ethical behaviour that are "known" within the culture may be acquired by an outsider through technical learning; however, they are often appreciated by a neophyte only when a transgression has occurred and corrections to, or sanctions for, the behaviour have been imposed. There is an innate human capacity for developing an ethical stance to life that emerges through this process.

Leininger (1978; 1984) and Tripp-Reimer (1987) speak of culture in terms of values, beliefs, customs, and behaviours that are learned within and shared by a group of interacting persons. Because values are *learned* within the context of a particular culture, moral values are culturally relative (Gostin, 1995). This suggests that a value such as individual autonomy may be regarded highly in a culture that prizes independence and individualism. However, the same value may be considered contrary to the norm in a society in which persons are defined by their relation to others or in a more communication way. Fowler (1981) notes that "we are formed in social communities and that our ways of seeing the world are profoundly shaped by the shared images and constructions of our group or class" (p. 105). Understandings of principles such as justice and care may vary in different cultures. In the ensuing discussion regarding stages of values development, it is important to be aware that the norms described have been derived primarily from Anglo-American and Anglo-European populations and, for the most part, are values that exist in a Western World tradition. Although significant work has been done, there is a need for further validation of the models within a transcultural context.

Ask Yourself

How Did I Learn My Values?

Think about a professional or personal situation in which you were faced with an ethical dilemma.

- What made it a dilemma for you?

(Continued)

- How did you decide the best course of action?
- What factors did you consider in making your decision?
- What values or principles guided you in this process?
- When and how did you learn these values or principles?
- Consider how you might have approached this same problem five or ten years ago. What, for you, has changed? Why?

THEORETICAL PERSPECTIVES OF VALUES DEVELOPMENT

Discussions of moral development found in current literature flow primarily from frameworks developed by Kohlberg (1981) and Gilligan (1982). An overview of the work of each of these scholars is presented in this section, followed by discussion of how they contribute to understanding moral reasoning within nursing. Fowler's (1981) work on faith development is briefly discussed regarding insights relative to values development. Kohlberg's theory, which suggests that cognitive development is necessary though not sufficient for moral development, draws upon Piaget's (1963) work on cognitive development in children. Thus, a brief review of Piaget's theory is included here. As you review the models highlighted here, remember that **theory** is a proposed explanation for a class of phenomena. A given theory is not necessarily truth or reality, but it may shed light on truth. Engage critical thinking and intuitive knowing as you read, being attentive to what rings true in your own experience. At the same time, use your critical thinking skills to consider other perspectives on moral development.

Piaget's Stages of Cognitive Development

Piaget's (1963) description of stages of cognitive development addresses how the mind works, that is, the development of intellectual capacities through the time of childhood, from birth to about fifteen years of age. He notes that cognitive development progresses through four stages, provided there is an intact neurological system and appropriate environmental interaction and stimuli. Although Piaget suggests specific ages for each stage, there may be variation due to environmental factors or innate intellectual capacities. Piaget's stages are:

- Sensorimotor (birth to 24 months), includes six substages;
- Preoperational (age 2–7), includes preconceptual and intuitive stages;
- Concrete operations (age 7–11);
- Formal operations (age 11–15).

Piaget believes that there are no further quantifiable changes in cognitive abilities after age fifteen. According to his theory, cognitive development progresses from thought dominated by motor activity and reflex, through development and use of symbolic representations such as language, to logical thought applied to concrete and then to abstract situations.

Kohlberg's Theory of Moral Development

Kohlberg's (1981) theory of moral development was derived initially from interviews conducted with boys distributed in age from early childhood to late adolescence. In these interviews he asked participants to respond to hypothetical ethical dilemmas, such as a man considering stealing a drug to save his dying wife because he cannot afford the drug and has exhausted other possibilities of paying for it. The pattern of the responses that he observed, coupled with inferences about the reasoning behind the responses, suggested a progression in moral reasoning spanning three levels, each of which includes two stages. These levels and stages are summarized as follows:

Level I.   The Preconventional Level has an egocentric focus and includes two stages. In Stage 1, *the stage of punishment and obedience*, rules are obeyed in order to avoid punishment. In Stage 2, *the stage of individual instrumental purpose and exchange*, conformity to rules is viewed to be in our own interest because it provides for rewards. Fear of punishment is a major motivator at this level.

Level II.   The Conventional Level is focused more on social conformity and includes two stages. In Stage 3, *the stage of mutual interpersonal expectations, relationships, and conformity*, concern about the reactions of others is a basis for decisions and behaviour, and being good in order to maintain relations is important. In Stage 4, *The Stage of Social System and Conscience Maintenance*, we conform to laws and to those in authority because of duty, both out of respect for them and in order to avoid censure. For persons in this level, fulfilling our role in society and living up to expectations of others are important, and guilt is more of a motivator than the fear of punishment noted in Level I.

There is a transitional phase between Stages 4 and 5 in which emotions begin to be recognized as a component of moral reasoning. This transition includes an awareness of personal subjectivity in moral decision making and a recognition that social rules can be arbitrary and relative.

Level III.   The Post-Conventional and Principled Level has universal moral principles as its focus. It includes two stages. In Stage 5, *the stage of prior rights and social contract or utility*, the relativity of some societal values is recognized, and moral decisions derive from principles that support individual rights and transcend particular societal rules such as equality, liberty, and justice. In Stage 6, *the stage of universal ethical principles*, internalized rules and conscience reflecting abstract principles of human dignity, mutual respect, and trust guide decisions and behaviours. Persons at this level make judgments based on impartial universal moral principles, even when these conflict with societal standards.

This model proposes a linear movement through hierarchical stages, whereby each stage presupposes having completed the prior stage and is the basis for the subsequent stage. It is the pattern of a person's utilization of a particular level of reasoning that determines the stage, noting that each successive stage requires more advanced levels of moral reasoning. Research utilizing this framework indicates that not everyone moves through all the stages, and that few people actually progress to the post-conventional level (Colby & Kohlberg, 1987). Within this framework, women tend to focus on relational stages, such as Stage 3. Men tend to focus on adherence to duty and the rules of authority, as highlighted in Stage 4. Kohlberg's model is generally considered to be an ethic of justice, because it is an approach to ethical decision making based on objective rules in which choices are made from a stance of separateness or individuality. Kohlberg's work highlights and informs the debate on an ethic of care versus an ethic of justice, in which the former is viewed as an approach that encompasses notions of relationships and responsibilities to others. The latter, an ethic of justice, is more focused on notions that are more concerned with social conformity and clear hierarchies (Gremmen, 1999).

Gilligan's Study of the Psychological Development of Women

Gilligan (1982; 1987) and Gilligan et al. (1988), a former student of Kohlberg, studied the psychological development of women, arguing that women approach moral decision making from a different perspective than men. In contrast to the justice ethic described by Kohlberg, in which personal liberty and rights are prime, Gilligan noted that women utilize an **ethic of caring**, in which the moral imperative is grounded in relationships with and responsibility for one another. "Women's construction of the moral problem as a problem of care and responsibility in relationship rather than of rights and rules ties the development of their moral thinking to changes in their understanding of responsibility and relationship, just as the conception of morality as justice ties development to the logic of equality and reciprocity" (Gilligan, 1982, p. 73). Gilligan's research did not say that most women think in the care perspective, while most men think in the justice perspective. Rather, as Little (2000) points out, she identified the default perspective that women use, the perspective they feel most comfortable with and that they would turn to first. She noted that many women think in the justice perspective, about one-third of the population are mixed between them, and, when pressed, all people can shift to the other perspective. However, women tend to start off from the care perspective, so if you leave women out of the study, you leave out the care perspective.

Gilligan's research suggests a progression of moral thinking through three phases, each of which reflects greater depth in understanding the relationship of self and others, and two transitions that involve critical reevaluation of the conflict between responsibility and selfishness. The sequence described proceeds from an initial concern with survival, to focusing on goodness, to reflectively understanding care as the most adequate guide for resolving moral dilemmas.

Phase 1. In this phase, *the concern for survival*, the focus is on what is best for the self, and includes selfishness and dependence on others. The *transition* to Phase 2 involves an appreciation of connectedness, and that responsible choices take into account the effect they have on others.

Phase 2.   The phase of *focusing on goodness* includes a sense of goodness as self-sacrifice, in which the needs of others are often put ahead of self, and there is a sense of being responsible for others, so that one is regarded positively. This focus on goodness reflects an awareness of relationship with others and may be used to manipulate others through a "see how good I've been to you" attitude. In the *transition* to Phase 3 there is a shifting from concern about the reactions of others to greater honesty about personal motivation and consequences of choices and actions. Responsibility to self is taken into account, along with responding to needs of others.

Phase 3.   The phase of *the imperative of care* reflects a deep appreciation of connectedness, including responsibility to self and others as moral equals, and a clear imperative to harm no one. We take responsibility for choices, in which projected consequences and personal intention are the motivation for actions, rather than concern for the reactions of others.

Although Gilligan does not clearly associate particular ages with each phase of development, she suggests a linear process moving from one phase to the next through the transitions. This process may be associated with cognitive and emotional development as they interface with experiences of connectedness. Gilligan's model is generally considered an ethic of care.

Fowler's Stages of Faith Development

Fowler's (1981) discussion of faith development incorporates reflections on the development of values. His insights offer another perspective on the process of moral development. Fowler refers to **faith** as "a generic feature of the human struggle to find and maintain meaning . . . a dynamic existential stance, a way of leaning into and finding or giving meaning to the conditions of our lives" (pp. 91–92). He notes that faith is not synonymous with religion and that it may or may not find religious expression. He suggests that faith development flows from an integration of ways of knowing and valuing. This perspective is different from the work of Piaget and Kohlberg who conceptually separate cognition or knowing from emotion or affection, suggesting that logical knowing is separate from other important modalities of knowing. Fowler writes that "in moral judgments the valuations of actions and their consequences as well as evaluations of self in relation to the expectations of the self and others are difficult to conceive, even in formal and structural terms, apart from inherent affective or emotive elements of knowing" (1981, p. 102).

Fowler (1981) proposes six stages of faith, beginning with an intuitive faith in early childhood and progressing to universalizing faith. He notes that movement through the stages may not be limited to a linear pattern, recognizing that spiralling back to earlier stages may occur in response to various life experiences.

Stage 1.   Occurring after the undifferentiated faith of infancy, *intuitive projective* faith is image and fantasy filled. The child's understandings and feelings toward the ultimate conditions of life are intuitive and shaped by stories, actions, moods, and examples of those around them.

Stage 2. *Mythic-literal* faith reflects beliefs and moral rules and attitudes that symbolize belonging within a community or family and that are taken on with literal interpretations. Story provides a major source of meaning, and a world view based on reciprocity and fairness is developed.

Stage 3. *Synthetic-conventional* faith reflects a movement into a world beyond the family in which values and beliefs derive from experiences in interpersonal relationships. Expectations and judgments of significant others are very influential in determining the values one holds. Although a personal clustering of values and beliefs is emerging in this stage, reliance on those in traditional authority roles or on the consensus of a valued group for validation of beliefs and actions is common. Fowler notes that although this stage arises in adolescence, many adults remain in this stage.

Stage 4. In the stage of *individuative-reflective* faith, persons must begin to take responsibility for their own beliefs, values, and commitments, differentiating personal identity and world view from that of others. In this way one's own values become recognized as factors in judgments on and reactions to actions and decisions of self and others.

Stage 5. *Conjunctive* faith requires an opening to our inner depths in which we are able to recognize values, beliefs, and myths developed within our particular cultural, social, or religious tradition that separate one from others. This stage requires an attitude of openness to that which formerly might have been perceived as threatening, different, and *other*, appreciating that although our own values provide a framework for ascribing meaning, they are only relative and partial apprehensions of transcendent reality.

Stage 6. With *universalizing* faith, the imperatives of absolute love and justice become prime, and we focus energy on transforming the present reality toward a transcendent actuality inclusive of all beings. Fowler notes that persons in Stage 6 are quite rare, frequently being honoured more after death than in life.

Ask Yourself

Where Are You in Your Values Development?

- Where do you think you fit in each of the frameworks discussed?
- Where would you place your parents? Classmates? Friends? Government officials?
- Where would you place the following noteworthy spiritual leaders Gandhi, Mother Teresa, the Dalai Lama or Martin Luther King Jr.?
- Based on your critical thinking and intuitive knowing, which framework rings most true for you?

- What are the implications of a model that suggests many adults still rely on authority figures or general consensus to validate beliefs?
- What are the implications of Fowler's model, when considering the development of moral autonomy?

Kohlberg and Gilligan suggest that values development moves from a focus on self and survival, through responding to external forces such as perceived authority or opinions of others, toward being motivated and guided by universal considerations. They, like Fowler, also note that it is more common to find adults functioning in the middle phases of relying on external authority as guideposts for moral decisions than to find adults who base their actions and decisions on internalized universal guides that transcend codified rules. Fowler's model acknowledges that both reason and emotional response are factors in moral decision making, and includes the suggestion that development may follow a pattern more spiral than linear. Within this pattern it is conceivable that, in response to life-changing experiences, persons may spiral back to an earlier stage and move through the stages again from a renewed perspective.

Thomas's Levels of Moral Response

When we consider difficult moral or ethical situations in which we are required to respond or act, our moral development and our subsequent level of moral autonomy inform our decisions, reactions, and actions. Thomas outlines three levels of moral response: the expressive level, the pre-reflective, level and the reflective level (Thomas, 1990). Consider asking someone why they oppose the legalization of abortion or euthanasia.

At an expressive level, while the person does express an opinion, the response is usually embedded in personal preferences, feelings, or emotional expressions. In and of themselves, these preferences and opinions are not reasons that are based on active reflection, research, and consideration of multiple perspectives. An example might be "I am against abortion because I don't like to think of anyone or anything being killed."

At a pre-reflective level, the rationale for the voiced opinion is usually provided in terms of unanalyzed values that have not been critically examined. Often the reasons for one's choice might be a reference to a widely held religious or cultural belief or a professional code of ethics. While this is considered, by some, to be more reflective than an expressive level of moral reasoning, others see this as representing a less-developed sense of moral reflection as it is viewed as the "blind following of standards set by somebody else." (Thomas, 1990, p. 5). These kinds of sets of conventional rules and codes are helpful to establish norms and guidelines for behaviours within particular contexts; however, it is also important for there to be personal and critical reflection on how these norms, rules, and codes are integrated with our own personal moral convictions. In other words, there needs to be some internalization of these kinds of rules along with an evaluation of their relevance, importance, and moral justification. At a pre-reflective level, according to Thomas, this has not yet occurred. At example of a pre-reflective moral response might be, "I oppose euthanasia because my professional duty precludes the taking of a life in any way."

Finally, at a reflective level, reasons or justification of moral views are provided based on rules, values, or principles that have been internalized, critically examined and, reflected upon. They may be rules or values espoused in a code of ethics or a widely held belief; however, instead of a blind acceptance of these rules, without critical analytical consideration of their relevance, there is some consideration of whether or not these are the kinds of rules and values by which individuals should be expected to live. An example of a statement at a reflective level might be, "I oppose euthanasia as the sanctity of all life and the principle of nonmaleficence takes precedence over the autonomy of the individual person to choose." Note the complexity of the reasoning and articulation of that process of reasoning through a difficult and often emotionally driven moral dilemma.

CASE PRESENTATION

Three Nursing Students

Pat, Tanya, and Kuan are discussing experiences they had in clinical today. Tanya describes her distress because her dying patient wanted to see her six-year-old granddaughter, which she thought would be very therapeutic, but her preceptor said absolutely not because there were strict rules against children under twelve visiting that unit. Pat notes that she did not have time to even change her patient's bed, but that the sheets were clean so she just straightened them out and the instructor did not even notice. She said the nurses on that unit do that sometimes when they are busy, so it was okay. Kuan says she had gotten behind too, but decided she had better get everything done the right way so she would get a good grade and not get into trouble.

Think About It

Indicators of Values Development

- What insights into the values of each of these students can you glean from this discussion?
- How do you think the theorists noted above would describe the level of development of each of the students?
- How do you think you would have responded in the situations described by the students? What values would guide your response?
- Consider each nursing student's decision and rationale. Then decide at what level of moral reasoning each one is functioning, in these examples.

SOME NURSING CONSIDERATIONS

Gilligan (1982; 1987) and others (Gilligan, Ward, Taylor, & Bardige, 1988; Kittay & Meyers, 1987; Larrabee, 1993; Noddings, 1984; Little, 2000) have suggested that there are gender differences in approaching moral decision making: women tend to utilize a care or relational perspective, whereas men more frequently use the justice perspective. These authors note that Kohlberg's perspective on moral development tends to portray women's choices as deficient in terms of moral capacity. Many authors claim that research related to differences in ethical decision making based on gender is inconclusive and that the justice perspective is used by both women and men (Colby & Kohlberg, 1987; Duckett, Rowan-Boyer, Ryden, Crisham, Savik, & Rest, 1992; Walker, 1993). When considering developmental norms for moral development, nurses must be alert for gender and cultural factors, norms, and bias in order to avoid erroneously classifying particular groups as lacking in moral capabilities.

The literature offers an ongoing deliberation about the ethic of care versus the ethic of justice. A comparison of the two perspectives reveals that the justice framework requires choices to be made from a stance of separateness, based on objective or universal rules and principles to ensure fair treatment of all persons (Botes, 2000). The care perspective arises from natural relatedness with particular others in which the choice is contextually bound and requires responding to others in their terms, developing strategies that maintain connections when possible, and striving to hurt no one. Moral concern within the ethic of justice is with rights and responsibilities; in the ethic of care the concern is with competing needs and responsibility in relationship. Fowler's model suggests that both are important factors in making moral decisions. Although much of the discussion in the literature focuses on the dichotomy between the two, we recognize that, rather than negating each other, the perspectives of justice and care offer different foci from which to examine problems. Offering balance to each other, these perspectives broaden the view from which to see the situation as a whole, and collectively constitute a more comprehensive moral perspective (Cooper, 1989; Little, 2000). Hekman (1995) suggests that a paradigm shift is occurring that requires a reconceptualization of morality and moral language away from the notion of universal morality toward a recognition of a plurality of moral voices. Furthermore, there are some who argue that viewing each of these perspectives as "mutually exclusive opposites" (Gremmen, 1999, p. 516) is an exercise that holds little value and functions to only try to resolve any discussion or debate by deciding "which is best." Instead of an attempt to decide which approach is "best," an exercise that is of little value, some theorists have instead proposed that by viewing the two perspectives as complementary, integrated, or comprehensive when considered together, a more relevant and fruitful discussion may ensue instead of a debate on the comparative value of each approach (Botes, 2000; Davis, 1992; Gremmen, 1999).

Because of nursing's concern for relational caring, an ethic of care may more thoughtfully reflect nursing's experience than a primary focus on justice (Cooper, 1989). Little (2000) notes that one of the lessons the ethic of care offers to health care professionals is the directive to meet the needs of *particular* others, recognizing that these needs are not always clear. This means caring about persons as individuals, and developing processes to help them figure out what they need. Part of this process, she suggests, is developing, through caring, a recognition that emotions are a constitutive part of the moral life. Considering the politics of caring, she speaks to the need of restructuring our health care systems to value caring through supporting and justly compensating those who do the sometimes emotional and taxing caring work.

It has also been suggested that nursing move beyond current models of biomedical ethics to a model that encompasses at least the concepts of care and justice (Cooper, 1990). One study exploring whether nurses deal with moral decisions using the justice or the care perspective found that both perspectives were utilized, with care being predominant overall (Chally, 1992). In this study, older nurses with more professional experience were more likely to utilize the care perspective than younger nurses with less experience. The author proposed a possible developmental process through which growth in experience leads from a reliance on rules to guide one's choices to a focus on the needs of patients and families, which is reflective of the care perspective. In their research exploring holistic ethics, Victoria Slater and colleagues (personal communication, November 13, 2000) discovered that holistic nurses blend the justice and care ethics. She notes that the pure justice ethic is about autonomy, whereas the pure care ethic is about relationships and nonviolence. The way holistic nurses blended them is seen in their sense that violating a person's autonomy (valued from an ethic of justice perspective) implies a lack of care toward that person. They came to their ethical decision based on experience and intuition. They fit their ethical decision to the situation with a focus of maintaining the patient's autonomy, which, for these nurses, was a form of nonviolence.

We need to understand that there are different perspectives from which moral decisions are made, so that we can better appreciate our own and our patients' approaches to ethical dilemmas. We need to identify honestly our own phases of values development and ethical perspective in order to better understand personal responses to situations and to recognize more effectively how our approaches may differ from those of colleagues or patients. Acknowledging differences and similarities may prevent making inappropriate judgments about another's moral capabilities, and make possible better communication and collaboration in care.

CASE PRESENTATION

A Difficult Decision

Reba's eighty-two-year-old father has been hospitalized with a stroke that has left him severely incapacitated, requiring total care. She has been informed that her father is ready for discharge, and the physician is suggesting that he go to a nursing home. Reba feels that she should take him home with her because her faith says to care for her parents, but the house is small and would need a bathroom added to the first floor. She also has concerns about performing her father's care because she works full time and has three small children. She has considered quitting her job, but the family needs her income because her husband's work is seasonal. When visiting her father, she tells the nurse, Moira, that she does not know what is best for him, noting that her sister in another province told her it is her duty to care for their father, but her husband says it is too much to take on with all her other family responsibilities. She asks Moira what she should do.

Think About It

Justice or Care—Is One Way Better?

- What values has Reba clearly articulated?
- What factors and forces do you think weigh most heavily in this situation?
- How would you respond if you were Moira?
- How would you approach this situation from the perspective of justice? From the perspective of care? Do you think one approach is better than the other? Explain.
- How would you describe Reba's phase of moral development? Her husband's? Her sister's?

SUMMARY

This chapter has presented an overview of theoretical perspectives related to values development, the importance of recognizing that values and beliefs are culturally relative, and nursing considerations related to moral development. Students are encouraged to explore and critique each model of values development in order to formulate a personal knowledge base to guide their own processes of development. Each perspective provides insight into what is true.

CHAPTER HIGHLIGHTS

- Human values development, which is a product of our sociocultural environment, reflects the content and process of learning what is right and wrong within the culture.
- Values development moves from a focus on self, through responding to external forces, toward being guided by universal considerations.
- Moral values are culturally relative.
- Current models of values development need further transcultural and transgender validation.
- Kohlberg's model, often referred to as an ethic of justice, suggests that choices are based on objective rules and principles and are made from a stance of separateness.

- In Gilligan's model, often referred to as an ethic of care, the moral imperative is grounded in relationship and mutual responsibility. Choices are contextually bound, requiring strategies that maintain connections and a striving to hurt no one.
- The notion of a plurality of moral voices, which recognizes that perspectives of both justice and care are factors in moral decision making, is an important consideration for nursing.
- Understanding varying perspectives from which moral decisions are made enables nurses to appreciate their own and their patients' approaches to ethical dilemmas and to avoid making inappropriate judgments about another's moral capabilities.

DISCUSSION QUESTIONS AND ACTIVITIES

1. What does it mean to say that moral values are culturally relative?

2. What factors would you consider in determining a person's phase of moral development?

3. Explore the model that you think best reflects the process of values development. Discuss it with classmates, giving rationale for your choice.

4. Identify stages of values development of three patients of different ages.

5. Compare and contrast the ethic of care and the ethic of justice, and discuss this topic with classmates. Which perspective do you think is most appropriate for nursing? Why?

6. Why is it useful for nurses to be aware of phases of values development for themselves, patients, and colleagues?

REFERENCES

Botes, A. (2000). A comparison between the ethics of justice and the ethics of care. *Journal of Advanced Nursing, 32*(5), 1071–1075.

Chally, P. S. (1992). Moral decision making in neonatal intensive care. *Journal of Obstetrics, Gynecology, and Neonatal Nursing, 21*(6), 475–482.

Colby, A., & Kohlberg, L. (1987). *The measurement of moral judgment volume I: Theoretical foundations and research validation.* Cambridge, MA: Cambridge University Press.

Cooper, M. C. (1989). Gilligan's different voice: A perspective for nursing. *Journal of Professional Nursing, 5*(1), 10–16.

Cooper, M. C. (1990). Reconceptualizing nursing ethics. *Scholarly Inquiry for Nursing Practice, 4*(3), 209–221.

Davis, K. (1992). Toward a feminist rhetoric: The Gilligan debate revisited. *Women's Studies International Forum, 15,* 219–223.

Duckett, L., Rowan-Boyer, M., Ryden, M. B., Crisham, P., Savik, K., & Rest, J. R. (1992). Challenging misperceptions about nurses' moral reasoning. *Nursing Research, 41*(6), 324–331.

Fowler, J. W. (1981). *Stages of faith: The psychology of human development and the quest for meaning.* San Francisco: Harper & Row.

Gilligan, C. (1982). *In a different voice: Psychological theory and women's development.* Cambridge, MA: Harvard University Press.

Gilligan, C. (1987). Moral orientation and moral development. In E. F. Kittay & D. T. Meyers, eds., *Women and moral theory* (pp. 19–33). Savage, MD: Rowman & Littlefield.

Gilligan, C., Ward, J. V., Taylor, J. M., & Bardige, B. (1988). *Mapping the moral domain.* Cambridge, MA: Harvard University Press.

Gostin, L. O. (1995). Informed consent, cultural sensitivity, and respect for persons. *Journal of the American Medical Association, 274*(10), 844–855.

Gremmen, I. (1999). Visiting nurses' situated ethics: Beyond "care versus justice." *Nursing Ethics, 6*(6), 515–527.

Hall, E. T. (1973). *The silent language.* Garden City, NY: Anchor Press.

Hekman, S. J. (1995). *Moral voices, moral selves.* University Park, PA: Pennsylvania State University Press.

Jameton, A. (1993). Dilemmas of moral distress: Moral responsibility and nursing practice. *AWHONN's Clinical Nurse, 4*(4): 542–551.

Kittay, E. F., & Meyers, D. T. (1987). *Women and moral theory.* Savage, MD: Rowman & Littlefield.

Kohlberg, L. (1981). *The philosophy of moral development.* New York: Harper & Row.

Lao Tsu. (1972). *Tao Te Ching* (Gia-fu Feng & Jane English, trans.). New York: Vintage Books.

Larrabee, M. J., ed. (1993). *An ethic of care.* New York: Routledge.

Leininger, M. (1978). *Transcultural nursing: Concepts, theories and practice.* New York: John Wiley & Sons.

Leininger, M. (1984). *Transcultural care diversity and universality: A theory of nursing.* Thorofare, NJ: Slack.

Little, M. (2000). Introduction to the ethics of care. Presentation at *New century, new challenges: Intensive bioethics course XXVI*, Kennedy Institute of Ethics, Georgetown University, Washington, DC, June 10, 2000.

Noddings, N. (1984). *Caring: A feminine approach to ethics and moral education.* Berkeley, CA: University of California Press.

Piaget, J. (1963). *The origins of intelligence in children* (M. Cook, trans.). New York: Norton.

Thomas, J. (1990). *Ethical frameworks for decision making.* Peterborough, ON: Broadview Press.

Tripp-Reimer, T. (1987). Cultural assessment. In J. P. Bellack, & P. A. Bamford, eds., *Nursing assessment: A multidimensional approach* (pp. 226–246). Boston: Jones & Bartlett.

Walker, L. J. (1993). Sex differences in the development of moral reasoning: A critical review. In M. J. Larrabee, ed., *An ethic of care* (pp. 157–176). New York: Routledge.

CHAPTER 6
Ethical Decision Making

OBJECTIVES

After completing this chapter, the reader should be able to:

1. Describe and differentiate ethical dilemmas, moral uncertainty, practical dilemmas, moral distress, and moral outrage.
2. Describe the process of making thoughtful decisions.
3. Discuss the nursing process as a decision-making model.
4. Discuss similarities between scientific process and ethical decision making.
5. Describe the role of emotions in ethical decisions.
6. Examine the process of ethical decision making.
7. Apply the ethical decision-making process to clinical case situations.

INTRODUCTION

Everyone makes decisions as part of everyday living. Some decisions seem routine, such as what to have for lunch or what to wear to work. Other decisions, like where to go to college or university, which job to accept, or whether to marry, call for more deliberation. Nurses constantly make decisions. We decide matters related to patient care, institutional policy, or how to collaborate or initiate referrals. Often we make decisions without conscious awareness of the process but have an innate sense of *knowing* what to do.

Ethical decision making may not seem as clear-cut as decisions made in other areas of life. How do we decide whether to remove life support measures for a parent or whether to cut funding for childhood immunizations in lieu of other, equally important programs? What factors are involved in an ethical dilemma that makes "the right choice" either evident or obscure? This chapter defines the concept of ethical dilemma, relates ethical decision making to nursing process, and presents a guide for ethical decision making.

MORAL/ETHICAL PROBLEMS

Jameton (1984) describes three different types of moral problems: *moral uncertainty*, which occurs when the nurse identifies a moral problem but is unsure of the morally correct action; *moral dilemma*, which occurs when two or more mutually exclusive moral claims clearly apply and both seem to have equal weight; and *moral distress*, which arises when the nurse knows the morally correct action and feels a responsibility to the patient, but institutional or other restraints make it nearly impossible to follow through with appropriate action (p. 6). Wilkinson (1987–88) added another category to Jameton's typology: *moral outrage*, which occurs when someone else in the health care setting performs an act the nurse believes to be immoral.

Moral Uncertainty

Moral uncertainty occurs when we sense that there is a moral problem, but are not sure of the morally correct action, when we are unsure what the moral principles or values apply, or when we are unable to define the moral problems (Jameton, 1984). This happens to us when we have a sense that something is not quite right. We are uncomfortable with a situation, but can't quite articulate the problem. Jameton (1984) offers the example of a nurse caring for an older patient who is somewhat neglected, with little attention being given to the patient's problem. The nurse feels dissatisfied with the patient's treatment, but is unable to pinpoint the nature and cause of the inadequacy.

Moral/Ethical Dilemmas

A dilemma exists when a difficult problem seems to have no satisfactory solution or when all solutions to a problem appear to be equally favourable (Davis, Aroskar, Liaschenko, & Drought, 1997). An **ethical dilemma** occurs when there are conflicting moral claims. Dilemmas present in at least two ways. According to Beauchamp and Childress (2001), a conflict can be experienced when there is evidence to indicate that a certain act is morally right and evidence to indicate that the act is morally wrong, but no evidence is conclusive. An example of this can be seen in the example of a terminally ill patient. While most would think it is morally right to preserve life, many would also believe it is morally wrong to prolong suffering. A dilemma may also occur when the agent believes that one or more moral norms exist to support one course of action, and one or more moral norms exist to support another course of action, and the two actions are mutually exclusive. Health care providers face this type of dilemma, for example, when they must decide who gets the critical care bed. Should they make the decision relative to who is most deserving, who arrives first, who is younger, or who has the best chance of survival? Different people perceive or conceptualize conflicts in different ways. Conflicting moral claims can be said to occur, for example, between obligations, principles, duties, rights, loyalties, and so forth.

Let us examine different perceptions of conflicting moral claims. The nurse might perceive a conflict between adherence to two different principles, such as wishing to avoid the suffering a patient experiences as a result of hearing a bad prognosis, while at the same time respecting the patient's right to know. In this instance, the nurse might perceive a direct conflict between the principles of nonmaleficence (the wish to do no harm) and autonomy (assuring that the patient is self-governing). In another instance, the nurse might perceive a conflict of duties. This type of conflict can occur, for example, when nurse managers must make decisions regarding staffing patterns. The nurse manager will recognize a duty to the institution, but will also feel a duty to meet the needs of individual patients and nurses. This will often result in a conflict, when the needs of the institution do not allow for meeting the needs of individuals.

There are instances in which the nurse might feel conflicting loyalties. For example, in providing care for a patient who is HIV positive, who admits to you that she is sexually active and not using protection against transmission of the virus, the nurse may experience a conflict between being loyal to the patient and being loyal to others or society at large. In this instance, the nurse could experience a conflict between doing that which seems morally right and avoiding that which carries legal consequences. This situation can also be conceptualized as a conflict between the nurse's duty to maintain confidentiality and the duty to warn those at risk. All of these examples portray ethical dilemmas that nurses commonly experience. These moral problems offer conflicting moral claims, and solutions that appear at once to be both favourable and unfavourable.

Think About It

Facing Ethical Dilemmas

Put yourself in the position of the nurse in each of the examples noted in the discussion of ethical dilemmas above.

- How would the situation present a conflict for you?
- How do you think you would respond in each situation?
- Why would you respond in that manner?
- Think about a personal experience of a moral dilemma and describe why it was a dilemma for you.

Practical Dilemmas

One must be careful to differentiate between **moral and practical dilemmas**. Occasionally, situations present themselves in which moral claims compete with nonmoral claims. Nonmoral claims can often be identified as claims of self-interest (Beauchamp & Childress, 2001). Consider, for example, the nurse who must to work overtime, caring for a gravely ill patient. The nurse might perceive a dilemma because she made a promise to take her children to the movies. Though the nurse might say that her duty to the children conflicts with her duty to care for the patient, it can be argued that the duties are not of equal moral weight. The duty to keep the promise to her children is a practical duty that is grounded in self-interest rather than having a moral claim. In decisions that involve practical dilemmas, moral claims have greater weight than nonmoral claims. Differentiating moral and practical dilemmas is an important facet of decision making.

Moral Distress

Occasionally, nurses face situations that present moral problems that seem to have clear solutions, yet they are unable to follow their moral beliefs because of institutional or other restraints. Nurses in these predicaments are said to experience **moral distress** (Jameton, 1984). These situations can be differentiated from those that present moral dilemmas. When moral distress occurs, there are no conflicting moral claims. The *right* action is clear, yet institutional or other restraints make it nearly impossible to pursue this course of action. It is important to note that nurses who experience moral distress often feel a personal responsibility to the patient. The distress occurs when the nurse violates a personal moral value and fails to fulfill perceived responsibility. For example, nurses in the hurried atmosphere of a particular hospital's same-day surgery report that they are expected to have sedated patients sign consent forms, recognizing that the physicians have often neglected to explain the scheduled procedures fully. The nurses know that this practice is one that does not respect patients' rights to informed consent and thereby violates the patients' autonomy. However, they feel they have neither personal authority nor access to decision-making channels, and therefore believe themselves to be powerless to make the necessary changes. Jameton points out that in situations of this sort, it can be personally risky for staff to criticize a practice that is felt to be in the best interests of the institution at large.

Situations in which nurses feel moral distress may represent practical, rather than ethical, dilemmas. Nurses may face the choice of continuing to participate in a system that they feel is ethically flawed, resigning, or acting in a manner that they believe is correct but that could jeopardize employment. Moral distress will undermine integrity if it is easier for the nurse to comply with policies that are believed to be morally wrong than to pursue the ethically correct action.

Though moral problems of all types are difficult, situations involving moral distress may be the most difficult moral problems facing nurses (Nathaniel, 2000). Reports of the number of nurses who experience moral distress vary. Nearly fifty percent of nurses in one study report that they had acted against their consciences in providing care to the terminally ill (Rushton, 1995). Studies have shown that as many as thirty percent to fifty percent of nurses either leave their units or leave nursing altogether as a result of moral distress (Wilkinson, 1987–88; Millette, 1994; Redman & Fry, 2000).

Other studies show that moral distress causes nurses to have physical and psychological problems, sometimes for many years. Some relate "burnout" to their experience of moral distress, and suggest that many nurses leave the profession as a result. More important, there is anecdotal evidence that nurses' moral distress affects quality of patient care and subsequent health outcomes (Nathaniel, 2000).

The consequences of moral distress may be profound. There is evidence that, as a result of moral distress, some nurses lose their capacity for caring, avoid patient contact, and fail to give good physical care. Hamric (2000) calls moral distress, "a powerful impediment to nursing practice" (p. 201). Nurses may physically withdraw from the bedside, barely meeting the patient's basic physical needs, or may leave the profession altogether (Fenton, 1988; Hefferman & Helig, 1999; Kelly, 1998). Loss of nurses from the workforce is an indirect but strong threat to patient care. The nursing shortage is compounded by a health care system in which increasingly complex technology is used to care for patients who are very old, very young, or very sick. Those in society with the greatest need may be the ones who suffer more acutely when nursing care is affected (Nathaniel, 2000).

Unrelieved moral distress over a period of time can erode the nurse's values and affect confidence and self-esteem. Unfortunately, there is no assurance that following what one considers to be the morally correct course of action will mean employer or legal support. Nurses should view these situations as practical dilemmas. Ethical decision making assures that moral claims hold greater weight than nonmoral claims. Thus, in the example offered above, the moral claim of respecting the right to informed consent constitutes greater weight than the nonmoral claim of system efficiency. The decision-making guide described in this chapter can be used to help nurses make practical decisions when facing moral distress.

Ask Yourself

Have You Experienced Moral Distress?

Moral distress occurs in situations that present moral problems which seem to have clear solutions, yet institutional or other restraints prohibit morally correct action. Consider a situation in which you experienced moral distress.

- What were the circumstances?
- How did you feel?
- How did you resolve the distress?

Moral Outrage

Moral distress and moral outrage share the common element of feelings of powerlessness (Jameton, 1993). **Moral outrage** occurs when someone else in the health care setting performs an act the nurse believes to be immoral (Wilkinson, 1987–88). In cases of moral outrage, nurses do not participate in the act, and therefore do not believe they are responsible for wrong, but perceive that they are powerless to prevent it or act upon it. The nurse is more likely to be on the fringes of the moral situation rather than directly involved. For example, the charge nurse on a medical/surgical floor on the evening shift is working at the desk when the nursing supervisor comes to the floor to use the telephone to call a hospital administrator. The charge nurse overhears the supervisor describing a situation in which a patient was endangered when a physician insisted on performing a surgical procedure in the patient's room. The surgeon was in a hurry and felt the patient would be safe, even though there were violations of patient privacy, informed consent, and safety. The charge nurse has no involvement in the situation, but recognizes a grave moral problem. Whistleblowing may be a response to moral outrage but in most cases, is considered to be a last resort. There are usually more constructive and meaningful ways to try to resolve issues, even those that lead to moral outrage, that can help to change-institutions and practices. Whistleblowing should be considered only when all other options have been exhausted.

MAKING DECISIONS

The process of making thoughtful decisions follows a similar pattern in most circumstances. This pattern includes gathering data, comparing options, using some criteria for weighing the merit of each option, and making a choice. Evaluation of outcomes or circumstances surrounding the choice provides more data regarding the *rightness* of the choice. A simple example of this process is how you choose what clothes to wear today. The data you gather includes such things as where you are going, what you will be doing, the weather, what is clean or handy, your mood, the colours you prefer, and the style of clothing you anticipate others will be wearing. You may narrow choices to several options that would be acceptable or appropriate, and you compare these based on some criteria. The criteria may be what is least wrinkled, or feels most comfortable, or makes you look or feel more confident, or is more appropriate for weather conditions, or a combination of such considerations. Using the criteria, you narrow down options and make a choice. As you move through the day, you gather more data about the *rightness* of your decision. For example, are you comfortable? Do you feel dressed appropriately for the meeting? Are you warm enough? Does the colour seem to make you stand out? Your evaluation of whether you made the right decision provides information about the strength or validity of the criteria you used to guide your decision, and whether to use these same criteria to guide similar decisions in the future.

Nursing Process and Ethical Decision Making

As nurses we commonly use the **nursing process** model for decision making. Utilizing both logical thinking and intuitive knowing, the nursing process is a deliberate activity that provides a systematic method for nursing practice. The nursing process directs nursing practice, standardizes nursing care, and unifies nurses (Christensen &

Kenney, 1990). Familiar to most nurses, the process generally includes the following interactive and sequential steps: problem identification based on assessment of subjective and objective data; development of a plan for care, guided by desired outcomes; implementation of interventions; evaluation of the outcomes; and revision of the plan over time. Criteria used in making nursing care decisions derive from areas such as knowledge of normal anatomy, physiology, psychology, pathophysiology, therapeutic communication, family dynamics, pharmacology, microbiology, nursing and other theories, human energy fields, familiarity with standards of care and protocols, experience related to what has worked in similar situations, and intuitive knowing. The process is systematic and involves both logical thinking and intuitive knowing.

Scientific Process and Ethical Decision Making

The process of decision making in ethics follows a procedure that is similar to the scientific process. "A comparison between the giving of good reasons in science, which is called 'explanation,' and the giving of good reasons in ethics, which is called 'moral justification,' reveals striking procedural similarities bordering on identity" (Gibson, 1991, p. 3). Gibson notes similarities between the scientific process of explanation, which moves from *observation → hypothesis → law → theory*, and the moral justification process of ethics, which moves from *assessed ethical dilemma → rule → principle → theory*. A strong knowledge base regarding societal rules, ethical principles and theories, and professional codes and standards is as important to making ethical decisions as knowledge of principles related to physical, psychological, social, and human science is to other nursing judgments.

ETHICAL DECISION MAKING

We often approach ethical problems with a problem-solving frame of reference. Similar to both nursing process and scientific inquiry, the ethical problem-solving process generally includes the following steps: (1) defining the problem, and collecting information, (2) identifying objectives to be achieved, (3) listing alternatives for meeting objectives, (4) evaluating each objective, and (5) choosing the best alternative.

Differences of culture or values among the various participants involved in ethical decision making often become an important issue. In this regard, defining the problem includes both determining the ethical issue at hand and identifying the value systems of those involved. Consider, for instance, parents who wish to terminate life support for a seriously injured child hospitalized with no hope of recovery. The parents believe that life support is causing harm by interfering with what they refer to as the natural process of death, while the physician feels that removing life support constitutes murder. The problem includes both the issue of terminating life support and the conflicting values between physician and family. Although both parties might identify what is best for and least harmful to the child as the ultimate objective, the list of potential options would be different for the family and the physician. Determining which principles and theories guide the people involved enables the nurse to help clarify the issue and facilitate the process of coming to an ethical decision.

Emotions and Ethical Decisions

Many approaches to ethical decision making describe a primarily cognitive process in which emotions are subordinated to reason. In a holistic view of people, however, both thinking and feeling are credible ways of knowing, each having a legitimate role in ethical decision making. Callahan (1995) suggests that heart and mind should not be viewed as antagonistic in the moral arena; rather, both reason and emotion should be active and in accord as we come to an ethical decision. Noting that emotions should influence reason while reason is monitoring emotions, she describes emotions as personal signals providing information regarding both inner processes and interactions with the environment.

It is important to appreciate not only what you *think* about what is right or wrong in a situation, but also what you *feel* in relation to the circumstances and decision to be made. If you are feeling discomfort, even though reason is pointing in a particular direction, it is wise to further explore both the arguments posed through reason and your reactions to them. Callahan (1995) writes:

> In our technological culture perhaps the greatest moral danger arises not from sentimentality, but from devaluing feeling and not attending to or nurturing moral emotions. Numbness, apathy, isolated disassociations between thinking and feeling are also moral warning signals . . . the absence of emotional responses of empathy and sympathy become critical bioethical issues. (pp. 30–31)

In the same way that people may approach an issue with differing moral reasoning, their emotional responses might be quite different from your own. In such situations you might see validity in the other's response and broaden your own view. On the other hand, you may recognize that the chasm between the two is too deep to bridge. Callahan suggests that such social conflicts and challenges present new ethical problems that may require dealing with the consequences of an ethical decision by repeating the decision-making process.

? Think About It

The Role of Emotions in Decision Making

Consider your emotional response to the following situations and how it would affect your dealing with and caring for the people involved.

- You work in a busy urban clinic primarily serving new immigrants to the country, and you hear one of your coworkers comment that "it's a waste of time trying to do health education, because these people just don't understand, and are just a drain on the system."

- You are working in an emergency department at the local hospital, where a two-year-old child dies as a result of injuries sustained while being "disciplined" by the mother's boyfriend. The child had previously been placed in foster care due to neglect, and had been returned to the mother's care only a week prior to this event.

- You are the head nurse in a coronary intensive care unit. You receive a call from a cardiologist from another hospital who is desperate to get a bed in your unit for a young pregnant woman in congestive heart failure. An hour prior, your last available bed was taken by a forty-two-year-old chronic cocaine user, who has had another myocardial infarction.

PROCESS OF ETHICAL DECISION MAKING

The nature of the ethical problem requires a decision-making process in which key facets are revisited from evolving perspectives, even as you move toward a decision or resolution. Many models for decision making describe step-by-step processes that are linear in nature, not reflecting the potential for an evolving perspective. The guidelines presented here provide a framework for entering a decision-making process that requires an ongoing evaluation and assimilation of information. Keep in mind, though, that no model for ethical decision making is a substitute for reflection and thoughtfulness or a guarantee of a good decision or outcome (MacDonald, 2002). Rather, an ethical decision-making guide helps us to consider multiple views, perspectives, and important steps in the process of working through an ethical dilemma. Furthermore, no ethical decision-making guide is meant to be applied in a purely linear fashion. The decision-making process is iterative and dynamic in nature, with each step being revisited as often as is required and moulded by the dynamics of changing facts, and contexts, evolving beliefs, unexpected consequences, and participants who move in and out of the process. Before we outline the steps in an ethical decision-making process, it is important to note that, on an ongoing basis, as ethical practitioners, we must always be attentive to morally problematic situations (McDonald, 2001). We must be aware of what a moral dilemma is and what a practical problem is as well as the differences between them. Being aware and being sensitive to moral and ethical dilemmas is a key foundational attribute of ethical practitioners. Without this "moral intuition" (McDonald, 2001), we cannot begin to enter into an ethical decision-making process as we may have difficulty identifying what kinds of situations are truly ethically or morally problematic. We must be able to recognize that the particular problem, in fact, has a moral dimension (MacDonald, 2002). The following describes the steps involved in the process of ethical decision making.

Gather Data and Identify Conflicting Moral Claims

When an ethical problem occurs, gather information or facts in order to clarify issues. Identification of the conflicting moral claims that constitute the ethical dilemma is the first part of the process. You should examine the situation for evidence of conflicting obligations, principles, duties, rights, loyalties, values, or beliefs. Additionally, data provide an understanding of the ethical components, principles of concern, and the various perceptions of issues and principles by those involved in the situation. You must pay attention to societal, religious, and cultural values and beliefs. In order to situate the problem, you must explore the context of not only the problem but also the context of decision making. Clinical issues and the stated, inferred, or known preferences of all involved (primarily the patient, but the preferences of family members and the health care team may well be relevant) must also be considered. Often, a situation you initially think constitutes an ethical dilemma will actually turn out to be a practical dilemma. This recognition allows the participants to appropriately weigh choices and expedite decision making. One important part of this stage of decision making is to identify what you know and admit what you do not know (McDonald, 2001). You may not have the perspectives or views of all involved and it may be difficult for you to acquire them. Alternatively, you may not have enough time to gather adequate information in one area or from one perspective. In this case, we must then attend to and be articulate and transparent about what we don't know, as much as we would about that of which we are sure. In order to begin to work through the dilemma, the values, benefits, and burdens need to be identified (MacDonald, 2002). This requires actively seeking this kind of information from a number of perspectives.

Identify Key Participants

Identify the key persons involved in the decision-making process and delineate each person's role. Determining rights, duties, authority, context, and capabilities of decision makers is a critical component of the process (Curtin & Flaherty, 1982; Husted & Husted, 1995). The focal question is, "Whose decision is this to make?" Identification of the principal decision maker or decision makers is sometimes all that is needed to facilitate the process. Recognition that one has the legitimate authority to make an important decision is an empowering event. Once the principal decision maker is identified, the roles of the other participants can be explicitly outlined. As MacDonald (2002) notes, examining relationships between key participants is also an important step. For example, nurses often feel the burden of difficult ethical decisions, even though the responsibility for the decision lies with the patient or the nearest relative. In these instances, the nurse serves as a resource for information, a source of emotional support for those making the difficult decision, and a facilitator of the decision-making process. Nurses must also be carefully attuned to the dynamics of relationships between patients, relatives, friends, and caregivers.

Determine Moral Perspective and Phase of Moral Development of Key Participants

Knowledge of moral development and ethical theory may provide a helpful framework for understanding participants and their perspectives and responses in the process. Assess how those involved fit into paradigms of moral development. It is valuable to recognize, for instance, whether the principal decision maker is at a developmental level in which choices reflect a desire to please others, and is thus susceptible to choosing an alternative solely on the basis of seeking approval. (See Chapter 5 for an in-depth discussion of moral development.) It may also be worthwhile to try to reflect upon the level of moral response that each key player articulates in relation to the problem. Establishing that a response is expressive, pre-reflective, or reflective may help you gain insight into the reasons behind the moral convictions of others as well as assist you in exploring their perspective and reasoning in a way that is relevant to them, and most facilitative for the decision-making process. In the following text box (Figure 6–1), we revisit the levels of moral response, as outlined by Thomas and Waluchow (1998).

Figure 6–1 **Examining Moral Responses**

Thomas and Waluchow (1998) examined the way that people respond to a moral problem or question. They identify three levels of response or reflection.

- At an expressive level, responses to moral problems are uncritical or unanalyzed. Usually cited in personal experience or emotions, the response may not, on its own, provide justification for the person's position on the moral problem.

    An example of an expressive statement might be: "Withdrawal of nutrition and hydration should never happen because it is murder."

- At a pre-reflective level, reasons behind one's position are often references to rules, laws, or principles accepted without question or critical analysis. They may refer to the status quo, i.e. a conventional community standard that is usually agreed upon by many. At this level, reference to these kinds of rules is often not done alongside critical reflection on whether or not these rules or standards are actually good, but it is done with what may be blind acceptance of rules without question.

    An example of a pre-reflective statement might be: "I disagree with the withdrawal of nutrition and hydration because it will directly cause death. The Catholic Church prohibits this on the basis of protecting sanctity of life and I am Catholic."

- At a reflective level of moral response, moral judgments and responses are based on "principles, rules and values to which we ourselves consciously subscribe." (Hardingham, 2001, p. 2). At this level, one is able to offer clear, thoughtful reasons about one's position on a moral problem.

    An example of a reflective statement might be: "Withdrawal of nutrition and hydration is a difficult concept to accept for many because of the social values we place on food and water. However, in some cases, with clear consent, a careful examination of the values of the patient, a negative prognosis and a demonstrably poor quality of life, it may be carefully considered with measures taken to minimize and ease any suffering."

It is crucial to identify the participants' ethical perspectives and explicitly stated values and beliefs. For example, if one of the major participants involved in discussions relative to discontinuing life support believes that it is always wrong to take a life (see discussion of deontology in Chapter 2), the process of negotiation with those who believe differently is likely to be frustrating. It would be more beneficial under those circumstances to begin the discussion by defining the point at which death actually occurs, thus finding common ground. When those involved present with diverse values, your role may be to facilitate their coming to a consensus around goals and the understanding of principles.

At this point, and throughout the process, we must always be "checking in" with ourselves, to see how we are feeling about the situation, how we are responding to the views and values of others, and our kind of moral response. No one can be a completely detached ethical decision maker. We always have our own views, values, and beliefs, which may affect how we approach the problem. "Checking in" with ourselves and our "moral barometer" on a consistent basis is an important part of any ethical decision-making process.

Determine Desired Outcomes

Identifying the desired outcomes and their potential consequences is a substantial step in the decision-making process. At this point, participants will exclude those outcomes that are totally unacceptable. As with the nursing process, implementation of a plan of action cannot logically occur without explicit knowledge of the desired outcome. Likewise, evaluation of the success or failure of the plan is measured by the degree to which the outcome is met. Clarifying the outcomes and their anticipated consequences enhances the understanding of options and alternatives.

Identify Options

Having determined the desired outcomes, participants should identify possible options for action. Various options begin to emerge through the assessment process. Participants must consider legal and other consequences. They must also determine which alternatives best meet the identified outcomes and fit their basic beliefs, lifestyles, and values. In addition to attending to the basic values, lifestyles, and beliefs that are held by those most affected in a decision, one must also be able to identify factors in each alternative that are "morally significant" (McDonald, 2001). Consider an alternative in which we would be breaking an important promise previously made to a patient. Would this breach of trust significantly harm the patient? Would it exploit them or treat them in a paternalistic way, thus limiting their autonomy? Would it cause indelible damage to the fidelity that exists between you and the patient?

To help in identifying morally significant factors in proposed alternatives, we must each have a good working knowledge of ethical theories and principles. Additionally, we must be sentient of the values, norms, and beliefs of our institutions, professions, and workplace cultures through review of policies, mandates, and mission and vision statements. We can use the resources around us to help identify morally important factors: clinical ethics consultants or research ethics consultants, formal ethics case conferences, research ethics boards or ethics committees, mentors, and those we have identified in our own professional life as persons of high moral integrity (McDonald, 2001). Our own judgments, along with the deliberation of those in the workplace for whom we have great deference, are also very helpful elements within the process. Remember, though, that discussing a sensitive patient care situation involves serious professional and legal responsibilities for protecting the privacy and confidentiality of others that must always be respected. This process helps to narrow the list of acceptable alternatives. It is critical to eliminate all unacceptable alternatives and begin the process of listing, weighing, ranking, and prioritizing those that are found to be acceptable. Participants must make a choice among options with both head and heart; taking time to dwell with remaining alternatives, recognizing that there is rarely a good solution. Remember that when considering possible options, as a nurse, you must try to bear in mind that there may be consequences of options that are farther reaching than one patient or one clinical situation. There may be implications for families, other professionals, institutions, or groups of patients. Many may be affected by a decision, including yourself. As McDonald notes, we must be honest about our "own stake in particular outcomes and encourage others to do the same" (McDonald, 2001). Once the selection is made, the decision makers must be willing to act upon the choice.

Act on the Choice

Taking action is a major goal of the process, but can be one of the most difficult parts. It can stir numerous emotions laced with both certainty and doubt about the rightness of the decision. Participants must be empowered to make a difficult decision, setting aside less acceptable alternatives. Chapters 19 and 20 discuss empowerment in more depth. It is important to be attentive to the emotions involved at this point of the process.

Think About It

Before acting upon a specific alternative, we can ask ourselves a few simple but important questions. These might include questions like:

- What would get you to change your mind, and act differently from this alternative?
- Are you setting a good moral example to others?
- Are you doing what you would think a good or virtuous person would do? If not, why? Which other alternative would the good person choose, then?
- From a Kantian or deontological perspective, consider the alternative as a universal maxim for anyone in a similar situation. Would you want the alternative to be such a maxim?
- Have you breached confidentiality or caused harm to any trust relationships?
- After all these questions, are you still content with the identified alternative?

Adapted from *A framework for ethical decision making:* Version 6.0 (McDonald, 2001)

Evaluate Outcomes of Action

After acting upon the decision, participants begin a process of response and evaluation. As in all decision making, reflective evaluation sheds light on the effectiveness and validity of the process. Evaluate the action in terms of the effects upon those involved. Ask, "Has the original ethical problem been resolved?" and "Have other problems emerged related to the action?" As the situation changes and new data emerge, participants must identify subsequent moral problems and adjust the course of action based upon both new information and responses to the previous decision.

Figure 6–2 is a guide for ethical decision making. Questions may need to be revisited several times and may emerge at various points as the process unfolds and new data are presented. For example, information about options may begin to emerge before all the parties involved are identified, and data regarding ethical perspectives of the various parties may be clarified only at the point when options are being discussed. No matter how much information the participants gather, they may make the decision with an awareness that they would like to have still more data, although having a long list of viable options may actually make it more difficult to come to a decision.

Figure 6–2 **A Guide for Ethical Decision Making**

Gather Data and Identify Conflicting Moral Claims

- What makes this situation an ethical problem? Are there conflicting obligations, duties, principles, rights, loyalties, values, or beliefs?
- What are the issues?
- What facts seem most important?
- What emotions have an impact?
- What are the gaps in information at this time?

Identify Key Participants

- Who is legitimately empowered to make this decision?
- Who is affected and how?
- What is the level of competence of the person most affected in relation to the decision to be made?
- What are the rights, duties, authority, context, and capabilities of participants?

Determine Moral Perspective and Phase of Moral Development of Key Participants

- Do participants think in terms of duties or rights?
- Do the parties involved exhibit similar or different moral perspectives?
- Where is the common ground? The differences?
- What principles are important to each person involved?
- What emotions are evident within the interaction and with each person involved, including oneself?
- What is the level of moral development of the participants?

Determine Desired Outcomes

- How does each party describe the circumstances of the outcome?
- What are the consequences of the desired outcomes?
- What outcomes are unacceptable to one or all involved?

(Continued)

Identify Options

- What options emerge through the assessment process?
- How do the alternatives fit the lifestyle and values of the person(s) affected?
- What are legal considerations of the various options?
- What alternatives are unacceptable to one or all involved?
- How are alternatives weighed, ranked, and prioritized?

Act on the Choice

- Be empowered to make a difficult decision.
- Give yourself permission to set aside less acceptable alternatives.
- Be attentive to the emotions involved in this process.

Evaluate Outcomes of Action

- Has the ethical dilemma been resolved?
- Have other dilemmas emerged related to the action?
- How has the process affected those involved?
- Are further actions required?

APPLYING THE DECISION-MAKING PROCESS

Application of the decision-making guide in clinical situations is illustrated in the following case and discussion:

> A couple is pregnant with their second child after numerous unsuccessful attempts with artificial insemination. During a routine ultrasound at 28 weeks gestation, the physician discovers that the fetus is anencephalic. The life expectancy of an anencephalic baby is only a few days to weeks after birth. The couple struggles with the choice to terminate the pregnancy at this time or to carry the child to term.

Gathering Data and Identifying Conflicting Moral Claims

One conflict relates to the principle of nonmaleficence (the wish to do no harm). Terminating the pregnancy can be perceived as harmful to the baby, while carrying it to term may result in emotional or physical harm to the mother. Another conflict relates to the duty to preserve life, allowing the pregnancy, birth, and death of the baby to take its natural course, versus the duty to alleviate the suffering that carrying the pregnancy to term might impose on the mother. Some of the important facts in this situation include knowing the life expectancy of a baby born with anencephaly, knowing the parents' attitudes toward abortion, appreciating the feelings that this news brings forth, and knowing the meaning of this pregnancy to the parents.

Identifying Key Participants

Valuing input from the physician and others, both parents have the moral and legal right and the responsibility to make the decision. They may want to consult family or friends, and they may request a second opinion. Though competent, the parents may have difficulty making a decision soon after receiving the painful news. Since this is not an emergency, the nurse and others should allow time and provide support, while the parents process the information and deal with emotions. If, for example, one parent wants the pregnancy terminated and the other is strongly opposed, participants should further explore who has the right to make the ultimate decision.

Determining Moral Perspective and Phase of Moral Development of Key Participants

It is important to consider whether the stance of both parents is the same. Are they thinking about the rights of the infant versus the rights of the mother, or the duty to preserve the family integrity? If one parent thinks the pregnancy should be terminated and the other feels that the baby has a right to life, no matter how short it may be, can a common ground be reached? Do the parents seek guidance from those in authority, or from beliefs regarding right and wrong in this situation? Do they talk of a relationship with the baby in utero and the impact of choosing to end its life—on the baby, its sibling, or their relationship?

Determining Desired Outcomes

Through discussion of outcomes, more insight into ethical theory may emerge. In this situation, participants could describe the desired outcome as prevention of unnecessary suffering for the mother and the baby. Further exploration might reveal the sense that carrying the baby to term would create such anguish for the mother that her emotional health, and even family integrity, would be threatened. In that instance, terminating the pregnancy would be more compassionate than prolonging the suffering of the mother and allowing the inevitable, yet slow, natural death of the baby. Legal considerations would include laws related to abortion.

Identifying Options

In this case, the physician presented the options at the outset: the parents could terminate the pregnancy, or allow it to go to term. One might well look at the risks for the mother involved in both choices. Participants need to clarify beliefs regarding life, abortion, family responsibility, duties, and the like. If carrying the pregnancy to term presents a health risk for the mother, an additional dilemma would arise regarding responsibility to the older sibling and family integrity versus responsibility to the baby.

If either carrying the pregnancy to term or terminating it now is acceptable, participants have the task of determining factors that may weigh one alternative more strongly than the other. They may decide that the grieving process of the baby's death has already begun and would be only intensified if the pregnancy were carried to term. With this in mind, they might decide to end the pregnancy.

Acting on the Choice

Deciding to terminate the pregnancy, the parents move toward action. As logistics of scheduling and preparing for the termination proceed, it is important to attend to the parents' emotional response and to ensure that they have other needed support.

Evaluating Outcomes of Action

The parents resolved the dilemma of whether to terminate the pregnancy or carry it to term by choosing to proceed with termination. Reactions to the choice may emerge in the forms of guilt, depression, acceptance, or always wondering how things might have been different if the other path had been chosen. If the parents have long-term reactions, such as deep guilt or depression, they might come to a point of saying that, faced with such a situation again, they should decide to carry the pregnancy to term. On the other hand, they may examine issues surrounding the emotions with the awareness that the decision to terminate the pregnancy helped them deal with these issues and that, in spite of the pain, they made the best decision at the time.

? Think About It

Various Responses to Terminating Pregnancy

Consider which areas of the "Guide for Decision Making" in Figure 6–2 may have to be revisited in the following variations of the case presented above.

- The mother indicates that she thinks she will "go crazy" if she carries the pregnancy to term, and the father says "no one is going to kill my child."

- The local hospital has a religious affiliation that does not permit abortions. The parents feel that terminating the pregnancy is the better decision, but the closest hospital that could perform the procedure is a four-hour drive and their parents and support network would not be present.

- The mother refuses to consider any alternatives, stating that "Allah will make the baby fine."

SUMMARY

Ethical decision making requires knowledge and attention to many factors. Determining the existence of an ethical dilemma is the beginning step in the process, which includes defining the problem, identifying desired objectives, listing and evaluating alternatives, choosing the best course of action based on one's knowledge and the current circumstances, and evaluating the outcomes of the action taken. One must consider both reason and emotion in making ethical decisions. Nurses are encouraged to utilize the decision-making process described in this chapter as a guide in dealing with dilemmas encountered in clinical settings. As with every other nursing skill, comfort and competency with ethical decision making comes with repeated practice.

CHAPTER HIGHLIGHTS

- Dilemmas exist when difficult problems have no satisfactory solutions or when all the solutions appear equally favourable.
- In decisions involving practical dilemmas, moral claims hold greater weight than nonmoral claims.
- Making thoughtful decisions in any arena follows a pattern that includes gathering data, comparing options based on particular criteria, making and acting on a choice, and evaluating outcomes or circumstances surrounding the choice.
- One's value system affects how one defines and deals with an ethical issue; thus, resolution of ethical dilemmas requires determining the ethical issue at hand and identifying the value systems of those involved.
- Both emotion and reason have legitimate roles in ethical decision making.
- Ethical decision making requires ongoing evaluation and assimilation of information, with revisiting of various steps in the process as often as required by the dynamics of changing facts, evolving beliefs, unexpected consequences, and participants moving in and out of the process.
- Familiarity with and practice in applying ethical decision making enables the nurse to develop competence and confidence with the process.

DISCUSSION QUESTIONS AND ACTIVITIES

1. Search an on-line database for full-text articles related to nurses' ethical decision making. How do other models compare to the one presented in this text?
2. Working in small groups, discuss ethical and practical dilemmas that you have experienced, then choose an example of each type of dilemma to illustrate for the class.
3. Describe a situation in which you or someone you know experienced moral distress, noting moral and nonmoral claims in the situation.
4. Talk with practising nurses about their experiences of ethical dilemmas. Identify their approaches to dealing with such dilemmas, including their processes of ethical decision making.
5. Debate the role of reason and emotion in ethical decisions with classmates.
6. Use the ethical decision-making process to revisit an ethical dilemma that you have encountered in the past, or to guide you through a current dilemma. Examine your sense of comfort with each part of the process, noting areas of strength and areas needing more practice.
7. Discuss the interaction among moral development, moral perspective, and ethical decision making.
8. How would you approach an ethical dilemma in which the parties involved exhibit different moral perspectives?
9. How might legal considerations affect the process of making ethical decisions?

REFERENCES

Beauchamp, T. L., & Childress, J. F. (2001). *Principles of biomedical ethics* (5th ed.). New York: Oxford University Press.

Callahan, S. (1995). The role of emotions in ethical decision making. In J. H. Howell & W. F. Sale, eds., *Life choices: A Hastings Center introduction to bioethics.* Washington, DC: Georgetown University Press.

Christensen, P. J., & Kenney, J. W. (1990). *Nursing process: Application of conceptual models* (3rd ed.). St. Louis, MO: Mosby.

Curtin, L., & Flaherty, M. J. (1982). *Nursing ethics: Theories and pragmatics.* Bowie, MD: Brady.

Davis, A. J., Aroskar, M. A., Liaschenko, J., & Drought, T. S. (1997). *Ethical dilemmas and nursing practice* (4th ed.). Norwalk, CT: Appleton & Lange.

Fenton, M. (1988). Moral distress in clinical practice: Implications for the nurse administrator. *Canadian Journal of Nursing Administration, 1,* 8–11.

Gibson, J. (1991). An introduction to the study of ethics and ethical theories. In B. R. Furrow, S. H. Johnson, T. S. Jost, & R. L. Schwartz, eds., *Bioethics: Health care, law, and ethics* (pp. 1–6). St. Paul, MN: West.

Hamric, A. B. (2000). Moral distress in everyday ethics. *Nursing Outlook, 48,* 199–201.

Hardingham, L. (2001). Reflective practice. *Alberta RN* (May/June 2001). Retrieved January 25, 2009, from http://findarticles.com/p/articles/mi_qa3929/is_200105/ai_n8941245/pg_1?tag=artBody;col1.

Hefferman, P., & Heilig, S. (1999). Giving "moral distress" a voice: Ethical concerns among neonatal intensive care unit personnel. *Cambridge Quarterly of Healthcare Ethics, 8,* 173–178.

Husted, G. L., & Husted, J. H. (1995). *Ethical decision making in nursing.* St. Louis, MO: Mosby.

Jameton, A. (1984). *Nursing practice: The ethical issues.* Englewood Cliffs, NJ: Prentice-Hall.

Kelly, B. (1998). Preserving moral integrity: A follow-up study with new graduate nurses. *Journal of Advanced Nursing, 28,* 1134–1145.

MacDonald, C. (2002). *A guide to moral decision making.* Retrieved January 26, 2009, from http://www.ethicsweb.ca/guide/.

McDonald, M. (2001). A framework for ethical decision making. Version 6.0 Ethics [Shareware]. Retrieved January 25, 2009, from http:www.ethics.ubc.cq.

Millette, B. E. (1994). Using Gilligan's framework to anlayze nurses' stories of moral choices. *Western Journal of Nursing Research, 16*(6), 660–674.

Nathaniel, A. K. (2000). A concept analysis of moral distress. Unpublished manuscript.

Redman, B., & Fry, S. T. (2000). Nurses' ethical conflicts: What is really known about them? *Nursing Ethics, 7*(4), 360–366.

Rushton, C. H. (1995). The Baby K case: Ethical challenges of preserving professional integrity. *Pediatric Nursing, 23*(1), 16–29.

Thomas, J. & Waluchow, W. (1998). Well and good: A case study approach to biomedical ethics. *Ad Edition.* Peterborough: Broadview Press.

Wilkinson, J. M. (1987–88). Moral distress in nursing practice: Experience and effect. *Nursing Forum, 23*(1), 16–29.

PRINCIPLED BEHAVIOUR IN THE PROFESSIONAL DOMAIN

Part III examines various categories of issues that affect the profession of nursing and the everyday practice of individual nurses. Recognizing nursing as a profession, the chapters describe nurses' responsibility related to ethical, legal, professional, and practice issues. These issues are examined in light of ethics and contemporary nursing. This part includes chapters discussing legal issues affecting nurses; professional issues such as autonomy, authority, and accountability; issues related to the relationship between nurses and the health care system; issues related to technology and self-determination; and scholarship issues.

CHAPTER 7

Legal Issues

OBJECTIVES

After completing this chapter, the reader should be able to:

1. Recognize the difference between ethics and the law, and discuss the relationship of each to the other.
2. Describe sources of law.
3. Distinguish between constitutional law, statutory law, administrative law, and common law.
4. Describe the difference between public and private law.
5. Define tort, and distinguish between unintentional and intentional torts.
6. Discuss the notion of consent and important elements.
7. Describe the importance of the right to privacy in Canada.

INTRODUCTION

Up to this point, the focus of this book has been upon values, morals, and ethics. You will recall from Chapter 2 that moral thinking, though influenced in great measure by prevailing cultural tradition, is essentially an individual enterprise. Ethics are rules of behaviour produced by moral thinking and may be either informal or formal rules of actions. Professional organizations, such as the Canadian Nurses Association, the American Nurses Association, and the International Council of Nurses, provide documents outlining a formal set of ethical guidelines. These guidelines offer some general rules that are intended for use as a tool to guide professional behaviour but are not, in themselves, fully enforceable. Laws, on the other hand, consist of enforced rules under which a society is governed. Many laws either directly or indirectly affect the practice of nursing. Highly publicized issues such as termination of life support and "do not resuscitate" status indicate a recent trend toward involving the legal system in issues that were previously thought to be ethical in nature. This chapter discusses the relationship between ethics and the law, general legal concepts, areas of potential liability for nurses, and recent legal trends. The legal regulation of nursing is addressed in Chapter 8.

RELATIONSHIP BETWEEN ETHICS AND THE LAW

Law is the system of binding rules of action or conduct that governs the behaviour of people in respect to relationships with others and with the government (Guido, 1997; Rhodes & Miller, 1984). Laws, meant to reflect the moral beliefs of a given population, are devised by groups of individuals serving in official capacity. There are four basic functions of the law in society: (1) to define relationships among members of society, and to declare which actions are and are not permitted; (2) to describe what constraints may be applied to maintain rules, and by whom they may be applied; (3) to furnish solutions to problems; and, (4) to redefine relationships between people and groups when circumstances of life change (Kozier & Erb, 1992).

The law establishes rules that define our rights and obligations, and sets penalties for people who violate them. Laws also describe how government will enforce the rules and penalties. In Canada and the United States, there are thousands of federal, provincial, state, and local laws. Among others, these laws ensure the safety of citizens, protect property, promote nondiscrimination, regulate the professions, provide for the distribution of public goods and services, and protect the economic and environmental interests of society.

How are ethics and laws related? Laws are intended to reflect popular belief about the "rightness or wrongness" of particular acts and are, like ethics, built upon a moral foundation. In most countries laws represent an attempt to codify ethics. Law can serve as the public's instrument for converting morality into clear-cut social guidelines, and for stipulating punishments for offences (Beauchamp, 2001). One would expect that laws would be congruent with the prevailing moral values of a society; indeed, they usually are, at least in most democratic societies. For example, most people would agree that the murder of an innocent person is an immoral act. Laws that prohibit murder reflect this ethical standard. Murder of the innocent is both ethically and legally prohibited in every culture. As society's needs and attitudes evolve, laws emerge to reflect these changes. Occasionally, however, governments create and enforce laws that many people believe to be unjust or immoral. In a democratic society, constitutional law provides mechanisms to change or abolish unjust or unpopular laws.

Some authors of nursing ethics texts take the view that professional ethical standards are congruent with the law, that is, that which is legal is also ethical, and vice versa. These authors imply that following a set of ethical guidelines, such as those provided by the Canadian Nurses Association, the American Nurses Association, and the International Council of Nurses, provides nurses a legal safety net. This is usually, but not necessarily, true. Laws exist that can be considered (by some at least) to be unethical. Some illegal acts are considered by many to be ethical.

? Think About It

Consider the following examples of situations that are illegal but arguably ethically fine:

- Breaking the speeding limit to rush a sick child to hospital;
- Breaking and entering into an isolated mountain cabin, if you are lost and suffering from exposure;
- Stealing a life preserver from someone else's boat to throw to a drowning person;
- Physically injuring someone in order to restrain them from imminently injuring someone else.

Consider the following situations or actions that are unethical but legal:

- Lying in almost any situation except in court or in advertising;
- Cheating on your spouse;
- Discriminating against someone for his or her race, gender or age;
- Gossiping about someone else.

What are some reasons for the possible discrepancy between that which is legal and that which is ethical? First, there are differences between ethical points of view. Deontology and utilitarianism, for example, offer quite opposite answers to some basic ethical questions. While the utilitarian perspective would allow consideration of euthanasia, for example, to provide for the good of many, deontological views might require that life be protected regardless of circumstance. Thus, a law thought to be ethical by the utilitarian might be considered unethical by the deontologist. Second, human behaviour and motivation are more complex than can be fairly reflected in law. Think back to Chapter 4. Individuals may consider the same act either right or wrong, depending to some extent on their stage or level of moral development. For example, acts of civil disobedience, such as those committed by Mahatma Gandhi and Martin Luther King, Jr., although considered at that time to be illegal, are generally considered to be motivated by high ethical standards. In his letter from the Birmingham Jail, Martin Luther King, Jr. wrote, "there are two types of laws: just and unjust. I would be the first to advocate obeying just laws. One has not only a legal but a moral responsibility to obey just laws. Conversely, one has a moral responsibility to disobey unjust laws" (1996, p. 574). Third, the legal system judges action rather than motivation. For example, nurses following personal moral convictions or professional ethical codes can find themselves at odds with policies or practices of employing institutions. In certain instances, the legal system may determine that an employing institution has the right to dismiss or discipline a nurse for laying aside institutional policy in favour of ethical considerations. Fourth, depending upon the political climate and other variables, laws change. Recent examples of laws that have changed and evolved over time include those related to expanded roles of nurses, abortion, fetal tissue use, organ transplantation, self-determination, privacy, informed consent, and legal definitions of death. As defined in Chapter 3, integrity is fidelity in adherence to moral norms sustained over time. One should be able to predict that nurses with integrity will not alter their basic moral beliefs in response to changes in the law. Thus, there are several valid circumstances in which there may be a discrepancy between that which is legal and that which is considered ethical.

GENERAL LEGAL CONCEPTS

Nurses need to familiarize themselves with the law and legal system for several reasons. First, the law authorizes and regulates nursing practice. Nurse practice acts and regulatory acts of the individual provinces and territories describe both the activity of nurses and their scope of practice. Chapter 8 discusses the legal regulation of nursing in greater depth. Second, the legal system scrutinizes nursing actions and omissions. The profession is in a dynamic state of change: advanced practice nurses are expanding the traditional boundaries; critical care nurses are performing complex and vital tasks; staff nurses are caring for older and sicker patients; and many nurses are practising in new settings. Working in such a dynamic and quickly evolving health care environment, nurses must have basic knowledge about enduring and new laws and legal processes. This knowledge will help ensure that our actions are consistent with legal principles, and that we can advocate effectively for the profession and patients, while remaining within the confines of the law. Knowledge of legal principles is a necessary component of ethical decision making. In order to make informed choices, nurses, physicians, patients, and families must be able to identify potential or real legal implications.

Sources of Law

There are at least four different sources of law that are relevant to the practice of nursing: constitutional law, statutory (legislative) law, administrative law, and common law. The foundation of Canada's legal system is developed from common law (except for Quebec's system which is based on civil law). Law can be divided into two main branches—private law and public law. Some laws are made by legislation, some by rule-making bodies, and some by judicial precedent. There is frequent overlap between the sources and branches of the law.

Constitutional Law refers to formal sets of rules and principles that describe the powers of a government and the rights of the people. The principles set out in a constitution, coupled with a description of how these principles are to be interpreted and carried out, form the basis of constitutional law. Many times, constitutional law is noted in reference to the United States because of the strength of its written constitution. Many countries and states, in fact, have constitutions. The format of them is highly variable—they may be written (e.g., United States, Australia, Japan) or unwritten (United Kingdom). They may be codified, meaning they are contained in a single document—again, the United States is a good example of a codified and written constitution—or they may be uncodified, meaning that they are contained in several documents. Israel and New Zealand have uncodified constititutions.

In Canada, our constitution is unique. It is partly written in several documents rather than one overarching constitutional document. Additionally, it is partially unwritten and partly rules of common law developed by the courts. In Canada, constitutional law is highly complex. Our most important constitutional document is the *British North America Act* (1867). This act was revised many times and finally renamed the *Constitution Act* in 1982. Part one of the *Constitution Act* is the **Charter of Rights and Freedoms**, which guarantees rights to individuals and groups and that you can read in full in Appendix B. The subsequent parts of the act note other rights and powers to groups like Aboriginal persons as well as noting further amendments to the original act. At the same time that the *Constitution Act* was being passed (1982), the *Canada Act* was also being passed, which essentially severed Canada's dependence on the United Kingdom to pass legislation, a process sometimes referred to as "patriation."

The *Charter of Rights and Freedoms,* however, is the document with which most people are familiar. It also is a document most people describe as a truly Canadian document—representing notions of human rights and dignity. As nurses, we should be especially familiar with the *Charter of Rights and Freedoms,* its meaningfulness in all realms of practice and professional life, and how our role as advocate for individuals and groups is supported by the kinds of values articulated in the *Charter,* which are considered by many to be values that, as a country, we embrace and embody.

Statutory/Legislative Law.   Formal laws written and enacted by federal, provincial, or local legislatures are known as **statutory** or **legislative laws**. Parliament passes many laws each year; these are added to the volumes of federal and provincial statutes already in force. Because many people think that every problem in society can be solved by passing a law, legislatures make more and more laws to satisfy the demands of society and special-interest groups. Provincial health care, professional regulatory acts, nonsmoking health acts, statutory recognition of nurses in advanced practice (including prescriptive authority), and proposed health care reform legislation are all examples of statutory or legislative law. For more information on how laws are passed through legislative processes, see Chapter 14.

Administrative Law. **Administrative law** involves the operation of government agencies. Federal, provincial, and local governments set up administrative agencies to do the work of government. These agencies regulate such activities as education, public health, social welfare programs, and the professions. Administrative law consists mainly of the legal powers granted to administrative agencies by legislative bodies and the rules that the agencies make to carry out their powers. Provincial regulations bodies for nursing are examples of this type of agency. These regulatory bodies are granted the authority to execute the intent of provincial statutes by creating, implementing, and enforcing comprehensive and appropriate rules and regulations. As administrative bodies, the role of colleges of nursing is to protect the public, rather than advocate for nurses. Rules promulgated by the individual provinces' regulatory bodies carry the same weight as other law.

Types of Law

Law can be divided into two different types: public and private. Recall that law is a system of enforceable principles and processes that governs the behaviour of people in respect to relationships with others and with the government. In general, legal problems related to the relationship between people and the government are the domain of public law, and problems occurring as a result of relationships between people are the domain of private law.

Public Law. **Public law** defines a person's rights and obligations in relation to the government and describes the various divisions of government and their powers. One important branch of public law is **criminal law**. Criminal law deals with crimes— that is, actions considered harmful to society. Even though a crime might be committed against a particular person, the government considers the commission of a serious act, such as murder, to be harmful to all of society. In Canada, the federal government presides over criminal law. The documents that outline and define aspects of criminal law include primarily the *Criminal Code of Canada* but also acts such as the *Youth Criminal Justice Act* (2003) and the *Controlled Drugs and Substances Act* (1996). While these are federal documents, the provincial governments are given the power to administer the criminal justice system, enforce laws, and prosecute offenders. Laws are enforced by the police, the courts, and the penal system, all under provincial and municipal jurisdiction. Crimes range in seriousness, from public drunkenness to murder. Criminal law defines these offences and sets the rules for the arrest, the appropriate procedures to ensure due process, and the punishment of offenders.

In the course of practice, nurses can be accused of a variety of criminal offences. For example, nurses can be accused of directly injuring a patient, either intentionally or unintentionally. Nurses can also be accused of crimes related to their actual relationship with the government. These include such actions as falsifying narcotic records, failure to renew licences, and fraudulent billing. In most countries that have a common law system, as Canada does, crimes are delineated according to seriousness as either indictable offences or summary offences.

Indictable offences are serious crimes that carry significant fines and jail sentences. Examples include first- and second-degree murder, arson, burglary, extortion, kidnaping, rape, and robbery. These crimes are punishable by jail terms. Nurses are rarely accused of felonies in the course of practice. However, this can occur. For example, it is possible that those participating in the unauthorized removal of life support from a terminally ill patient could be accused of first-degree murder, because of the intentional nature of the act which resulted in death. This could occur even though the act might be viewed as beneficent by a majority of people. A nurse who unintentionally causes the death of a patient by administering a medication to which a patient is allergic could be charged with second-degree murder (manslaughter).

A summary offence is a less serious crime, usually punishable by a fine, a short jail sentence, or both. In the United States system, these crimes are known as misdemeanors. Examples of summary offences include disturbing the peace, solicitation, assault, and battery (assault and battery are also considered intentional torts and can be decided by private or civil law). A nurse slapping a patient or giving an injection without consent can be accused of the summary offence of battery.

Private Law. **Private law** is also called **civil law**. It determines a person's legal rights and obligations in many kinds of activities that involve other people. These activities include everything from borrowing or lending money to buying a home or signing a job contract. There are a number of branches of private law, including contract and commercial law, tort law, property law, labour law, inheritance law, family law, and corporations law. Private or civil law often is representative of a society's attitudes toward issues like family, marriage, property ownership, labour laws, small businesses, and privacy. In Canada, privacy is of particular concern, and protection of personal information is considered an important priority of both individuals and agencies that hold our personal or private information. There are a number of federal and provincial statutes that help to protect privacy, and these will be discussed later in the chapter. The branches of private law that are most applicable to nursing practice are contract law and tort law.

Contract Law. **Contract law** deals with the rights and obligations of people who make contracts. A **contract** is an agreement between two or more people that can be enforced by law. Contracts may be either written or oral; however, in the presence of both a written and oral contract, the written contract takes precedence. In health care, contracts may be either expressed or implied. Expressed contracts occur when the two parties agree explicitly to its terms, as in an employment contract a nurse signs when she begins employment at a hospital or agency. Implied contracts occur when there has been no discussion between the parties, but the law considers that a contract exists (Kozier & Erb, 1992). The nurse–patient relationship is essentially an implied contract with which the nurse agrees to give competent care.

Tort Law. A **tort** is a wrong or injury that a person suffers because of someone else's action, either intentional or unintentional. The tortious action may cause bodily harm; invade another's privacy; damage a person's property, business, or reputation; or make unauthorized use of a person's property. The victim may sue the person or persons responsible. Tort law deals with the rights and obligations of the persons involved in such cases. Many torts are unintentional, such as damages that occur as a result of accidents. But if a tort is deliberate and involves serious harm, it may also be treated as a crime. The purpose of tort law is to make the person whole again, primarily through the award of monetary damages. Because it can involve negligence and malpractice, tort law is the branch of law with which nurses are most familiar. There are three types of torts (or wrongs): unintentional, intentional, and liabilities.

Unintentional torts occur when an act or omission causes unintended injury or harm to another person. The majority of lawsuits against nurses and other health care professionals are unintentional torts, usually claims of negligence. Nurses are familiar with the unintentional torts of negligence and malpractice. **Negligence** is "the omission to do something that a reasonable person, guided by those ordinary considerations which ordinarily regulate human affairs, would do, or doing something which a reasonable and prudent person would not do" (Creighton, 1986, p. 141). Often the terms "negligence" and "malpractice" are used interchangeably, as negligence can imply care or treatment that falls below the standard of a reasonable and prudent nurse.

As part of ensuring the safety of citizens, the law requires that every person is accountable for behaving in a reasonable way, particularly if the welfare of others is jeopardized. For example, there is certainly no law against throwing rocks into the air. However, throwing rocks off a bridge into highway traffic is not the act of a reasonable or prudent person. The resultant injury that might ensue (and has, in a number of cases in Canada and the United States) would be considered to be negligent, as the person would have not acting in a reasonable way toward others.

The word "negligence" is rooted in the Latin term "negligentia," which literally means, "not to pick up," or to neglect. To neglect is not *necessarily* the same as to commit an error or be careless (although instances of careless or erroneous nursing actions might be classified as negligent) because someone might be using as much care as possible, but still their actions fall below the standard to which we would hold them. Take, for example, a case of a nurse who has been in active practice for many years, but has not taken part in any professional development activities or continued learning activities. Within her professional practice, she may, on an individual level, try hard to provide high-quality, competent care to her patients. However, although she may not be "careless" per se, her lack of updated skills and knowledge may contribute to negligent care. Most provincial regulatory bodies are now paying attention to how much continued learning and professional development licensed nurses are conducting, and requiring it as evidence of continued competent practice.

Standards of competent care are set out by various mechanisms: Nursing education and accreditation of nursing programs and curricula, up-to-date textbooks and peer-reviewed evidence-based articles outlining practices, provincial nursing certification examinations, nursing practice standards, and best practice guidelines all act to set standards of nursing care at a particular level. Individual hospitals and agencies require certification in particular skills or roles—nurses often must be certified on an ongoing basis, for example, to give chemotherapy or to insert an intravenous or a central line. If a nurse fails to meet the standard of care, either through not attending to his or her practice or by failing to ensure certification or qualification, then that nurse can be considered to be negligent.

In most cases of negligence, the injured person (also called the **plaintiff**) would likely sue the accused offender (also called the **defendant**) through civil litigation, for damages or compensation. However, this would require that the case go through a court process. In order for a case of negligence to be heard by the court, the case must have four important attributes (Morris, Ferguson, & Dykeman, 1999). First, a duty to care must exist. **Duty to care** is an important overarching legal principle in nursing and it refers to the legal obligation imposed on someone to act or refrain from acting in a way that would cause harm to another (Keatings and Smith, 1999; Potter and Perry, 2008). Briefly, this means that nurses have a duty to act in a way that does not harm their patients. Furthermore, they should act to prevent foreseeable harm. Second, there must be evidence that the defendant has failed to comply with that duty to care. In other words, their care must be shown to fall below the level of care required to maintain the duty of care. Third, there must be demonstrable suffering or injury to the plaintiff. Finally, the suffering or injury must be shown to be a result of the negligent conduct of the defendant.

Tort law in relation to negligence has a very specific goal—to compensate the injured party for harm. In this instance, the law does not punish the defendant. The courts, in this case, function to establish that negligence has in fact occurred, by examining each case for the four components noted above and then attaching a compensatory amount to the injury or harm caused by either intentional or unintentional negligence.

Anyone can be sued for negligence. A storeowner who fails to clear a significant amount of ice from his sidewalk may be sued for negligence if someone slips and becomes injured. A bicycle rider might sue someone for negligence who opens their passenger side car door and knocks the cyclist off of the road, injuring them. Omissions can also be considered negligent—in other words, failure to do something that a reasonable person might do. Failure to warn persons that there is spilled liquid on the floor of the grocery aisle might result in a negligence suit if someone unknowingly walks through the liquid, slips, and falls, sustaining an injury. So while anyone potentially can be found to be negligent, nurses, physicians, and other health care professionals are held to higher standards. **Foreseeability** is a significant part of assessing whether negligence occurred or not, in many health care cases. Foreseeability is having the knowledge that one's actions or omissions might result in harm or injury. Nurses have special knowledge about medication administration, procedures, and treatments, which includes knowledge regarding the foreseeable potential harms or injuries of those medications, and treatments. While someone trained as a car mechanic might not have knowledge of the potential harms of an improper dressing change, a nurse is expected to understand the potential harms of not maintaining sterility and cleanliness. As a more specific example, an untrained layperson caring for her bedridden elderly mother at home without assistance might not know the dangers from lying in one position all the time. However, a nurse in a long-term care setting is expected to have knowledge of properly turning and positioning patients in order to maintain skin integrity and prevent skin ulcers and serious subsequent complications. Standards of care and practice standards outline the kinds of specialized knowledge that nurses must have and that contribute to nurses' unique ability to be able to foresee potential benefits, harms, and risks of particular actions or omissions. Thus, when a nurse fails to do this, she or he can be considered to be negligent.

In 2004, a group of Canadian researchers published the *Canadian Adverse Events Study* in the *Canadian Medical Association Journal*. It was the first pan-Canadian study examining the rate of adverse events in Canadian hospitals (Baker et al., 2004). Adverse events in the study were defined as those injuries or complications caused by health care management rather than the condition or disease of the patient. Notably, a number of the adverse events relate to nursing care, either directly or indirectly. One out of every thirteen patients admitted to a Canadian hospital, at the time of the study, experienced an adverse event. The three main areas in which adverse events occurs were surgery, medication, and infection. Nursing care is at the front line in every aspect of hospital care, and while the researchers did not point a finger at nursing, the implied message was that nurses are responsible for much of the delivery of patient care in hospitals and may also be responsible, even in part, for some of the adverse events that patients experience. Therefore, nursing, as a profession, must be attentive to the kinds of adverse events reported and ways in which they can be monitored and, eventually, completely prevented. Would increased education or continued professional development help? Could the systems of communication in the hospital be improved? Are there policies in place that are helping or hindering nurses in the delivery of care? Are the physical environments amenable to delivering competent care or are there marked limitations, such as lack of resources or continued understaffing that might contribute to the inability of nurses to deliver competent care? Reports like this one need to be translated into close examinations of practice, environments, and institutional structures, not just individual professionals. However, nothing this, each individual nurse is responsible for providing safe and competent care. Additionally, nurses in most jurisdictions have a professional responsibility to report cases of unsafe or incompetent care, negligence, or malpractice. So as nurses, we have both individual and collective responsibilities to prevent negligence.

Think About It

A very common area for nursing liability involves medication errors. There are many ways that nurses can make errors of medication preparation and administration. The nurse can give the wrong medication, or the wrong dose, at the wrong time, by the wrong route, or to the wrong patient. Because of the frequency and likelihood of medication error and the potentially serious consequences that can result, nurses need to be especially careful in administering medicine. Nurses are responsible for safe and appropriate administration of medication, regardless of physician orders, workload, unusual circumstances, or institutional policy. There

(Continued)

are many examples of medication errors cited in the literature. It is not unusual for damages to be awarded to victims or families when medication errors occur. Again, however, medication errors need to be examined from both an individual and an institutional perspective. Staffing mixes with increased numbers of higher levels of regulated nursing staff (i.e., RNs) have been shown to affect rates of medication errors (Doran et al., 2001). It makes sense that units with lower nurse-to-patient ratios might have lower rates of medication errors, because nurses can afford the proper amount of time to administer medications.

- What other factors do you see that might influence rates of medication administration errors on a nursing unit?

- How do you see technology either helping or hindering the administration of medication? Think about where you work. Are there persons who fill the medication carts or are they automatic or computer driven?

- What kinds of improvements could a nursing unit put in place to help prevent medication errors?

- Think about a medication error you might have made, nearly made, or noted another nurse making. What happened? What did you learn? How did the unit nurses and administrators handle the event? What kinds of factors contributed to that error?

Intentional torts are "willful or intentional acts that violate another person's rights or property" (Catalano, 1991, p. 69). A tort must include three elements to be considered intentional: the act must be intended to interfere with the plaintiff or his property; there must be intent to bring about the consequences of the act; and the act must substantially cause the consequences. There is no legal requirement that damages or injury actually result from the act; proof of the defendant's intention is sufficient (Catalano, 1991). Examples of intentional torts include fraud, invasion of privacy, assault, battery, false imprisonment, slander, and libel.

Fraud is a deliberate deception for the purpose of securing an unfair or unlawful gain. Although nurses are seldom accused of fraud, when this occurs it is usually prosecuted as a crime. Examples of potential areas of nurses' fraud include falsification of information on employment applications, false representation of health states in order to access services or secure insurance funds, and falsification of patient records to cover up an error. Fraud is a concern in Canada related to health insurance billing. The website for the Ontario Ministry of Health and Long Term Care has a section devoted to the discussion of health card fraud, which is an ongoing problem (Ontario Ministry of Health and Long Term Care, 2002). As is true with some other intentional torts, fraud can lead to both civil and criminal proceedings. Because of the deliberate nature and potential harm of fraudulent acts, court decisions tend to be harsh. Fraud is a more significant concern in the United States, where complex billing procedures and inequality of reimbursement set the stage for not only errors but also opportunities to gain funds or access to medical care through misrepresentation or other forms of deception. In the United States, an incident of fraud in health care can result in up to five years imprisonment, up to $25 000 in fines, and exclusion from reimbursement from both Medicare and Medicaid for up to five years (Mazzocco, 2000).

The **right to privacy** is the right to be left alone or to be free from unwanted publicity. Individuals have the right to withhold themselves and their lives from public scrutiny. The intentional tort of **invasion of privacy** occurs when a person's privacy is invaded. In Canada, protection of privacy is now not only an individual priority, but also a governmental priority. Various complex legislations have been put in place, at both a federal as well as provincial and territorial levels of government, to ensure that individuals' personal information as well as private health information are protected. More on the protection of privacy and the supporting legislation follows at the end of this chapter. Fiesta (1988) outlines four types of invasions of privacy: intrusion on the patient's physical and mental solitude or seclusion; public disclosure of private facts; publicity that places the patient in a false light in the public eye; and appropriation of the patient's name or likeness for the defendant's benefit or advantage (p. 160). There are many cases involving invasions of privacy. The following American case outlines how privacy can be invaded in a most serious and inappropriate manner, as noted in Fiesta (1998, p. 160), in the case *Bethiaume v. Pratt*, a dying patient being treated for cancer of the larynx was repeatedly photographed at the direction of his surgeon. On the day of his death the patient asked not to be photographed, but nevertheless the physician photographed him after lifting his head to place a pillow under it. A court decided that the physician should be held liable for invasion of privacy.

In another invasion of privacy case, Earl Spring, a senile seventy-eight-year-old man, was residing in a nursing home where he was undergoing kidney dialysis. In an attempt to discontinue dialysis treatments, his legal guardians, his wife and son, were involved in a prolonged court battle. In opposition to the family's position, and without their consent, the nursing home staff permitted right-to-life advocates to interview the senile man. Interviews with the patient and four nurses were published. After winning a Superior Court ruling regarding discontinuing the dialysis, Mrs. Spring sued the nursing home and the four nurses for $80 million in damages. She claimed that her husband's right to privacy had been violated. Although the attorney for the nursing home maintained that the patient had become a "public figure," the jury found in favour of Mrs. Spring, awarding her $2.5 million.

The terms "*assault*" and "*battery*," though usually used together, have different legal meanings. Both are intentional torts. **Assault** is defined as the unjustifiable attempt or threat to touch a person without consent that results in fear of immediately harmful or threatening contact (Bernzweig, 1990). Touching need not actually occur. **Battery** is the unlawful, harmful, or unwarranted touching of another or the carrying out of threatened physical harm. Battery can include any willful, angry, violent, or negligent touching of a person's body or clothes, or anything held by or attached to the person (Creighton, 1986; Guido, 1997). In the course of everyday activities, nurses have been accused of both assault and battery. For example, if a nurse threatens to give an injection to an unruly or noncompliant adult patient without consent, actionable assault has occurred. Battery is often thought of as such actions as slapping, shoving, or pinching, but the courts have upheld battery charges in actions that were much more subtle. Regardless of intent or outcome, *touching without consent is considered battery*. Even when the intention is beneficent and the outcome is positive, if the act is committed without permission, the nurse can be charged with battery. Surgical procedures that are performed without informed consent are the most common example of battery occurring in the hospital setting. Common defences to charges of battery arise from two other legal concepts: necessity and consent. **Necessity** refers to the privilege granted to a person to touch another person. A physician or a nurse may touch a person in order to provide care or direct medical aid to them in an emergency situation. **Consent** implies express or implicit permission to another to touch you. A nurse may not ask directly each time he takes a patient's blood pressure to "touch" the patient, but by asking if he can take the patient's blood pressure, he is essentially asking for permission to touch the patient's arm. By agreeing to have one's blood pressure taken, one implicitly agrees to being touched. An example of express permission would be signing a consent form for an invasive procedure, such as a liver biopsy or a surgery.

False imprisonment is the unjustifiable detention of a person within fixed boundaries, or an act intended to result in such confinement, without consent and without authority of law (Creighton, 1986; O'Keefe, 2000). Such acts can include physical restraint of the person, or acts intended to accomplish confinement, such as refusing the patient clothing or car keys. If false imprisonment is accompanied by forcible restraint or the threat of restraint, assault and battery may also be charged. There may be special cases in which persons may be detained for a limited period of time or held by authorities without explicit consent. Some examples include being detained by the police, being detained for capacity assessment or assessment of suicidal risk, and quarantine.

Defamation is any statement that represents a false claim against or a derogatory remark about an individual, group, product, company, government, or nation that would lead to a falsely negative image. Defamation tort law is designed to protect the esteem and positive image of subjects. It is, however, a difficult tort to prove and because of this, very few cases of defamation have been tried in civil courts. In a landmark 1970 case, *Murphy v. LaMarsh* (13 DLR 3d 484), the BC Supreme Court classified defamation as follows:

> … a shameful action is attributed to a man (he stole my purse), a shameful character (he is dishonest), a shameful course of action (he lives on the avails of prostitution), (or) a shameful condition (he has smallpox). Such words are considered defamatory because they tend to bring the man named into hatred, contempt or ridicule. The more modern definition (of defamation) is words tending to lower the plaintiff in the estimation of right-thinking members of society generally.

Defamation must be demonstrated to be harmful, must be aimed at the person or his or her reputation and must be conveyed to others, either verbally (also called slander) or in writing (libel). **Slander** and **libel** can occur in nursing and health care. By making value judgments or voicing that a patient is uncooperative, malingering, unintelligent, or drug seeking, a nurse may be committing actionable slander. Nurses may also be accused of slander as a result of inappropriate defamatory remarks voiced against another professional. Nurses can risk accusations of libel when writing information in patients' charts that can be damaging. Judgmental, critical, or speculative statements made in patients' charts such as "The patient is drug seeking" or "The patient is very uncooperative" can lead to an accusation of libel, particularly if the patient has reason to believe that the words adversely affect the care given by others.

Nurses have also been the object of defamatory remarks. A physician accused his office nurse of having mixed up reports on a patient's chart and lying about it. He fired her the next day and called a meeting of his office employees. He told his staff that he couldn't work with anyone who was a liar, untrustworthy, and disloyal. A jury awarded the nurse $125,000 in damages (Creighton, 1986).

Defences against accusations of defamation include truth telling (i.e., the remark or statement is accurate or true), statements made in good faith (i.e., with the belief that they were, in fact, true), statements provided to a third party that are negative but justified (i.e., a negative remark on a job or academic reference), privilege (i.e., statements made by a person to his or her spouse, on a legislature floor, or in a court room), and opinion (as opinion is a subjective notion and cannot be proven to be "true" or "untrue." Furthermore, there may be a legal or moral duty to pass on defamatory information in certain circumstances. A nurse has a duty to report child abuse, a director of nursing service has the duty to report truthfully the character and qualifications of nurses seeking employment references elsewhere, and peer review disciplinary groups are required to discuss privileged information for the purpose of disciplining others and following due processes. Nurses have a professional obligation to report incompetent or illegal practice of others. To avoid accusations of defamation, prudent nurses will take care to observe appropriate channels of communication when making reports of this nature. In the absence of privileged communication, truth is a good defence for defamation.

Intentional infliction of emotional distress (also called "intentional infliction of mental distress" or the "tort of outrage" in some jurisdictions) is a relatively new tort claim. This allows for a claim to be made against someone who acts in a heinous, reckless, or extreme way, to bring about emotional distress in a plaintiff. This tort claim was created to allow for instances when a threat is not imminent or the threat of harm is in the future—as this could not be considered as assault. (In order for a claim of assault to be made, the threat has to be fairly imminent, causing harm.) This new tort claim allows for claims against persons who cause emotional distress to others, and for compensation to be granted to the plaintiff.

Some examples might include failing to tell an estranged spouse the whereabouts of her or his child for many years or lying to someone about your death or the death of another person. In health care, unfortunately, we might be able to think of examples of cases in which the intentional infliction of emotional distress might be claimed by patients against nurses, especially those patients who are more vulnerable, homeridden, and dependent upon visiting nurses, or institutionalized. On a positive note, this is not, at this time, a common tort claim in the general public or in health care.

Think About It

It is important that nurses be aware of the legal system in relation to their practice. While the rate of litigation for malpractice or negligence against nurses and health care professionals is lower in Canada than in the United States, there are still cases in which nurses have been charged with this serious crime.

In 1998, Lisa Shore, an otherwise healthy ten-year-old girl, was admitted to the Hospital for Sick Children in Toronto, Ontario, for relief of pain due to reflex sympathetic dystrophy syndrome resulting from a leg fracture earlier in the year. This syndrome is results in extreme pain and sensitivity of the affected area. On admission, Lisa was given a steady a dose of morphine and within approximately twelve hours, was found to be in respiratory and cardiac arrest, and was pronounced dead shortly after that. Her death was noted to be caused by the administration of morphine with other medications and insufficient monitoring. The coroner's report classified Lisa's death as a homicide and the nurses who were caring for her were charged with negligence in 2001. The charges of negligence were withdrawn in 2003. Two years later, the two nurses went through a disciplinary hearing at the College of Nurses of Ontario and were found guilty of professional misconduct with a suspension of licensure for a period of one month, which was suspended.

In another case at the Hospital for Sick Children, Sanchia Bulgin, a seventeen-year-old girl with sickle cell anemia, died after routine gallbladder surgery. Sanchia was given morphine post-operatively, a drug to which she had a known sensitivity. She also was inadequately monitored for signs of bleeding and shock, and hemorrhaged to death. There were a number of recommendations made by the coroner regarding prevention of any further deaths like this one, including better communication between members of the nursing and medical team; better training for nurses about vital signs, shock, and sickle cell disease; as well as monitoring post-operative patients.

Nurses do not go to their jobs with intentions to do harm or to make fatal errors. Incompetence, carelessness, or lack of knowledge may, unfortunately, exist in nursing and certainly may lead to errors, some of them serious. On the other hand, even well-intentioned, competent, and careful nurses can make mistakes.

(Stewart, 2002).

- Read more about the coroner's recommendations made after reviewing the Lisa Shore and the Sanchia Bulgin cases. Discuss the recommendations in light of your current workplace and practice.

- Coroner's verdicts and summaries can be found at: http://www.mcscs.jus.gov.ca/english/office_coroner/verdicts_and_recs/verdicts_and_recs_intro.html

- What are your feelings as you read the cases and coroner's recommendations?

- Reflect on any situations that may have made you feel that you were unable to practise safely or competently. What did you do?

- How would you react today if you were asked to do something that you considered to be beyond your level of competence or skill?

- How much should family members or patients be told about mistakes or errors that may have occurred while they were in the health care system?

Consent

Consent is a complex legal and ethical notion, arising from notions of dignity and autonomy. It is entrenched in the idea that persons have the right to decide what can and cannot be done to them. In law, it is often referred to as the right to be free from interference.

Before health care treatments of all kinds can be provided, consent of the patient must be obtained. An exception is made in cases of emergencies and other extenuating circumstances. However nurses should practise with the ever-present idea that patients must consent to be touched, to have treatments administered, to undergo surgery, to be given medications, to allow testing to be done, and to have even low-risk procedures carried out. Many treatments and skills that nurses carry out on patients can arguably be considered to be low risk, such as bathing, positioning, taking vital signs, and physical assessments. Other activities, such as dressing changes, venipuncture, wound irrigation, and catheter insertions are considered as somewhat higher risk. With the increasing scope of nursing practice, more nurses are able to do higher-risk procedures, treatments, and examinations of patients. But the most important point to note is that even the low-risk procedures, such as bathing and the taking of vital signs, must be consented to by the patient before the activities can be carried out. As noted earlier in the chapter, the intentional tort of battery involves touching of a person without the person's consent. Much of nursing care involves touching, so patient consent to touch must be sought in these circumstances.

Consent is a provincial jurisdiction and most provinces and territories have distinct statutes in place describing consent; for example, the *Health Care [Consent] and Care Facility [Admission] Act of British Columbia* (1996), Manitoba's *Health Care Directives Act* (1992), and Prince Edward Island's *Consent to Treatment and Health Care Directives Act* (2002). In Ontario, there are two pieces of legislation around consent: the *Health Care Consent Act* (1996) and the *Substitute Decisions Act* (1992). The *Health Care Consent Act* helps to protect patients' decision-making autonomy by facilitating communication with health care providers and patients, and helping to include family members as appropriate when a patient is incapable of making his or her own decisions. The *Substitute Decisions Act* addresses decision making regarding personal care and care of property in the case of a person who is deemed to be incompetent (College of Nurses of Ontario, 2008).

These documents and their specific directives vary from province to province; however, for the most part, they espouse similar values, which include protection and promotion of patients' autonomy, and authority over their health care decisions. They also usually outline the necessary elements of consent. In Ontario's *Health Care Consent Act,* the elements of consent are as follows [1996, c.2, Sched. A, s. 11 (1).]:

- Consent must relate to the treatment
- Consent must be informed
- Consent must be given voluntarily
- Consent must not be obtained through misrepresentation or fraud

These elements are, for the most part, reflected in other provincial and territorial legislative acts describing consent, alongside notions of capacity to consent. In a jurisdiction in which there is no specific legislation regarding consent, these elements are usually noted when defining a valid consent: The consent must be voluntary, informed, and refer to both the treatment and the provider. Furthermore, the patient must have the capacity to consent.

In most discussions of consent in health care, we are usually referring to consent of a patient to allow a treatment or procedure. For the purposes of discussion, in the following sections, while we acknowledge that consent is required in a variety of circumstances and contexts, we will refer to consent, usually, as consent for treatment.

Consent can be explicit or implied. **Explicit consent** is either verbal or written consent specifically articulating the patient's agreement to a particular treatment or procedure. Implied consent is less concrete—but quite often encountered. It is inferred from a person's presence and actions as well as the context of the situation. In other words, a pregnant woman who admits herself to the hospital to give birth under the care of her obstetrician implies consent for the obstetrician to examine her. **Implied consent** does not infer, however, that the person's consent should be taken for granted or assumed. Just as a patient in the post-operative cardiac ward might not give express consent to have his vital signs taken every six hours, it is still important for the nurse to ensure that the patient is willing to have his vital signs taken when she enters the room to do so.

Voluntary Consent

In order for consent to be considered valid, it must be provided freely, without coercion or undue influence. In other words, it must be provided by the patient of his or her own free will, without feelings of obligation, urgency, or necessity unrelated to the treatment. This has implications regarding which member of the health care team obtains consent, when, and how. Consent should be obtained by the appropriate health care provider with a nonjudgmental, skillful, and thorough approach. Nurses often do not obtain informed consent for surgical procedures or other invasive procedures, such as wound debridement, lumbar punctures, or biopsies. Usually surgeons or physicians obtain such consent. However, nurses often are the persons to whom patients turn when they have questions about the consent that they provided. Some patients may voice to the nurse that they felt unable to "say no" or ask for more time to make the decision as they didn't want to displease the physician who was providing their care. While the physician may well have approached the consent process in a facilitative, approachable, and relaxed way, patients may still feel intimidated by the role of the physician and the process of providing consent. In this case, nurses must be attuned to patients' needs and whether or not the consent was voluntarily given.

Informed Consent

Consent is informed if the person receives information about the proposed treatment that any reasonable person would want to know in the same situation in order to make a similar decision. Additionally, the person must have received answers to her questions or requests for additional information.

Information must include the condition for which she is being treated; the nature of the treatment; the expected benefits of the treatment; the known, anticipated, or foreseeable risks and/or side effects of treatment; alternative options for treatment; and the likely outcomes if no treatment is provided. Information should be provided to patients at an appropriate level, keeping in mind patients' age and developmental stage. Medical jargon and highly technical terms should be avoided as much as possible, and, if used, should be defined and explained thoroughly to patients. Opportunity should be provided for patients to think about the options provided to them along with the risks and benefits, in order to formulate questions and recognize where they require more information in order to be fully informed.

Informed consent is not a panacea. It is impossible to list every possible risk, every potential benefit and sometimes, every known accessible or real alternative option. Furthermore, some people quite mistakenly believe that lay persons cannot ever fully understand the implications of all the possible benefits, risks, and side effects of proposed treatments, and they conclude that the process of obtaining informed consent is, therefore, ineffective or useless. All this, however, should not deter health care professionals from providing as much accurate, appropriate, and thorough information as possible to patients and allowing them the time and freedom to make an informed, voluntary decision.

Treatment and Provider

Consent, when given, is usually specific to a treatment or procedure as well as a particular provider. This element of consent is noted to be a response to the kind of "blanket" consents that used to exist in many health care contexts. For example, patients used to sign blanket consents when entering hospital for any and all testing and investigations. Today, a patient would provide informed consent for each individual test and investigation to be carried out.

When a patient consents to have one treatment, he is not implying consent, in any way, for other related or unrelated treatments. For example, when a patient consents to have his blood taken for a complete blood count, differential and electrolyte measurement—all common blood tests—he is not providing consent to also have a blood test for human immunodeficiency virus (HIV). Consent to have an HIV test must be taken separately, with an entirely different kind of discussion. Furthermore, in many cases, consent is attached to a specific provider. For surgical procedures, this is almost always the case. A patient signs a consent to allow a particular surgeon to perform the surgery and has, in the case of elective or urgent surgery, usually met and discussed the procedure with the surgeon already. In emergent cases; this might not be the case; however, even a signed consent in an emergent surgical situation would usually refer to a particular surgeon. So if the surgery is then performed by a less qualified person (such as a trainee or resident) or an alternative physician without seeking explicit permission, this would not be in keeping with the patients' original informed consent.

Capacity to Consent

When we talk about capacity, we are usually talking about a legal capacity to provide consent. In general, capacity refers to the ability to learn, gather, retain, and apply knowledge. In law, it is the ability to understand the significance of behaviours or decisions and the influences upon those behaviours or decision-making abilities. The legal notion of capacity formally refers to the age and mental competence of the person to understand information provided to her along with the risks, benefits, and value of alternatives along with the consequences of the decision once made (Downie and Caulfield, 2002). As age and mental competence are the two key concepts in capacity, the two groups for whom consent becomes a more difficult or complex matter are adults with questionable capacity (due to disability or mental health issues) and children.

Children and Capacity to Consent

Consent is not an "all or nothing" concept. Many persons have evolving capacities in many areas of their lives, and the ability to learn and retain knowledge for purposes of making decisions is one area in which capacity may be developing. It is not the case, that on their eighteenth birthday, young adults are suddenly able to make decisions for themselves that they were incapable of making the day prior. Most adolescents have evolving capacity to decision make alongside their evolving moral agency.

As children, our **values** and decisions are mostly dictated by those of our parents or guardians. The food we eat, the school we attend, the church where we may worship or the lack of religion in our lives—all these things are not usually based on autonomous choices we make as children, but on the choices our parents make for us, based on their values, beliefs, and ideas about what constitutes our best interests. As we grow and expand our social world, our ideas about our values and beliefs we held as children and usually attributed to our parents now include ideas from our friends, our teachers, mentors, and community members. Additionally, during adolescence, most young people tend to want to find their own "identity" or worldview, which may differ from their parents and may be more strongly aligned to that of peers and mentors. Through this process, we learn, as we reach adulthood, what our own values and beliefs are, usually influenced by a combination of those instilled in us through our parents, guardians, families, culture, environment, socioeconomic status, neighbourhood, school, teachers, religion, community groups, etc., and those that we find and internalize ourselves. What this demonstrates, though, is that capacity to consent is as dynamic as one's own moral agency, developing over time and with experience and exposure to decision making and different circumstances.

Some children and adolescents, however, have a more advanced level of understanding, and may be deemed to be "mature minors." Usually a mature minor is a young person above the age of thirteen; however, there have been instances in which children as young as seven or eight have been found to be mature minors. The notion of a mature minor is part of common law and not statutory law—in other words, decisions about whether a child can be considered a mature minor are not made by referring to statutes or legislation. Rather, these decisions are made by an ad hoc or a "case-by-case" decision by judicial law, taking into consideration the child's age, intelligence, education, and previous experiences.

In a 2006 Manitoba case, heard at the Supreme Court of Canada in 2008, *A.C. et al. v. Director of Child and Family Services*, a fourteen-year-old Jehovah's Witness was forced to undergo a blood transfusion to replace blood lost in complications from Crohn's disease, against her explicit and articulately stated objections to this procedure, based on her deeply held spiritual beliefs. The case focuses specifically on older minors who are forced to accept treatment, even though they have the mental capacity to make treatment decisions.

❓ Think About It

The Case of Tyrell Dueck

Tyrell Dueck was a thirteen-year-old boy diagnosed with osteosarcoma in Saskatchewan. Tyrell's parents refused to consent to traditional treatments for osteosarcoma, which include chemotherapy and surgery for amputation. In most cases of osteosarcoma, early treatment with chemotherapy can lead to a significant chance of recovery with a year. Without chemotherapy, Tyrell had a very small chance of recovery beyond a year. In many cases, children of Tyrell's age would be included in the decision-making processes, as much as their developmental stage would allow. It was noted that Tyrell was highly uninvolved in decision making for his care as his parents made the decisions for him. This concerned the health care team, who started a legal process to assume guardianship of Tyrell. Two issues were key in this case and both have legal and ethical implications. The first important issue was determining the best interests of Tyrell. The second important issue was determining if Tyrell had the developmental capacity to make decisions for his own care.

Eventually the health care team was awarded guardianship of Tyrell and chemotherapy was started. During his treatment with chemotherapy, Tyrell then voiced that he did not want further chemotherapy; however, he also did not want

(Continued)

his leg amputated. This choice demonstrated, to some, the inability of Tyrell to understand the situation at hand because without these options, patients with osteosarcoma ultimately succumb to the disease. So the health care team returned to the court system to help determine if Tyrell was a "mature minor," in other words, could he be deemed capable of making his own decisions without parental involvement?

Adding to the concern of the health care team was the fact that they felt Tyrell's father did not allow any health care staff to approach or talk to Tyrell without his presence. In a return to the courts, it was deemed that Tyrell did not have the decisional capacity of a mature minor, that he was strongly influenced by his father, and that he likely had not obtained information about the risks and benefits of options for treatment as much of the information he did receive was "filtered" through his father. During the court proceedings, it was determined that the cancer had in fact spread to his lungs and at this point, any further treatment was futile.

Tyrell died soon after this.

(Nelson, 1999)

- How do you think the best interests of Tyrell should have been determined? What do you think was in his best interests?
- This case involves differences in values. How should health care professionals approach persons who have different values that affect care?
- What is different about a competent adult refusing treatment for him- or herself compared to an adult refusing treatment for his child?
- Discuss the notion of a "mature minor." What kinds of things should a child or young person demonstrate in order to be considered a mature minor?

Adults with Diminished Capacity

Normally, we expect that adults will have decisional capacity. However, there are many factors that can interfere with the ability of an adult to be competent to take part in decision making about their care. Disease processes, disabilities, developmental delays, dementia, and neurological injuries are some examples.

Again, remember that capacity is not an "all or nothing" concept. Persons may have diminished capacity for a temporary period, if they experience, for example, post-operative delirium or disorientation due to a medication. Furthermore, persons who have limited capacity may be able to consent to certain things but for other kinds of decisions, may require assistance, support or a substitute decision maker.

Legislation exists in most provinces and territories regarding the ability of persons to appoint valid substitute decision makers or proxies, and create advance directives for care, in the event that they are unable to decision make by virtue of diminished capacity. In this case, it is important that nurses and other health care providers attend to the previously stated wishes of persons articulated through advance directive documents as well as through proxies. Substitute decision makers are

> person or persons with the best knowledge of the patient's specific wishes, or of the patient's values and beliefs, as they pertain to the present situation. In general close relatives are preferred as substitute decision makers in the belief that they will know the patient well enough to replicate the decision that the patient would make if he or she were capable. (Lazar et al., 1996, p. 1436)

In some cases, such as a person with a chronic disability or development delay, there are directives and substitute decision makers in place before an event or decision that requires urgency or efficiency in decision-making processes. In other words, a person who may have had limited capacity since childhood may, more often than not, have these kinds of things in place to help when care decisions must be made. However, for someone who is competent who sustains an injury, or has a stroke or neurological event that leads to diminishment of their decision-making capacity, it is ideal when their wishes have been previously documented using advance directives. This makes it much easier for substitute decision makers and the health care team to act in a way that the patient would have also wanted, if she were able to contribute to the decision. Nurses should educate patients about the advantages of having a living will or advance directive and the positive benefits of having discussed these issues with those closest to them.

If an adult's capacity is questioned, this activates a process of determining capacity that involves multiple persons, over time. Take the example of a woman found on the street late at night with some minor injuries, who is disoriented and possibly delusional. The woman is brought to the emergency room and, before treatment of her minor injuries and a full assessment of any further injury or illness, consent is sought. However, in this case, as the woman has no identification and seems to be disoriented and delusional, her capacity to consent for her own care is questioned by the health care team. Before a "one-off" decision can be made, for the sake of efficiency, a formal process to assess capacity must be undertaken.

CASE PRESENTATION

Marc is a forty-two-year old man with advanced AIDS, living at home with his partner of ten years, Charles. Charles and Marc have discussed the future and, together, have written a living will for Marc. Charles is Marc's substitute decision maker. Recently, Charles has noticed that Marc is becoming forgetful and behaving oddly. He suspects that it is the early stages of AIDS-related dementia. Marc has also been investigated for AIDS-related lymphoma as he has had frequent fevers, night sweats, and extreme weight loss with lymph node swelling.

When Marc's physician informs them that Marc does in fact have lymphoma, the physician notes that the disease may have spread to the brain, which may account for some of Marc's changing behaviours. While noting that the lymphoma

(Continued)

has spread, the physician recommends treatment immediately, noting the burden that it will pose, but assuring both Marc and Charles that it may be possible, through timely treatment, to arrest the rate of the spread of the malignancy. Previously, Marc has clearly expressed to Charles that he would not want to have any burdensome treatment just to extend a life in which he could not participate fully. Charles isn't sure if this is what Marc meant but he is unable to get Marc to discuss this, as Marc's episodes of forgetfulness and disorientation are rapidly increasing in frequency and intensity.

Lucille is an elderly woman diagnosed with Alzheimer's disease over 15 years ago. She lives in a residential seniors centre in Vancouver with advanced medical care. Both her daughters are listed as joint substitute decision makers. One daughter, Maggie, lives in the city and visits her mother almost daily. She is highly involved in her mother's care. Hannah, Lucille's other daughter, lives on the East Coast and gets out west twice a year to spend a few days with her mother. Recently, Lucille's physical condition has deteriorated and she has becoming noticeably more frail. Her ability to take nutrition and hydration by mouth has worsened and she is quickly losing weight. The medical team approaches Maggie about placement of a feeding tube. Maggie quickly agrees but asks that she have time to consult with her sister. Two days later, Hannah arrives and promptly tells the medical team that her mother would never have wanted a "tube to feed her" and that they should not do the procedure as it would be in opposition to Lucille's wishes, which, she states, her mother discussed with her and not Maggie. Maggie is visibly upset and the two sisters appear to have a significant amount of tension between them.

Later in the day, Hannah again approaches the medical team, and tells them that Maggie is "too close" to the situation and she cannot make decisions in the best interest of their mother. Hannah tells them that Maggie is severely depressed, on medication, unable to work and that she has told Hannah her only reason for living is "to take care of mom." Without her mother, Hannah states, Maggie would have no reason for living.

? Think About It

Questions to Consider

1. In each of the cases, who should give consent for care?
2. What are some things that the health care team can do, in each of the above situations, to help facilitate substitute decision making?

Documentation

Nursing documentation is an important part of practice. It communicates to others not only the care and treatment of clients but also valuable information about assessments, evaluations, progress, and concerns related to client care. Nursing notes are part of patient's health record—a document that reflects the overall interdisciplinary care of a patient during a period of time, an admission to a health care institution, or the progress of an outpatient at a clinic or family doctor's office.

Being clear, accurate, concise, and nonjudgmental are important when making nursing notes. One must ensure that any information documented in health records reflects what actually occurred or was said. Patients' own words should be labelled as such, using quotation marks. Only actual events should be noted, not speculations about what might have happened or what may happen. Of course, there may be exceptions. For example, a nurse may document that over a shift, a patient become increasingly less oriented and note the concern for the immediate future. Clarity is important—using proper language and grammar so that others reading the health record at a later time have a full understanding of the events. Being concise or brief is also important. While it is necessary to document as completely as possible, being concise does not necessarily mean that one must compromise on quality of information. Additionally, legibility is important in hand-written records. As noted earlier in the chapter, making judgmental remarks might be seen as libelous. Noting that a patient is "uncooperative," "lazy" or "unwilling" are all judgments, and there is no place in nursing notes for these kinds of remarks. If a patient is, in fact, not willing to undergo, for example, a burdensome treatment, it should simply be noted that the patient refused the treatment. A competent and caring nurse would explore with the patient why she refused the treatment and try to help facilitate understanding about the importance of the treatment, while exploring the valid reasons the patient may have for not consenting to this particular treatment on this particular day. Those kinds of things may be noted in the nursing notes but a quick descriptor, "unwilling," not only is judgmental, but also does not allow for any kind of intervention or support for the patient.

Further supporting the need for clear, accurate, concise, and nonjudgmental documentation is the fact that nursing notes can be introduced as evidence in court proceedings or disciplinary hearings. Health records, which may include nursing notes and legal documentation in most provinces, are also known as "business records," i.e., records relevant to the operation of hospital or agency. In many jurisdictions, a nursing record can be called as evidence, therefore, documenting in a sloppy, careless or incomplete way demonstrates not only lack of accountability, but also a lack of professionalism.

There are many problems in nursing documentation that we see frequently. Sometimes there are significant gaps in the records, i.e., periods of time not accounted for or documentation about specific shifts that might be missing. It is always difficult, later on, to verify that something was done when no documentation exists. In terms of the use of documents in courts and hearings, complete documentation provides a way for nurses to "remember" the day or the event. When documentation is complete and accurate, it serves as a more effective cue to memory and a more reliable source of information. Documentation may be messy, difficult to read, or sloppy. There may be errors in the documentation or documentation by someone other than the nurse who provided the care. *The person who provided care* must document care accurately. In other words, a nurse simply covering for his colleague who is on a break cannot chart that the original nurse completed the morning care and gave medications. He can document only the care he gave during the relief time and nothing more. Finally, there may be cases in which documentation is falsified or facts and events misrepresented. In this case, a nurse may be considered negligent and certainly unaccountable for his actions.

In an important Canadian case, which originated in Ontario, in 1976, *Kolesar v. Jeffries,* the Canadian Nurses Protective Society (2007) notes that a patient who had undergone a spinal fusion was returned to a post-operative surgical unit. The morning after his surgery, he was found dead. Upon review of the nursing notes, there was found to be no nursing notes from the previous night at ten o'clock until five in the morning. According to the courts, this clearly established blame, i.e. liability, as the assumption was that if nothing was charted, nothing was carried out. In other words, no documentation implied no nursing care. Yet, in an interesting subsequent case, *Ferguson v. Hamilton* (1983), the notion that no nursing notes implies no care for that time period was rejected, with two caveats. First there must be clear evidence that there was care provided during the period of time. Second, there needs to be confirmation of a usual institutional practice not to chart for periods of time (College of Registered Nurses of British Columbia, 2003). The important message here is that, to the world outside of a hospital or agency, lack of adequate documentation leaves questions and concerns about quality of nursing care.

Technology and Documentation

Most hospitals and health care agencies have some form of computerized documentation. Many of these programs require special training and orientation to the programs and are complex, integrated, and a key part of the patient's health record. Electronic records have many advantages—they can be easily transferred (with explicit permission) between providers and institutions with a few simple keystrokes. If a patient's primary physician is in another country or halfway across the world, electronic records can easily be shared for efficient transfer of important information. Computerized documentation is standardized in terms of legibility and where to find it. In other words, there are no problems with reading persons' writing or trying to flip through pages in a paper chart looking for a test result or notation. Furthermore, electronic documentation can help with accuracy by automatically identifying who made the entry, the date and time the entry was made, and even the computer on which the entry was recorded.

The accuracy of computerized documentation can also identify improper access to information or records. For example, a nurse cannot access the computerized personal health records of her father-in-law, in the hospital on another unit. Another example might include accessing the record of a friend or colleague who is also a patient in the agency in which you might work as a nurse. While it might seem harmless to look up their blood tests for someone you know to tell them all is fine and reassure them, if they are not directly under your care as a patient, then it is unadvisable, even illegal, to access their health records through a computer.

Nurses' use of electronic communication raises a number of legal and ethical questions. What are the legal implications of electronic communication? What is our responsibility for maintaining patient confidentiality? Does this change with the use of electronic documentation? How does electronic documentation affect or change nursing practice?

Some provinces have updated their privacy legislation to reflect the ubiquity of computerized record keeping. Nurses should be familiar with not only institutional policies and procedures around electronic record keeping but also provincial privacy laws.

Privacy and Confidentiality

The right to privacy and the duty of confidentiality are two important concepts in law and ethics. They are often, mistakenly, used interchangeably. In health care, privacy is the right of the patient while confidentiality is what we owe to the patient, when we have intimate knowledge of their personal or health data. Privacy is considered a constitutional right in Canada and it may affect how other laws are enacted. Confidentiality, on the other hand, is a duty of a health care professional who has an obligation to not share that information. This obligation or duty may be ascribed by an institution or it may be implicit in the relationship between the person who provides the information and the person who then receives it and is expected to keep it confidential (Slowther & Kleinman, 2008).

In Canada, both federal and provincial legislation regulate the collection, storage, and dissemination or sharing of personal information by the government and agencies that hold or store such information. The laws describe how this kind of data can be collected, stored, and accessed or used.

At a **federal** level, two privacy laws exist: *The Privacy Act* (1983) and the *Personal Information Protection and Electronic Documents Act* (PIPEDA). *The Privacy Act* imposes obligations on how federal government departments collect, manage, use, and share personal information that they hold. It also provides individuals with the right to change or correct information held about them and outlines mechanisms to do so.

PIPEDA applies to personal information about customers that is collected, used, or disclosed by all organizations involved in commercial activities including the retail sector, the federally regulated private sector (e.g., banks, airlines, telecommunications), the service industry, and provincially regulated organizations (Office of the Privacy Commissioner of Canada, 2008). Oversight and enforcement of these laws is carried out by the Privacy Commissioner of Canada. This office also hears and investigates privacy complaints of individuals.

According to PIPEDA, personal information (e.g., identifiable information that may include your name, age, height, weight, medical records, income, purchases, spending, race, ethnic origin, skin colour, blood type, DNA, fingerprints, marital status, religion, education, address, and phone number) can be collected only by a company involved in commercial activities with the following guidelines:

- Information must be gathered with the explicit knowledge and consent of the person.
- Information must be gathered for a reasonable (relevant) purpose.
- Information must be used only for the specific purpose for which it was collected.
- Information must be kept accurate and current.
- Information must be accessible for inspection and correction by the individual.

- Information must be stored securely and destroyed appropriately.
- Policies regarding information in companies must be clear, and easy to understand and access.

Additionally, the law gives individuals the following rights:

- To know who within an organization is responsible for protecting your personal information
- To complain about how an organization deals with or manages your personal information or if you believe that your privacy rights have not been protected
- To be supplied with a product or service even if you refuse consent for the collection, use, or sharing of your personal information unless that information is necessary for the transaction.

Each **province** has legislation regarding privacy as well. Currently the only province that does not have legislation is Newfoundland and Labrador: That province's legislation has been passed but is not yet active. Provincial and territorial privacy legislation functions to govern the collection, use, and disclosure of personal information gathered, held, and used by government agencies. Oversight of this is again either by a provincial commissioner or ombudsperson.

Some provinces also have specific legislation regarding the collection, use, and sharing of personal health information. Alberta, Saskatchewan, Manitoba, and Ontario have each passed laws addressing personal health information. Alberta has the *Health Information Act* (2001) as well as the *Personal Information Protection Act* (PIPA) (2004). Ontario has the *Personal Health Information Protection Act* in addition to the *Freedom of Information and Protection of Privacy Act* (FIPPA) the *Municipal Freedom of Information and Protection of Privacy Act*. Saskatchewan has the *Health Information Protection Act.*

As you can see, privacy is a highly complex and highly legislated concept in Canada. As Canadians, we value this; privacy is entrenched in *Canadian Charter of Rights and Freedoms*. Although the term "privacy" is not used in the *Charter* document, Sections 7 and 8 outline the following rights:

7. Everyone has the right to life, liberty and security of the person and the right not to be deprived thereof except in accordance with the principles of fundamental justice.

8. Everyone has the right to be secure against unreasonable search or seizure.

Inherently understood in these sections of the *Charter* is the right to privacy of individuals, unless, as Section 7 notes, there is justification for not maintaining confidentiality and protecting the privacy of individuals.

Nurses have access to patients' personal and health information on a constant basis. We refer to records with personal health information in order to complete histories and assessments. We collect information from patients regarding their personal habits, health, diagnoses, treatments, and even views on health and illness. Maintaining this information in a confidential manner is incredibly important—both from a legal and a professional perspective. Most regulatory bodies overseeing nursing practice in each province have practice standards regarding privacy and confidentiality. Hospital acts in each province also reinforce the patients' rights to confidentiality in records held in hospitals. Nurses in all sectors—not just hospitals, however—have a professional responsibility to maintain patient confidentiality in all aspects of care. Nurses who do not respect this responsibility can be found guilty of professional misconduct.

There are some exceptions to maintaining confidentiality. They include the following:

- The client expressly consents that her information is shared to persons other than those named who can have access to the information.
- Situations that require mandatory reporting. These may include the mandatory duty to report child abuse or suspected child abuse, certain communicable diseases, and negligent or incompetent practices of other health care professionals.
- A court order is used to obtain health records for use in a court proceeding.

The complex nature of privacy and confidentiality, added to the increased use of electronic documentation to collect and store personal data, makes patients sometimes more vulnerable than they ever have been. Many people are confused and overwhelmed by the depth and degree of legislation around privacy and confidentiality, and are unsure of how the laws apply to them, either as private citizens or as patients in a health care environment. Even some health care professionals do not fully understand the concepts of persons right to privacy and the duty of professionals to maintain confidentiality. This is demonstrated by the number of disciplinary hearings related to breaches in privacy and instances of not maintaining confidentiality adequately. As the laws become more and more a part of our daily lives and we learn through experiences, both positive and negative, nurses can no longer say "I didn't know" when it comes to privacy and confidentiality of patients' personal and health information. It is the responsibility of individual nurses to learn about privacy legislation in their province or territory as well as institutional policies, professional standards, and expectations, and apply these to individual accountable nursing practice.

Accountability in Practice

Accountability in practice not only refers to legal accountability but also to professional accountability. Recall that expertise in practice is not only one hallmark of a professional but also a legal and ethical imperative. There have been monumental advances in knowledge and technology in the past several years. With the advent of health insurance in the post–World War II era and malpractice litigation in recent years, standards of care have become very stringent. Society's expectations of nurses' knowledge and abilities are high. Consequently, nurses must strive to maintain up-to-date knowledge and technical skills through professional development activities. Lack of knowledge is no defence in a court of law or during a professional disciplinary hearing. It is, in fact, tantamount to an admission of negligence. It is important that nurses know and uphold institutional, professional, and legal standards of practice and work within their scope of practice, never attempting to perform any task or administer any medication that is unfamiliar. Nurses' actions are examined in light of current information, professional or statutory scope of practice, and institutional and professional practice standards. Statements such as "Everyone does it that way," "That is what I learned in school twenty years ago," or "I did the best I could" will not protect a nurse from being found negligent.

Accountable practice also includes close attention to detail. Nurses make serious errors when they become overly tired or distracted, are called away from tasks, are inattentive to patients' changing health status, or do not take the time to document thoroughly. Attention to detail will eliminate many errors that result in charges of negligence. Ethics and the law are closely related in regard to attention to detail. Recall from Chapter 2 that deontological ethics requires that each person is seen as an end and not as a means only, and that one is compelled to fulfill one's duty to others, thus implying that nurses must focus clearly upon each patient and each task. Attention to detail will serve to improve patient outcomes and ensure that the profession continues to engender the public trust.

SUMMARY

As the enforceable system of principles and processes that govern the behaviour of people, laws reflect moral and ethical tradition. Though there is sometimes disagreement regarding the rightness or wrongness of certain laws, the laws are generally consistent with popular beliefs.

Laws can be constitutional, statutory, or administrative, and are divided into public and private realms. Public law deals with the relationship between persons and the government, and private law deals with the relationship between people. Nurses and other health care providers are more likely to be involved in liability cases related to tort law, a division of private law. Tort law includes unintentional torts, such as negligence and malpractice, and intentional torts, such as fraud, invasion of privacy, assault, battery, false imprisonment, defamation and intentional infliction of emotional distress.

Consent is an important overarching legal and ethical notion. Nurses must be aware of the four elements of consent—that it be voluntary, that it be informed, that it relate to specific providers and treatment, and that capacity to consent is assessed. Furthermore, they should be aware of consent legislation in the province in which they work. As advocates, nurses can help patients to understand the notion of substitute decision makers or proxies, and help patients in creating advance directives, in keeping with helping patients to maintain their autonomous wishes, even if they are unable to participate in decision making.

Persons are owed the right to privacy and, as professionals, we have a duty to maintain confidentiality. Numerous federal and provincial laws protect the privacy of individuals. Some of these are laws specifically addressing the collection, use, and sharing of personal health information. Nurses must be aware of not only federal and provincial legislation but also professional standards and institutional policies around maintaining confidentiality of patients' information.

CHAPTER HIGHLIGHTS

- Ethics is the foundation of law; however, because laws are created by individuals and there are differences in beliefs among people, ethics and the law are not always congruent.

- Statutory law is created through the law-making process in federal or provincial legislatures; it is also called legislative law.

- Administrative law consists mainly of the legal powers granted to administrative agencies by the legislature, and the rules that the agencies make to carry out their powers.

- Common law, also known as case law, is a system of law based largely on previous judicial decisions.

- Public law defines a person's rights and obligations in relation to government, and describes the various divisions of government and their powers.

- Private law, also called civil law, determines a person's legal rights and obligations in many kinds of activities that involve other people.

- A tort is a wrong or injury that a person suffers because of someone else's action, either intentional (willful or intentional acts that violate another person's rights or property) or unintentional (an act or omission that causes unintended injury or harm to another person).

- Consent is an important foundational ethical and legal notion.

- Nurses must take care to ensure patients' consent to care.

- Protecting the privacy of persons is a key priority in Canada.

- Both federal and provincial legislation exist to help protect the privacy of individuals.

DISCUSSION QUESTIONS AND ACTIVITIES

1. Discuss with classmates their opinions about the courts becoming involved in issues that have traditionally been considered ethical in nature.

2. Refer to Appendix B and read the *Charter of Rights and Freedoms*. How do these rights relate to patient care? How do they relate to nurses?

3. Discuss recent examples of federal or provincial legislation that create changes in the health care delivery system or in the practice of nursing.

4. In the common law system, how do previous court decisions affect the outcome of current cases?

5. Discuss instances in which nurses can be charged with crimes of public law, even though acts were committed without malice in the process of giving nursing care.

6. Discuss specific examples of unintentional torts.

7. How can you protect yourself from being accused of an unintentional tort?

8. In what instances can nurses be charged with intentional torts, even though they follow a professional code of ethics?

9. Discuss areas of potential liability for nurses and the present health care delivery system.

REFERENCES

A compendium of all provincial privacy legislation can be found on the following web page from the Office of the Privacy Commissioner of Canada. Retrieved January 29, 2009 from http://www.privcom.gc.ca/resource/prov/index_e.asp#001.

A.C. et al. v. Director of Child and Family Services. Manitoba, Canada. Retrieved January 29, 2009, from http://cases-dossiers.scc-csc.gc.ca/information/cms/case_summary_e.asp?31955.

Baker, G. R., Norton, P. G., Flinloft, V., Blais, R., Brown, A., Cox, J., Etchells, E., Ghali, W. A., Hebert, P., Majumdar, S. R., O'Beirne, M., Palacios-Derflingher, L., Reid, R. J., Sheps, S., Tamblyn, R. (2004). The Canadian Adverse Events Study: the incidence of adverse events among hospital patients in Canada. *Canadian Medical Association Journal 170*(11): 1678–1686.

Beauchamp, T. L. (2001). *Philosophical ethics: An introduction to moral philosophy* (3rd ed.). Boston: McGraw-Hill.

Bernzweig, E. P. (1990). *The nurse's liability for malpractice* (5th ed.). St. Louis, MO: Mosby.

British North America Act, Constitutional Acts. Retrieved January 2, 2009, from http://lois.justice.gc.ca/en/const/c1867_e.html.

Canadian Nurses Protective Society. (2007). Quality documentation: Your best defence. *Info: A legal information sheet for nurses.* Ottawa: Author.

Catalano, J. T. (1991). *Ethical and legal aspects of nursing.* Springhouse, PA: Springhouse.

College of Nurses of Ontario. (2008). *Practice guidelines: Consent.* Toronto: Author.

College of Registered Nurses of British Columbia. (2003). *Nursing documentation.* Vancouver: Author. Retrieved January 29, 2009, from http://www.crnbc.ca/NursingPractice/Requirements.aspx.

Creighton, H. (1986). *Law every nurse should know* (5th ed.). Philadelphia: Saunders.

Doran, D., McGillis Hall, L., Baker, G. R., Pink, G., Sidani, S., O'Brien Pallas, L., & Donner, G. (2001). Nursing staff mix and patient outcome achievement: The mediating role of nurse communication. *International Nursing Perspectives, 1*(2-3), 74–83.

Downie, J., & Caulfield, T. (2002). *Canadian health law and policy* (2nd ed.) Toronto: Buttersworth Canada.

Fiesta, J. (1988). *The law and liability: A guide for nurses* (2nd ed.). New York: John Wiley & Sons.

Furrow, B. R., Johnson, S. H., Jost, T. S., & Schwartz, R. L. (1991). *Liability and quality issues in health care.* St. Paul, MN: West.

Guido, G. W. (1997). *Legal issues in nursing* (2nd ed.). Norwalk, CT: Appleton & Lange.

Health Card Fraud. (2002). Ministry of Health and Long Term Care, Ontario. Retrieved January 29, 2009, from http://www.health.gov.on.ca/english/public/pub/ohip/card_fraud.html.

Keatings, M., & Smith, B. (1999). *Ethical and legal issues in nursing* (2nd ed.) Toronto: Elsevier.

King, M. L., Jr. (1996). Letter from the Birmingham jail. In J. Feinberg, ed., *Reason and responsibility: Readings in some basic problems of philosophy* (9th ed., pp. 572–580). Belmont, CA: Wadsworth. (Reprinted from M. King, Jr., *Why we can't wait*, 1963, John Davis Agency).

Kolesar v. Jeffries. (1976), 9 O.R. (2d) 41 at 48 (H.C.J.), varied 12 O.R. (2d) 142 (c.A.) aff'd (*sub nom, Joseph Brant Memorial Hosptial v. Koziol*) [1978] 1 S.C.R. 491. Retrieved January 29, 2009, from http://csc.lexum.umontreal.ca/en/1977/1978rcs1-491/1978rcs1-491.html.

Kozier, B., & Erb., G. (1992). *Concepts and issues in nursing practice* (2nd ed.). Menlo Park, CA: Addison-Wesley.

Lazar, N., Grenier, G., Robertson, G., & Singer, P. (1996). Bioethics for clinicians: 5. Substitute decision-making. *Canadian Medical Association Journal, 155*: 1435–1437.

Mazzocco, W. J. (2000). "Mixed" billing raises questions. *Advance for Nurse Practitioners, 24*–25.

Morris, J. J., Ferguson, M., & Dykeman, M. (1999). Canadian nurses and the law. Toronto: Buttersworth Canada.

Murphy v. LaMarsh (13 DLR 3d 484). From Martin, R. and Adam, G. S. (1994) *A Sourcebook of Canadian Media Law*, pp. 569–573. Ottawa: Carleton University Press.

Nelson, E. (1999). Law, ethics and consent to medical treatment. *In Touch, 2*(6). Alberta: Provincial Health Ethics Network.

O'Keefe, M. E. (2000). *Nursing practice and the law: Avoiding malpractice and other legal risks*. Philadelphia: F. A. Davis.

Potter, P., & Perry, A. (2008). *Fundamentals of nursing*. Toronto: Mosby.

Rhodes, A. M., & Miller, R. D. (1984). *Nursing and the law* (4th ed.). Rockville, MD: Aspen Systems.

Slowther, A., & Kleinman, I. (2008). Confidentiality. In P. A. Singer & A. M. Viens, eds., *The Cambridge textbook of Bioethics* (pp. 43–50). Cambridge, England: Cambridge University Press.

Stewart, A. (2002). Medical error—cautionary tales that leave us wondering about the system. *University of Toronto Medical Journal, 79*(2), 125–128.

The Personal Information Protection and Electronic Documents Act. (2000, with 2006 update). Retrieved January 29, 2009, from http://laws.justice.gc.ca/en/P-8.6.

CHAPTER 8

Professional Issues

OBJECTIVES

After completing this chapter, the reader should be able to:

1. Discuss the meaning of the term "professional," including traits commonly associated with professional status and the historical debate regarding the professional status of nursing.
2. Relate codes of ethics to professional status.
3. Discuss the relationships among the concepts of expertise, ethics, and professional status.
4. Discuss autonomy in terms of both the individual nurse and the profession of nursing.

5. Discuss the relationship between professional autonomy and ethics.

6. Discuss the concept of "*accountability*," including various mechanisms of nursing accountability.

7. Explain the relationship between accountability and professional status.

8. Define the concept of "*authority*," differentiating between professional and personal authority.

9. Discuss the concept of unity and its relationship to professional status in nursing.

INTRODUCTION

This chapter begins by examining the meaning and historical context of the term "profession," and then discusses the professional status of nursing and the selected characteristics of expertise, autonomy, accountability, authority, and unity in nursing.

PROFESSIONAL STATUS

Professions exist for the purpose of meeting the needs of society. The larger society determines its needs, and authorizes certain people to meet those needs. There is a uniform process by which professionals develop the values that lead to a type of social responsibility and desire to meet the needs of society (Aydelotte, 1990). Professionals contract with society by promising to meet a set of identified needs better than any other group of people. In turn, society grants the profession a monopoly over these particular services. Historically, professions have attempted to instill in their members a somber recognition of the profound nature of their responsibility through the recitation of pledges and oaths, such as the Hippocratic Oath for physicians and the Nightingale Pledge for nurses.

Since before the turn of the twentieth century, nurses and others have debated the professional status of nursing. Professions have been described in a number of ways. Gruending (1985) describes a **profession** as a complex, organized occupation preceded by a long training program. Professional education is geared toward the acquisition of exclusive knowledge necessary to provide a service that is either essential or desired by society. These attributes lead to a monopoly that provides autonomy, public recognition, prestige, power, and authority for the practitioner. Many other distinguishing attributes of professions have been proposed over the years. Among others, these can include expertise, accountability, the presence of systematic theory, ethical codes, a professional culture, an altruistic service orientation, competency testing, licensure, high income, credentialing, the description of a scope of practice, and the establishment of standards.

Ask Yourself

Is Nursing a Profession?

Most nursing programs have course content that is geared toward identifying the professional status of nursing through the use of identified traits or functions.

- Do you recall discussions in earlier courses about the professional status of nursing? If so, what do you recall from those discussions?
- What (or whose) criteria were used to judge professional status?
- Based upon what you recall, would you identify nursing as a profession, an emerging profession, a quasi-profession, or an occupation struggling to become a profession?

A classic source describing the criteria of professionals is Abraham Flexner. An educator, Flexner was well known for his 1910 evaluation of the professional status of medical schools. In 1915, Flexner listed traits that he observed in the established professions of medicine, law, and the clergy. He then proposed that in order to be recognized as professions, all occupations must meet these criteria. Following are six criteria that he utilized to identify professions:

1. Professions involve essentially intellectual operations.
2. Their activities are learned in nature and based on a unique body of knowledge.
3. Their emphasis is practical not necessarily theoretical.
4. They possess an educationally communicable technique.
5. They are well organized internally.
6. They are motivated by altruism. (Flexner, 1915, pp. 901–912)

Quinn and Smith (1987) further discuss the notion of altruism as a key attribute of a profession. They note that a profession is characterized by a commitment to the direct benefit of other human beings. While there is minimal societal control over the way that a profession carries out its responsibilities, there must be strong internal motivation and organization to ensure that the notion of direct benefits of others is and continues to be a priority. Additionally, the unique body of knowledge that a professional embodies must be used in a way that promotes this notion of direct benefit.

Unsolicited by the nursing community, Flexner evaluated nursing according to his criteria. He judged that nursing was not a profession but an occupation. Optimistically, he proposed that occupations could alter their status by developing these traits.

Subsequently, in 1945 and 1959, two educators, Genevieve and Roy Bixler, published landmark articles in the *American Journal of Nursing* (AJN) evaluating the professional status of nursing. These articles utilized criteria similar to those proposed by Flexner. They listed the following seven criteria of a profession:

1. A profession utilizes in its practice a well-defined and well-organized body of specialized knowledge which is on the intellectual level of the higher learning;

2. A profession constantly enlarges the body of knowledge it uses and improves its techniques of education and service by the use of the scientific method;

3. A profession entrusts the education of its practitioners to institutions of higher education;

4. A profession applies its body of knowledge in practical services which are vital to human and social welfare;

5. A profession functions autonomously in the formulation of professional policy and in the control of professional activity, thereby;

6. A profession attracts individuals of intellectual and personal qualities who exalt service above personal gain and who recognize their chosen occupation as a life work; and

7. A profession strives to compensate its practitioners by providing freedom of action, opportunity for continuous professional growth, and economic security. (Bixler & Bixler, 1959, pp. 1142–1147)

Predictably, the Bixler evaluations came to the same conclusion as Flexner: Nursing was deficient as a true profession.

Though both Flexner and the Bixlers had a tremendous lasting impact on nursing, none were nurses. Even though their lists of traits seem to have been chosen arbitrarily, their approach assumes that true professions will demonstrate all of the essential attributes. Fowler (1990) calls their lists of characteristics "an untidy aggregation of overlapping, arbitrarily chosen, or undifferentiated elements, lacking a unifying theoretical framework that explains their interrelationship" (p. 24).

Prior to the Flexner report, American nurses were secure in their identity as professionals. Even physicians and the judicial system recognized nursing as a profession. However, following the Flexner report and the subsequent Bixler articles, nurses began to question their status as professionals (Parsons, 1986). Like sixteenth-century women who came to believe the myth that women were intrinsically evil, nurses accepted the idea that nursing was not a true profession (Newman, 1990; Sleicher, 1981). The process of examining and evaluating, though, resulted in many positive changes for nursing. Striving to meet the criteria set by Flexner and the Bixlers, nurses became involved in research to create a unique body of knowledge for nursing, to move "professional" nursing education to the university setting, to become politically involved, to increase the autonomy of nursing, and to expand their scope of practice.

There are those who argue that the process used to identify traits of professions was flawed from the inception (Achterberg, 1990; Ehrenreich & English, 1973; Parsons, 1986). There are even those who suggest that the term "professional" is sexist, elitist, and racist. At the turn of the century, the three "professions" that were said to be universally accepted as such—medicine, law, and the clergy—were overwhelmingly male and Caucasian. As a result of the cultural and religious influences discussed in Chapter 1, by the time Flexner wrote his report, women had been systematically purged from both professional education and practice. Examining and describing traits of the male-dominated "professions," and subsequently using those findings as criteria to judge the professional status of other occupations may have effectively excluded all predominately female groups.

Nurses as Professionals

For lack of a better word, nurses continue to discuss their occupation in terms of a profession. Recognizing that there are a myriad of sources claiming to define the term "professional" by describing traits, attributes, functions, or characteristics, there will likely never be agreement about the professional status of nursing. Even though these discussions are important, for the purposes of this chapter, we propose that nursing is a true profession.

In many ways nurses, as professionals, are connected to each other and set apart from others. Professionals are connected to each other by common experiences, language, and body of knowledge. We are set apart from others by virtue of the prestige offered members of a profession, and by the personal, intimate, and spiritual experiences surrounding the beginning and the end of life.

Beletz describes a professional as "one bound by values and standards other than those of his or her employing organization, setting one's own rules, seeking to promote standards of excellence, and being evaluated and looking for approval from one's own professional peers" (1990, p. 18). Jameton further suggests that being a professional is similar to having a calling. He describes a calling as "something one feels called upon to do, perhaps by God, by some deep need in one's being, or by the demands of historical circumstance. A calling is central to one's life and gives it meaning" (1984, p. 18). Moving the discussion further, Reed (2000) declares that nursing is a spiritual discipline. She argues that regarding a discipline as spiritual enhances the meaning of a profession. Reed writes that there is a pragmatic and normative call to action which is freely chosen by its members—one in which the person is said to be "called" or "launched outward to others" (p. 132).

EXPERTISE

Expertise relates to the characteristic of having a high level of specialized skill and knowledge. It is a "composite of a knowledge base, gained through long years of study in an academic setting, and superior skill. Expertise is the primary distinguishing difference between professionals and nonprofessionals" (Beletz, 1990, p. 17). Professionals must have the knowledge and functional skills required to meet the needs of society and thereby fulfill the purpose of the profession. Regarding expertise, Jameton writes:

> Professions maintain their autonomy partly through their claim to maximal competence [expertise]. So long as people believe that the professionals are the only ones who fully understand their work, it is very hard to supervise or criticize them. (1984, p. 21)

We gain expertise in a variety of ways. Extensive educational requirements, intense guided practice, examination for licensure, certification, and mandatory continuing education are ways that we either attain, maintain, or assert expertise. Florence Nightingale recognized the importance of an education consisting of depth and breadth of general knowledge, combined with a very specific nursing focus. Today we have a knowledge base that is continually expanded through research. Having completed basic nursing education and successfully demonstrated a minimum level of competence through licensure examination, we are further required (both ethically or legally) to continue the learning process and maintain up-to-date knowledge and technical proficiency. Continuing-education programs assist us in this process. Our expertise is also advanced through graduate nursing education, specialty preparation, and the certification process.

Merely claiming expertise is not enough. Through the various mechanisms of accountability, we must prove to society that we are faithful to the promise the profession makes. In response, society grants us the authority to practise with a certain measure of autonomy. Thus, the professional realms of expertise, accountability, autonomy, and authority are interrelated.

Ask Yourself

When the Bottom Line Becomes Personal

Alex is an operating room nurse in a busy urban hospital. When his elderly, independent mother becomes ill, she is taken to the emergency room of an adjacent hospital. It is suspected that she has had a stroke and needs urgent intensive care. However, there are no beds in the intensive care unit, so she is admitted into the emergency department to wait for a bed there. Because of Alex's background, he is familiar with the kinds of medical and nursing interventions that his mother urgently requires. He notes that the nurses are too busy to advocate adequately for his mother for an intensive care bed along with necessary tests she requires, and even for help with activities of daily living that his mother requires. He has to return to work for some of his shifts and is very worried about the care his mother will get in his absence. He notes that her meals are placed out of her reach, as is her call bell. She cannot get up to the bathroom herself and becomes confused at night, trying to get up herself. Her room is far from the nursing station and he is concerned that no one might hear her call out in the busy, hectic atmosphere of the emergency room. He would like neurological and vital signs more regularly, but notes that they are being done only once or twice a shift, although his mother has frequent changes and shifts in her neurological status. She has not been washed or assisted with personal hygiene for two days and is confused and depressed.

- How would you feel if you were Alex?
- What do you think the very busy nurses' responsibilities are regarding their ability to adequately care for Alex's mother?

(Continued)

- What would you do if you were Alex? What are the challenges to the options available to Alex?

- In the context of this case, discuss your own beliefs about whether it is a true ethical obligation to maintain expertise in your areas of practice, as a nurse.

- An emergency room nurse has to have a broad foundation of knowledge in a number of areas. While it is not realistic to expect that every nurse knows "everything," should it not be expected that a professional nurse has the capacity for basic nursing care and skills of advocacy? Is this an ethical or professional obligation?

AUTONOMY

The word **autonomy** literally means "self-governing." The concept of nursing autonomy can be discussed on two levels: autonomy of the profession and autonomy of the individual practitioner. Self-regulation is the mark of collective professional autonomy. Individual autonomy involves self-determination, responsibility, accountability, independence, and a willingness to take risks. Autonomy is generally considered to be an important criterion in judging professional status of an occupation. People who are considered to be professionals have the power and authority to control various aspects of their work, including goals toward which to work, whether to work and with whom, details of how the work is to be done, choice of clientele, and so forth (Jameton, 1984). We continue to debate whether nurses have autonomy.

 Think About It

Regulation

In Canada, the goal of regulation of registered nurses is protection of the public (Canadian Nurses Association, 2007b). Professions can be regulated by an external body, such as the government, or from within, as nurses are. In each province and territory, the regulation and monitoring of professional registered nurses is delegated to the profession itself. Nursing regulates members through provincial and territorial regulatory bodies, e.g., Ontario College of Nurses, College of Registered Nurses of British Columbia, College of Registered Nurses of Nova Scotia. These regulatory bodies have a number of responsibilities, always with the overarching goal of protecting the public. While each college may articulate these goals and responsibilities in a slightly different way, they remain fairly consistent and include:

- Setting requirements for entering the profession;
- Making certain that standards for nursing practice are met, adhered to, and enforced;
- Ensuring the consistent competence of nurses and quality of care provided by nurses;
- Making decisions regarding disciplinary action for nurses who do not adhere to standards of practice.

Colleges of nurses in each province and territory are run and governed by nurses; in doing this, the profession remains autonomous. In most colleges, there are members of the public who sit on the advisory boards and disciplinary boards. Part of the responsibility of a self-regulating profession is transparency, so involving community members is an important part of maintaining trust and upholding the responsibility of the profession to society at large.

The profession of nursing in Canada is self-regulating and therefore can be said to be autonomous. The notion of self-regulation is one that explicitly recognizes that professions are in the most appropriate position to set standards and guidelines for practice and education, as well as ensuring that these standards are met, and taking suitable action, if they are not.

At provincial and territorial levels, the government has delegated the authority to self-regulate to a variety of health care professions, including nursing. Other self-regulated professionals include physicians, midwives, chiropractors, occupational therapists, pharmacists, social workers, and psychologists. In nursing, as with many other health care professions, the provincial and territorial governments provide professional colleges and associations the authority and responsibility to regulate members of the profession.

One mechanism of regulation is the protection of the title of "registered nurse." Other protected titles in nursing in Canada include "registered practical nurse," "RN," "Registered psychiatric nurse," and "licensed practical nurse." The protection of these titles implies that anyone identifying themselves in one of these categories is registered with a regulatory body to practise nursing in the capacity that is identified by the title.

Jameton (1984) implies that the profession of nursing maintains autonomy through the combination of a claim to maximal competence and a continuing monopoly over their work. He writes:

> Professions also maintain their autonomy by means of monopoly over their work. In our competitive culture, people do not achieve autonomy simply by declaring it or believing in it. Professions maintain their control over their work partly by keeping people with other skills and other ideas from doing the same work. Only nurses may legally practice nursing. Licensure, educational requirements, certification of schools, and the like help nurses maintain control over

nursing practice. This control is strengthened when nurses—rather than physicians and nonprofessionals—control the processes of licensure and certification. (p. 21)

No other group has the ability to do the work of nurses; consequently in Canada, as noted, there is a legal restriction barring non-nurses, i.e., persons who do not have a title of "registered nurse," from practising nursing or using the term "nurse" to describe their role. This legally sanctioned monopoly helps to establish autonomy.

Nurses are both legally and ethically required to practise autonomously. Autonomous practice serves as a safeguard for the patient, nurse, physician, and institution. Nursing codes of ethics support the nurse's autonomous decision making and responsibility. The Canadian Nurses Association *Code of Ethics for Registered Nurses* (2008a) and the International Council of Nurses *ICN Code of Ethics for Nurses* (2000) implicitly and explicitly reflect nursing autonomy and responsibility. The purpose of autonomy as described in these codes is to protect the patient from harm, and allow for the full benefit of professional nursing care.

We often hear questions about the autonomy of individual nurses. As a nurse, do you really have autonomy? Can you say that you are autonomous, even though you are required to follow physicians' orders? Are you autonomous, even though you can't get to know the patients because you have too many patients and too much work to do? Lyon defines autonomous nursing practice as "the diagnosis and treatment of phenomena that nurses have the self-directed authority to treat" (1990, p. 270). Furthermore, she writes that nursing has a social mandate for two different scopes of practice: the medical scope that requires physician authorization to initiate treatment, and the autonomous nursing scope that requires no authorization.

Hospitals and other health care institutions require qualified and knowledgeable persons to carry out physicians' orders and the medical plan of care. When we seek employment at these institutions, we are implicitly agreeing to perform the functions for which we are hired. This includes carrying out the medical plan of care alongside the provision of unique nursing care. Accepting a position implies this contract. Nevertheless, we are legally and ethically required to use independent judgment in making nursing decisions. The exercise of independent nursing judgment is valuable to health care institutions because of the safeguards that are afforded. Nurses are in fact responsible for their own practice, in providing both independent nursing care and in collaborative roles, such as transcribing a medication order written by a physician and administering the ordered drugs to a patient. While nurses are accountable for maintaining competency in their own practice, a nurse who, for example, transcribes a drug or a dosage ordered incorrectly by a physician and then administers it, is in fact, responsible for that medication error. Competency and accountability in nursing imply responsibility for all conduct and actions—even collaborative ones. A nurse transcribing a medication must have basic knowledge about the medication, dosage, safety, side effects, and how all these relate to the individual patient. This is a part of competent nursing care and is also what it means to be an autonomous health care professional with unique responsibilities working in a collaborative, interdisciplinary team environment.

Autonomy does not mean that we have absolute control of every facet of practice. Accepted as one of the three prototype professions, medicine, for example, no longer retains the measure of control it once enjoyed. Government regulations guide some facets of medical care such as salary rates or caps and length of hospital stays. Consequently, physicians, though continuing to maintain professional status, are experiencing less absolute control over patient care than ever before. In the past, some (including Abraham Flexner) based the argument that nurses were not autonomous on comparisons between the independent decision-making capacities of medicine and nursing. That comparison no longer illustrates a great degree of distinction.

It is clear that nurses do not always feel autonomous, and, in fact, some may not practise autonomously. Certainly there are nurses who spend each workday complying with physicians' orders without question and completing various nonautonomous tasks, never exercising independent nursing functions, nor making nursing judgments or initiating self-directed interventions. In the truest sense, these nurses are only marginally practising professional nursing and cannot be said to be autonomous. When we practise in this manner, we fail our ethical duty to make independent nursing judgments.

ACCOUNTABILITY

"Nurses are accountable for their actions and answerable for their practice." (Canadian Nurses Association *Code of Ethics for Registered Nurses,* 2008a)

According to the American Nurses Association (1985), "**Accountability** refers to being answerable to someone for something one has done. [It is] grounded in the moral principles of fidelity and respect for the dignity, worth, and self-determination of clients" (p. 8). Safe, autonomous practice is ensured through various processes of nursing accountability. Accountability is related to both responsibility and answerability. Because of the trust accorded nurses by society (gained through recognition of nurses' expertise) and the right given the profession to regulate practice (autonomy), individual practitioners and the profession must be both responsible and accountable. The annual Gallup poll on Honesty and Ethics of professions consistently has the public rating nurses as the most trusted of all professions (Gallup 2008). For the seventh year in a row, nurses have been named as the profession with the highest ethical standards and level of honesty. Added to the list of professions in 1999, nurses have consistently been the highest rated, with the exception of 2001, shortly after the September 11 terrorist attacks in the United States. That year, when the poll was conducted in November, firefighters were rated highest. With a rating of eighty-four percent in 2008 (which translates roughly as eighty-four percent of the public have the highest trust in nurses), nurses are followed by pharmacists (seventy percent), high school teachers (sixty-five percent), medical doctors (sixty-four percent), and police officers (fifty-six percent). At the bottom of the list are car salesmen (seven percent), telemarketers, and lobbyists (both with no positive rating). A high level of accountability goes hand in hand with sustaining the high level of trust that the public has in the profession of nursing.

Related to the concepts of autonomy and authority, accountability is an inherent part of everyday nursing practice. Each nurse is responsible for all individual actions and omissions.

Mechanisms of Accountability

Accountability is based upon the implicit contract between nursing and the larger society. The Canadian Nurses Association notes that self-regulation ensures that nursing, as a profession, continues to be one of the most trusted professions in Canada by making certain that the public receive "safe and ethical care from competent, qualified registered nurses" (Canadian Nurses Association, 2007b, p. 1). The profession of nursing has developed several mechanisms through which this relationship between nursing and society is made explicit, thereby acknowledging both the professional and the public the areas of nursing accountability. These mechanisms include codes of nursing ethics, standards of nursing practice, nurse practice acts, nursing theory and practice derived from nursing research, educational requirements for practice, advanced certification, and mechanisms for evaluating the effectiveness of nurses' performance of nursing responsibilities (ANA, 1985). In both a professional and a legal sense, it is necessary that we are familiar with various mechanisms of accountability.

Codes of Nursing Ethics. Nearly universally accepted as one criterion of a profession, a code of ethics is profoundly important to nursing. A **code of nursing ethics** is an explicit declaration of the primary goals and values of the profession that indicates the "profession's acceptance of the responsibility and trust with which it has been invested by society" (ANA, 1985, p. iii). Like other professions, nursing has developed and enforces specific obligations to ensure that members of society will find them to be competent and trustworthy. These obligations are correlative to the rights of individual patients and society as a whole (Beauchamp & Childress, 2001). Upon entrance into the profession, nurses make an implicit moral commitment to uphold the values and moral obligations expressed in their code. Nurses are called upon to base professional judgment upon consideration of consequences and the universal moral principles of respect for persons, autonomy, beneficence, nonmaleficence, veracity, confidentiality, fidelity, and justice (ANA, 1985). Examples of professional codes of ethics for nurses include the American Nurses Association *Code of Ethics for Nurses* (2001), the International Council of Nurses *Code of Ethics for Nurses* (2000), and the Canadian Nurses Association *Code of Ethics for Registered Nurses* (2008a) (see Appendices C, D, and A, respectively).

Standards of Nursing Practice. **Standards of nursing practice** are written documents outlining minimum expectations for safe nursing care. Standards may describe in detail specific acts performed by nurses or may outline the expected process of nursing care. We use standards to guide and evaluate nursing care. As part of establishing and sustaining the public trust in nurses, standards are in place and publicly accessible in order to clearly demonstrate the commitment of the profession to transparency and accountability as self-regulated professionals (Canadian Nurses Association, 2008b). Courts look to standards of nursing practice for guidance when malpractice cases are deliberated. The two basic types of standards of nursing practice are internal and external standards (Fiesta, 1988).

Internal standards of nursing practice are those developed within the profession of nursing for the purpose of establishing the minimum level of nursing care. They help to ensure that nurses are competent and safe to practise. These documents guide us in providing nursing care, and can be used as a consistent baseline to measure the practice of individual nurses. While outlining the minimal expectations for practice, standards are of vital importance. As outlined by the Canadian Nurses Association, nurses are the largest group of front-line health professionals in the country, caring for diverse groups and individuals in a variety of contexts and settings. Therefore, having standard expectations for practice assists not only nurses but also the public in having access to what kind of standards and best practices guide nurses in their professional activities and practice settings. Standards help protect the public, who are the recipients of nursing care (CNA, 2008b).

As nursing is a self-regulated practice, each province and territory has regulatory bodies that set the standards of practice and enforce professional practice and conduct. Alongside these standards is the Canadian Nurses Association *Code of Ethics,* which articulates the kinds of values that the nursing profession supports and embodies. Together standards and codes of ethics make up the basis for a practice in nursing in Canada (CNA, 2008a; 2008b).

In addition to nursing practice standards, the Canadian Nurses Association has a number of policy statements, publications, position papers, fact sheets, and position statements that all demonstrate accountability and are publicly available. Examples of these include the Canadian Nurses Association Joint Statement on Resuscitative Interventions (1995), the Position Statement on Nurses and Human Rights (2004), and the Position Statement on Emergency Preparedness and Response (2007).

External standards of nursing practice consist of guides for nursing care that are developed by non-nurses, the government, or institutions. These standards describe the specific expectations of agencies or groups that utilize the services of nurses. They serve some of the same functions as internal standards, including guidance and evaluation. Examples of external standards include such documents as the *Health Professions Act* in British Columbia (1996), the *Act Respecting the Protection of Confidential Disciplinary Proceedings of Health Professions* in Nova Scotia (2008), and the Regulated Health Professions Act in Ontario (1991). Nurses are responsible and accountable to know and follow the standards of care for the profession, the specialty (if applicable), the geographic area, and the institution in which they practise.

CASE PRESENTATION

The "Real World" of Nursing

Erinn is a new graduate nurse working on a large medical surgical unit. She wrote the Canadian Registered Nurses Examination (CRNE), passed, and now has a licence to practice. While she worked under her temporary licence, immediately after graduation, the unit manager ensured that she had lighter assignments and was paired up with a more experienced registered nurse, in order for Erinn to learn the policies and procedures of the unit, before getting used to having a full patient load on what is, traditionally, a very heavy unit.

(Continued)

When the unit manager and staff find out that Erinn has been successful in her CRNE and becoming a licensed registered nurse, they congratulate her heartily. The next night, Erinn returns to work to find that she has a very heavy assignment and is not paired up with anyone to help her. Up until now, she has had only four patients on night shift and has been able to cover one other nurse, while that nurse goes on break. Tonight, Erinn finds that she has been assigned nine patients. One patient requires careful monitoring as she becomes disoriented at night and is at risk for falls or wandering. There is no one available to provide constant care for the patient tonight. Another patient requires administration of a chemotherapy drug via a peripherally inserted central catheter (PICC) line. The report notes that the PICC line is not working well and may require reinsertion.

Erinn approaches James, the nurse in charge, to ask for help. She isn't sure how she can provide constant care for one patient, with eight others. Erinn is also very concerned about the patient with the PICC line who requires chemotherapy. The hospital has a policy stating that only nurses who have undergone special certification may administer chemotherapeutic agents. While she has flushed PICC lines, Erinn has not been certified to insert one.

James tells her that they are very understaffed tonight as the nursing supervisor pulled two of the unit nurses to cover in the intensive care unit. He suggests that Erinn first go and try to flush the PICC line and if it sticks, just push harder. He quietly adds that he knows the policies state not to do this, but it usually works, if you "do it just right." If it doesn't work, he adds, he'll show her how to insert one himself and she can do it. He also tells Erinn that he will prepare the chemotherapy drug but Erinn will have to give it. Finally he instructs Erinn to just try to look in on the patient requiring constant care once in a while, as often as she is able. "If something happens," he states, while shrugging, "we'll deal with it."

Erinn is well aware that her provincial regulatory body outlines seven standards of practice and that one of the standards, accountability, is demonstrated by "maintaining competence and refraining from not performing activities for which she/he is not competent" (College of Nurses of Ontario, Professional Standards, Revised, 2002).

James sees Erinn hesitating. "This happens all the time," he says to Erinn, "Welcome to the real world!"

Think About It

- What dilemmas does Erinn face?
- What are the alternatives available to Erinn?
- Can Erinn meet the standards and adhere to the policies of the institution?
- What role does James have in ensuring accountable and competent care? Has he met that standard?

- If something adverse happened to any patient on this shift, as a result of not adhering to policies and standards, who should be responsible?
- Do institutions have a role in ensuring competent, safe, and accountable care? If so, what is their role?
- Is there any way that Erinn can meet the standard of accountability, with James's advice?
- What would you do? How would you feel in this situation?
- What are the ethical implications for the institution, James, and Erinn?

Scope of Practice Statutes.   Each province and territory has laws or statutes respecting the regulation of nursing. While some statutes are more specific to nursing, such as the *Registered Nurses Acts* for Saskatchewan (1988) or Newfoundland (2008), others are "umbrella" types of legislation, such as the *Regulated Health Professions Act* in Ontario (1999), and the *Health Professions Act* in Alberta (1999), which cover a variety of health professions and are not restricted to the profession of nursing only.

These statutes outline legislation for how the **scope of practice** is outlined by the colleges that oversee regulation for each health profession (e.g., College of Nurses of Ontario, College of Registered Nurses of Nova Scotia, College of Registered Psychiatric Nurses of British Columbia, etc.). They provide frameworks outlining the way that colleges operate the regulation processes as well as the disciplinary processes that must be carried out if a complaint is received regarding the conduct of a health professional who is registered with a college in each province or territory.

Nurses are accountable to follow legislation that outlines scope of practice, as part of being accountable and maintaining the trust of the public. As one example, the *Regulated Health Professions Act* in Ontario (RHPA) (1999) outlines both the scope of practice for registered nurses along with a list of thirteen specific authorized controlled acts that only qualified persons can perform (College of Nurses, RHPA, Scope of Practice, Controlled Acts Model, 2008). Of these thirteen acts, registered nurses are authorized to conduct three, and these are carefully outlined in the RHPA. The scope of practice and controlled acts statements also address important notions of initiating, performing, and delegating controlled acts by registered nurses.

The Canadian Nurses Association, in conjunction with the Canadian Pharmacists Association and the Canadian Medical Association, notes that the following four principles must be included in any scope of practice statement. First, the statements should *focus* on care that is not only highly responsive to the needs of the patients and communities but also ethical, safe, and high quality. Second, there needs to be enough *flexibility* to allow health care professionals to practise at a level that relates to their education, skills, and competence. Third, there must be *cooperation* to engage in *interdisciplinary collaboration* as a means by which to provide high-quality care. *Coordination* and *patient choice* must always be a part of any scope of practice statement, as means of ensuring patient care is appropriate and relevant (Canadian Nurses Association, 2003).

Abiding by provincial and territorial legislation governing scope of practice and regulation, maintaining requirements for entry to practice, ensuring members are conducting ongoing competency evaluation, setting and monitoring standards for practice, and adhering to codes of ethics are all part of the responsibility and accountability of being a self-regulated nursing profession in Canada.

Nursing Theory and Practice Derived from Research. A frequently cited characteristic of professions is the existence of a unique body of knowledge derived from research. Recall that Genevieve and Roy Bixler's first two characteristics of a profession relate to a unique body of knowledge. The Bixlers' second characteristic calls for professions to constantly enlarge the body of knowledge by use of the scientific method (1959). In the past, authorities debated whether nursing's body of knowledge was unique to the profession, or was borrowed from behavioural and physical sciences and medicine. It seemed clear to some that nursing knowledge had been derived from the combination of experience and intuition, and by borrowing from other disciplines (Leddy & Pepper, 1989). Responding to arguments that nursing was not true profession because of this lack of a clearly unique body of knowledge, nurses in academic and clinical settings began gathering data and doing legitimate research. The process of theory building and research in nursing continues to increase the unique body of nursing knowledge. There are many unique nursing research peer-reviewed journals, interest groups, and conferences across Canada and around the world. More and more nurses are entering and continuing into graduate school, doing doctoral and post-doctoral research. At most schools of nursing, academic nurse educators also maintain clinical and research agendas in order to maintain currency and contribute to the growing body of unique nursing knowledge and research. The benefit of this process is twofold. First, the expanded knowledge base allows nurses to respond to the needs of society more knowledgeably and skillfully. Second, the presence of a clearly unique body of knowledge aids in validating nursing as a true profession.

AUTHORITY

The term **authority** in terms of nursing usually refers to the government's having legitimate power and sovereignty. The authority to practise nursing is granted by statute, based upon the contract the profession has with society. As part of being a self-regulated profession in Canada, the provincial and territorial governments grant authority, in turn, to the professional colleges and associations of nursing that exist in each province and territory. This is done with the mutual understanding that there are clear mechanisms for public accountability, transparency of processes, and acknowledgment of the rights and responsibilities of self-regulation. Authority assumes a certain measure of autonomy. Donabedian relates authority to both autonomy and accountability:

> Society grants the professions authority over functions vital to itself
> and permits them considerable autonomy in the conduct of their
> affairs. In return, the professions are expected to act responsibly,

always mindful of the public trust. Self-regulation to assure quality in performance is at the heart of this relationship. It is the authentic hallmark of a mature profession. (1976, p. 8)

In a practical sense, authority is granted by society in the form of the permission for the profession to exist, coupled with the privilege granted to individuals to practise the profession. Thus, as with autonomy, authority for nurses is two-tiered. As noted, provincial and territorial regulatory bodies have statutes that are designed to protect the public's health and safety. These statutes describe scope of practice and provide frameworks for regulatory processes carried out by provincial and territorial colleges or associations of nursing. Thus, the provincial and territorial regulatory bodies have the legitimate authority to regulate the practice of nursing within each jurisdiction.

Having specified requirements for entry into practice, defined nursing, and described the scope of nursing practice, nurse practice acts empower the provincial and territorial regulatory bodies to grant individual nurses the authority to practise. This authority is granted through the process of examination and licensure. Licensure benefits both the public and the professional. It protects the public from the unqualified, and it protects professionals' job territory by establishing a monopoly. The protection afforded by licensure enhances our status by authenticating the profession (Beletz, 1990). After meeting all requirements for entry into practice, we are granted the legal authority to practise nursing.

The authority given each nurse to practise is contingent upon the nurse's continuing to uphold the established standards of nursing. Provincial and territorial colleges of nursing have the power and responsibility to discipline nurses who do not follow established standards or who violate provisions of licensure law. Discipline can take several forms, including suspension or revocation of licence. Disciplinary processes must be made publicly accessible, to some degree. This is a significant part of maintaining accountability of the profession. In order to avoid appearances of impropriety or secrecy, disciplining members must not be seen as something that happens behind closed doors. As the goals of disciplinary processes are to protect the public and maintain trust in the profession, transparency and accessibility to the proceedings and outcomes are of utmost importance. In the case of suspected incompetence or professional misconduct, most disciplinary processes involve a formal hearing. Moreover, these hearings almost always involve members of the public, who serve as members of the panel and contribute to the proceedings.

UNITY

There is general agreement that one of the defining characteristics of a profession is a sense of unity among its members. This unity is multifaceted and based on what Aydelotte (1990) calls moral uniformity and class ideology among its practitioners. Most nurses believe that as a profession, we have shared values. Ideologies, or worldviews, are embedded in values and beliefs. While we have values and beliefs as individuals, many nurses share broad common values and ideas about what "ought" to be. These kinds of values are usually expressed in codes of ethics and mission statements. If we look at the Canadian Nurses Association *Code of Ethics* (2008a), some of the shared values expressed there include the provision of safe, compassionate, competent, and ethical care; the promotion of health and well-being; the preservation of dignity; the promotion of informed decision making; the maintenance of privacy and confidentiality; the promotion of justice; and accountability. Although these values are articulated in a Canadian context, many codes of ethics for nursing across the globe embrace similar values. Unity relates to the ability of nurses to organize for the purpose of fulfilling the profession's promises and the relationships that nurses have with one another.

It is only through unity that nursing is able to coherently standardize the professional characteristics of competence, autonomy, authority, and accountability. Through political and policy processes, we work together to meet the health care needs of society and to improve the status of the profession. The structural component of a professional community is realized through a professional association. The professional association provides a collective identity and serves as the voice of the profession to both the profession and society (Beletz, 1990). It fulfills four basic functions: to standardize services provided by its members; to provide a professional hub for members; to assist with educational needs of members; and to perform political, advisory, and policy functions. There is an expectation that professionals will be active members and leaders of their professional association. Across Canada, many professional nursing associations exist in every province and territory. Some examples include the Registered Nurses' Association of Ontario (http://www.rnao.org), the College and Association of Registered Nurses of Alberta (http://www.nurses.ab.ca), and the Association of Registered Nurses of Newfoundland (www.arnnl.nf.ca). Additionally, many special a interest groups exist for nurses with expertise, interest, and engagement in a particular area of practice, research, or education. Some examples include the Canadian Association for the History of Nursing, the Canadian Association for Neuroscience Nurses (www.cann.ca), and the Canadian Nursing Students' Association (http://www.cnsa.ca).

Although systematic organization of professional groups is necessary in fulfilling the professions' responsibilities, we also need unity among individual members. Unity involves showing sympathy, care, and reciprocity to those with whom one appropriately identifies, working closely with others toward shared goals, keeping promises, making mutual concerns a priority, sacrificing personal interests to the relationship, and attending to these over a period of time (Jameton, 1984). Beletz eloquently describes this type of unity:

> The professional's bond with colleagues emanates from relationships established by shared mysteries of a common technical language, educational background, rites of passage, styles of work, attire, and a consciousness of being set apart and insisting on being set apart from other occupational categories. Colleague relationships are expected to be cooperative, equalitarian, and supportive vis-à-vis clientele and peers. (1990, p. 19)

Though loyalty is a virtue, there are certain risks when we experience a strong sense of loyalty to each other. Jameton (1984) warns that nurses must be careful that their loyalty to each other does not supersede loyalty to patients. For example, mistakes that nurses or doctors make should be reported to patients. Because of a sense of loyalty and friendship that exists between coworkers, there is a risk that our duty to patients will be neglected. We are required to examine and prioritize conflicting loyalties closely. Jameton identifies nurses' main priorities as patients, nurses and the nursing profession, physicians, hospitals, other health professions, and society. Questioning which of these priorities should be central and which should be peripheral, he suggests that the best choices for first priority are patient, nursing, and society.

Ask Yourself

To Whom Should We Be Loyal? To What End Should We Be Loyal?

In 1994, twelve children died while undergoing or after having undergone cardiac surgery at the Children's Hospital of Winnipeg. Throughout these events, many health professionals involved in the treatment of these children voiced concerns about the conditions of the cardiac surgery department as well as the treatment of the children. A significant number of those voicing concerns included the intensive care and surgical nurses at the hospital.

A full review and eventual inquest was carried out to determine culpability, review processes and infrastructures that existed at the time in that hospital and department, and to avoid further deaths of children undergoing cardiac surgery.

During the inquest, it was found that while the nurses did voice their concerns to those in positions of authority, their concerns were trivialized at times and dismissed as being overly emotional reactions to the deaths of the children instead of valid concerns of knowledgeable professionals who function as part of a multidisciplinary team.

Some of the nurses were understandably hesitant and afraid to voice their concerns as their colleagues had been treated in a dismissive and patronizing manner. While they continued to care for children undergoing surgery, they did so with grave misgivings.

Today, we have the luxury of being able to be reflective about this case and others like it, by reading inquests and reports and learning from the challenges and tragedies of others. We must always remember, when reflecting on cases like this, that the individuals involved were undergoing significant challenges, conflicts, and anguish. Our own critique of these past situations must always include our own compassion and empathy for the difficulties endured by others.

(Continued)

To read more about this case, go to http://www.pediatriccardiacinquest .mb.ca.

- Imagine yourself in a situation in which you have grave concerns about the multidisciplinary care of the patient for whom you are responsible. How would you feel?

- How far would you go to have your concerns or voice heard? Would you put your own position "on the line"?

- What should the role of nursing administration be, in cases like this one? What about the role of regulatory bodies or professional associations? Do they have a role to play?

- Jameton (1984) discusses a priority of loyalties with the patient always coming first, and nursing and society falling after. In this case, the nurses did try to advocate for the patient by voicing their concerns. As these concerns were not heeded, what might they have done at that point?

Reflect on your own place of work. Do you feel that you have a voice to advocate for others or to challenge actions or decisions with which you do not agree? Why or why not?

SUMMARY

Because ethics is a commonly cited criterion for judging the professional status of an occupation, the study of ethics must include a discussion of nursing's professional status. In order to discuss professional issues in nursing rationally, one must examine the meaning and historical context of the term "professional." Beginning with Abraham Flexner's 1915 opinion that nursing did not meet his criteria for professional status, there has been continuing debate about this topic. Striving to create professional status for nursing, nurses have worked to solve the deficiencies that were identified by Flexner and others. There are those who believe that the original methods of determining professional status were flawed by a cultural and historical context of sexism, racism, and elitism. Though this debate will continue, there are a number of traits that are nearly universally accepted as belonging to professional groups. Expertise, autonomy, accountability, authority, and unity were discussed as professional characteristics of nursing.

CHAPTER HIGHLIGHTS

- Acknowledgment of professional status is dependent upon meeting particular criteria that include, but are not restricted to, expertise, autonomy, authority, accountability, and unity.

- Historical and cultural influences have affected the trait definitions commonly used for the term "professional."

- A system or code of ethics is generally accepted as one trait of professions.
- Because society allows professionals a monopoly over the services they provide, ethics demands that those services must be provided with expertise.
- Because it is self-regulating, the profession of nursing can be said to be autonomous.
- There are legal and ethical imperatives for individual nurses to practise autonomously.
- Autonomy does not mean full and absolute control over every aspect of practice.
- Grounded in the moral principle of fidelity, accountability refers to being answerable to someone for something one has done.
- Mechanisms of accountability include, but are not restricted to, codes of nursing ethics, standards of nursing practice, nurse practice acts, and nursing theory and practice derived from nursing research.
- Authority for nurses to practise is granted through the legal processes of society.
- Nursing unity relates to the profession's ability to organize for the purpose of fulfilling the promises made to society.

DISCUSSION QUESTIONS AND ACTIVITIES

1. Write your own definition of the term "professional." In your definition, include the characteristics of a profession.
2. List ten different occupations and compare their common characteristics. Which occupations meet your criteria for professional status?
3. Discuss the relationship between historical and cultural influences and Flexner's method of identifying professions.
4. Discuss the relationship between the concepts of fidelity, professionalism, and expertise.
5. Discuss the statement, "To be less than maximally competent is unethical."
6. Find recent examples of case law that relate to court opinions regarding autonomy in nursing.
7. Observe a registered nurse at work. List tasks that the nurse performs and categorize them as autonomous or dependent.
8. Read the nurse practice act in your province or territory. Evaluate your province or territory's law in terms of its usefulness as a mechanism of accountability.

REFERENCES

Achterberg, J. (1990). *Woman as healer*. Boston: Shambhala.

American Nurses Association. (1985). *Code for nurses with interpretive statements*. Washington, DC: Author.

American Nurses Association. (2001). *Code of ethics for nurses*. Washington, DC: Author.

Aydelotte, M. (1990). The evolving profession: The role of the professional organization. In N. L. Chaska, ed., *The nursing profession: A time to speak* (pp. 16–23). St. Louis, MO: Mosby.

Beauchamp, T., & Childress, J. (2001). *Principles of biomedical ethics* (4th ed.). New York: Oxford University Press.

Beletz, E. (1990). Professionalization: A license is not enough. In N. L. Chaska, ed., *The nursing profession: Turning points* (pp. 16–23). St. Louis, MO: Mosby.

Bixler, G. K., & Bixler, R. W. (1959). The professional status of nursing. *American Journal of Nursing, 59*(8), 1142–1147.

Canadian Nurses Association. (1995). Canadian Nurses Association Joint Statement on Resuscitative Interventions. http://www.cna-nurses.ca/CNA/documents/pdf/publications/PS21_Joint_Statement_Resuscitative_Interventions_1995_e.pdf. Retrieved July 15, 2008.

Canadian Nurses Association. (2003). *Joint position statement: Scopes of practice.* Retrieved January 2, 2009, from http://www.cna-aiic.ca/CNA/documents/pdf/publications/PS66_Scopes_of_practice_June_2003_e.pdf.

Canadian Nurses Association. (2004). Position Statement on Nurses and Human Rights. http://cna-aiic.ca/CNA/documents/pdf/publications/PS78_Human_Rights_e.pdf. Retrieved July 13, 2008.

Canadian Nurses Association. (2007a). *Position statement on emergency preparedness and response.* Retrieved January 2, 2009, from http://cna-aiic.ca/CNA/documents/pdf/publications/PS91_Emergency_e.pdf.

Canadian Nurses Association. (2007b). Understanding self-regulation. *Nursing Now, Issues and Trends in Canadian Nursing, (21).* Ottawa: Canadian Nurses Association.

Canadian Nurses Association. (2008a). *Code of ethics for registered nurses.* Author. Retrieved January 20, 2009, from www.cna-aiic.ca/CNA/documents/pdf/publications/Code_of_Ethics_2008_e.pdf.

Canadian Nurses Association. (2008b). *Standards and best practices.* Retrieved January 2, 2009, from http://www.cna-aiic.ca/CNA/practice/standards/default_e.aspx.

College of Nurses of Ontario. (2002). *Professional Standards.* Revised 2002. Toronto: Author.

College of Nurses of Ontario. (2008). *RHPA: Scope of Practice, Controlled Acts Model.* Toronto: Author.

Donabedian, A. (1976). Foreword in M. Phaneuf, Ed., *The nursing audit: Self-regulation in nursing practice* (2nd ed.). Norwalk, CT: Appleton & Lange.

Ehrenreich, B., & English, D. (1973). *Witches, midwives, and nurses: A history of women healers.* New York: The Feminist Press.

Fiesta, J. (1988). *The law and liability: A guide for nurses.* New York: John Wiley & Sons.

Flexner, A. (1915). Is social work a profession? *School Society, 1*(26), 901–911.

Fowler, M. (1990). Social ethics and nursing. In N. L. Chaska, ed., *The nursing profession: A time to speak* (pp. 24–31). St. Louis, MO: Mosby.

Gallup. (2008). Nurses shine while bankers slump in ethics rating. Retrieved January 2, 2009, from http://www.gallup.com/poll/112264/Nurses-Shine-While-Bankers-Slump-Ethics-Ratings.aspx.

Gruending, D. L. (1985). Nursing theory: A vehicle of professionalization. *Journal of Advanced Nursing, 10,* 553–558.

International Council of Nurses. (2000). *The ICN code of ethics for nurses.* International Council of Nurses, Geneva Switzerland. Retrieved January 23, 2001 from http://icn.ch/index.html/.

Jameton, A. (1984). *Nursing practice: The ethical issues.* Englewood Cliffs, NJ: Prentice-Hall.

Kozier, B., & Erb, G. (1994). *Concepts and issues in nursing practice* (2nd ed.). Menlo Park, CA: Addison-Wesley.

Leddy, S., & Pepper, J. M. (1989). *Conceptual bases of professional nursing* (2nd ed.). Philadelphia: Lippincott.

Lyon, B. (1990). Getting back on track; nursing's autonomous scope of practice. In N. L. Chaska, ed., *The nursing profession: A time to speak* (pp. 267–274). St. Louis, MO: Mosby.

Murphy, J. D. (1990). The legal perspective of nurse autonomy. In N. L. Chaska, ed., *The nursing profession: A time to speak* (pp. 32–39). St. Louis, MO: Mosby.

National Council of Boards of Nursing. (2000). *What are boards of nursing.* Chicago: Author. Retrieved January 31, 2001 from the World Wide Web http://www.ncsbn.org/.

Newman, M. A. (1990). Professionalism: Myth or reality. In N. L. Chaska, ed., *The nursing profession: A time to speak* (pp. 49–52). St. Louis, MO: Mosby.

Parsons, M. (1986). The profession in a class by itself. *Nursing Outlook, 34,* 270–275.

Quinn, C. A., & Smith, M. D. (1987). *The professional commitment: Issues and ethics in nursing.* Philadelphia: Saunders.

Reed, P. G. (2000). Nursing reformation: Historical reflections and philosophic foundations. *Nursing Science Quarterly, 13*(2), 129–136.

Sleicher, M. N. (1981, April). Nursing is not a profession. *Nursing & Health Care,* 186–218.

State Scan. (1996, March/April). *Nurse Practitioner World News, 1,* 22–23.

Zschoche, D. (1983). Letter calling for a national nurses' congress. In M. M. Styles, The anatomy of a profession. *Issues in Critical Care, 12,* 570–575. (Original letter December 29, 1972).

CHAPTER 9

Professional Relationship Issues

OBJECTIVES

After completing this chapter, the reader should be able to:

1. Identify relationships and potential conflicts that nurses face in the professional realm.
2. Characterize the nature of various conflicts.
3. Examine beliefs about the relative strength of various obligations.
4. Identify nurses' primary obligation.
5. Discuss issues related to nurses' relationships with other nurses, institutions, physicians, and subordinates.

INTRODUCTION

Armed with knowledge about the physical, psychological, social, and spiritual realms of nursing care, and proudly possessing a wide range of coveted technical and professional skills, new nurses expectantly enter the workforce. Anticipating respect for our opinions and encouragement to focus our efforts on giving excellent care, we soon realize that our attention must be divided between giving patient care and dealing with challenges among providers and within the institutional system. This dichotomy can present a confusing and frustrating challenge, forcing us to examine conflicting loyalties, question previously held values, make decisions based upon both practical and moral considerations, and test skills of negotiation.

The nurse continually affirms that each person is a moral agent, an autonomous being worthy of respect and having the duty to pursue solutions to problems of a moral nature. It is important that solutions consistently honour the uniqueness and value of each person and faithfully adhere to ethical principles. This process requires us to critically examine our own particular values and determine an ethically sound method of conflict resolution, even before conflict arises.

Recognizing that the profession of nursing struggles to overcome contextual barriers with cultural and historic overtones, we must enter professional relationships with attentiveness and skill. Rather than attempting to offer solutions to a comprehensive list of system-related problems, this chapter provides the opportunity to examine critically selected problems related to nurses' relationships within the health care delivery system. We suggest that students further prepare themselves to deal with conflict by learning morally sound skills of negotiation and conflict management.

PROBLEM SOLVING IN THE PROFESSIONAL REALM

Practical and ethical dilemmas are part of everyday nursing practice. Though many dilemmas involve patient-centred issues such as self-determination, confidentiality, and the like, we frequently encounter troubling moral questions related to professional relationships, conflicting role expectations, and patterns of interaction within the institutional setting. In the long run, problems of this nature can affect patient well-being both directly and indirectly and are, therefore, important to us on a professional level. These problems are often more troubling to us than problems directly involving patients. Recognizing that dilemmas of this sort are frequent and troubling, we must consider rational methods of solving problems before they occur. If we fail to try to solve conflict, we may add to the problem.

Although there is no absolute formula with which to solve conflicts, there are some general guidelines that can be helpful. First, we must maintain attentiveness to personal values and beliefs. Firm and consistent adherence to personal values allows us to approach problems with integrity. Second, we should construct a hierarchy of loyalty or obligation based upon both personal and professional values and beliefs. For example, do you owe a primary obligation to the physician, the institution, or the patient? Third, when conflicts arise, we should determine the nature of the problem. Is the dilemma ethical, or practical in nature? Is it a conflict of loyalty, obligation, duty, values, principles? Fourth, we should consider and weigh alternatives thoughtfully, including the degree of immediate harm or potential for harm, as well as the long-range effects that could occur with any given alternative. Although some alternatives may seem attractive initially, there may be long-term effects that are undesirable. Fifth, it is imperative to develop solutions that recognize each person as an autonomous being, worthy of respect. Utilization of these steps will help us resolve most professional conflicts.

Maintain Attentiveness to Personal Values

Prior to other considerations, we must both acknowledge and maintain our own personal values and beliefs. This attention to integrity is unrelated to self-interest and predicates action based upon coherent and integrated moral values. Integrity ultimately leads to trustworthiness and the respect of others. Beyond questions of loyalty or duty, we are compelled to maintain integrity in seeking to do the right thing. This is sometimes referred to as attention to matters of conscience. Childress (1978) distinguishes between **appeals to conscience** and appeals to self-interest or convenience in that appeals to conscience are personal and subjective beliefs, founded on a prior judgment of rightness or wrongness. These are motivated by personal sanction, rather than external authority. Institutions, in turn, must recognize the nurse as a person and encourage ethical autonomy. This enables us to act in ways that are rational, free from coercion or manipulation, and consistent with personally held values and principles (Benjamin & Curtis, 1986).

Acknowledging your own set of values and principles is a process that takes time. As we grow and develop, so does our moral autonomy, or our ability to identify our own beliefs and hold onto them, even in the face of adversity or conflict. This is a difficult skill to develop and, like any skill, becomes easier the more we practise exercising our own moral values and beliefs in everyday challenges. Institutions that encourage and facilitate our own ability to explore and hold true to our values and beliefs, while understanding and acknowledging the values of the institution, are ones that create positive morale-enriching environments.

In addition to enhancing professional relationships, the nurse's integrity aids patient well-being. Gadow (1980) asserts that only nurses who act with integrity can truly assist patients in reaching decisions that express their complex totality as individuals. Integrity is required of us since the welfare of patients is our primary obligation.

Clarify Obligation

Even nurses who possess a high level of integrity do not escape a sense of conflicting loyalty on occasion. When this happens, how do we determine the best course of action? We can be prepared by examining **obligations,** and devising a rational and consistent hierarchy. An obligation signifies being required to do something by virtue of a moral rule, a duty, or some other binding demand. Some obligations derive from a particular role or relationship (Honderich, 1995). We may believe an obligation is owed to any of the following (in no particular order as priorities may change depending on the context and situation): the patient, other patients who may be affected in the future by problems that occur in the present, the employer with which the nurse has an implied or expressed contract, the profession of nursing, peers and other coworkers, physicians, the broader society, family, and self.

Obligation to Patients. As a part of professional nursing practice, we have an obligation to patients above all others. Because nurses are professionals, we have a moral obligation to maintain fidelity—we must be faithful to the promises made to society, and thus give priority to meeting the needs of each patient. The International Council of Nurses *Code of Ethics for Nurses* (2000) makes clear that the nurse's primary responsibility is to the patient. By following established professional codes of ethics and maintaining integrity and loyalty to patients, we also fulfill related obligations to the broader society, the profession, and ourselves.

The duty that nurses and other health care professionals have to their patients is often described as a **fiduciary** relationship. Typically a legal term, a fiduciary refers to someone who has an ethical duty to act in the best interests of another. Simply put, it is the ethical obligation health care professionals have to act in a way that protects others, furthers their interests and their wishes, and, essentially, puts aside the agendas and competing priorities of the practitioner in favour of the patient's immediate and long-term needs. Consider this example: If, as a nurse, you are participating in the resuscitative efforts of someone in a cardiac arrest at exactly the same time you are entitled to be taking a coffee break, your fiduciary duty would dictate that you remain part of the life-saving efforts and delay your break. An obvious example, perhaps. Consider this example: A nurse, overtired from working too many night shifts in a row, who is also the primary caregiver for her elderly mother, arrives to work to find that she has been assigned a patient who, it is reported, after being cancelled for surgery, has been angry and aggressive with the nursing staff. When she enters the patient's room, she finds that he is refusing all medication and bloodwork. He is visibly upset, angry, and confrontational with the nurse. For a moment, she is tempted to return his anger and share with him her own frustrations, letting him know that everyone has problems. She is even tempted to just walk out of the room and leave him. However, realizing that, to some degree, her own frustrations must be put aside while she is in the role of nurse, she stays and voices to him her understanding of how frustrating it must be to have a surgical procedure cancelled. She asks him how she can help and after some discussion gets the patient to agree to take his medications and allow bloodwork to be done, in preparation for a possible surgical date tomorrow. While this does not ease her own frustrations, she can be assured that she has acted in his best interests, and not allowed herself an inappropriate opportunity to vent her own feelings of frustration and anger.

Obligation to the Institution Agency. Another obligation we have as nurses is to the Institution/Agency. By accepting and maintaining terms of employment and payment for services, we have both a legal and moral obligation to the institution or agency in when we work. This obligation, however strong, does not suggest that we should jeopardize personal integrity or subordinate loyalty to the patient. To succeed in the age of technological advancement, competition, and litigation, institutions need the services of nurses who express the professional characteristics of autonomy, integrity, and ethically based practice. Conflicts arise when the institution's goals are focused more on "bottom-line" economics than on moral responsibility and patient welfare. Conflict is inevitable when nurses, whose primary loyalty is to the welfare of patients, are employed by institutions that set priorities in a unilateral or authoritarian manner, without seeking input from "front-line" workers like nurses. Some examples of these kinds of decisions, often poorly received, include the following: elimination of important programs, employment of poorly qualified staff or inadequate numbers of staff, or other decisions that have a negative effect on patients' needs.

CASE PRESENTATION

When Economy Replaces Excellence

Western District Hospital was a busy acute care centre that serviced a distinct community in a highly urban environment. There were many unique programs and services that met the needs of the ethnically diverse community surrounding the centre. For many years, the hospital maintained excellent nursing care standards. After a period of difficult financial strain, the board of the hospital decided to amalgamate with two other large urban centres in the same city, to create a corporation that would, it was hoped, strengthen each centre and provide financial stability. Each of the three hospitals had a unique personality and set of special services and programs. After much enthusiastic publicity and positive hype, the amalgamation took place.

Immediately after the amalgamation, the hospital, under the auspices of the new corporation, began restructuring the delivery of care at the Western District Hospital, in order to cut back expenses. Important and well-used services were closed and nurses who provided services in these units were moved to other programs. The most junior nurses on the other units were dismissed, after more senior nurses were forced to take their positions. New mission and vision statements were introduced and the unique, highly patient-centred care at Western District was replaced by a clear orientation toward efficiency, episodic care, and an overarching concern for the "bottom line."

It was clear to many nurses that patients would no longer be receiving the excellent nursing care that had been the hallmark of the hospital for many years. However, many nurses felt trapped as they had worked for years in the same hospital and couldn't imagine working anywhere else, despite the current problems. They also felt powerless to change policies and priorities that were made without consideration for the best interests of the community.

❓ Think About It

How Do Nurses Respond to Bottom-Line Economics?

- What kinds of dilemmas are likely to occur in this situation?
- Recognizing that a nurse's primary responsibility is to patients, how does the new hospital arrangement affect the nurse–patient relationship?
- Can nursing practice maintain a patient-centred, ethically sensitive focus in this type of setting? Discuss your thinking.
- What alternative solutions to potential problems faced by nurses in this situation can you suggest?

Determine the Nature of the Problem

It is important that we are able to determine the nature of the problem. Is this a problem of moral uncertainty, moral distress, moral dilemma, or moral outrage? Is this a problem of a practical or ethical nature? Ethical considerations should carry more weight than matters of self-interest, though, clearly, we owe some consideration to our own needs. For example, with changing patient demographics and increasing hospital bed vacancies, we face being asked to "float" to unfamiliar settings. This practice redistributes the workload and offers the promise of improved nursing care. However, we frequently object to the prospect of being asked to float. Some nurses complain, "I've never worked there; I would be unsafe to practise in that setting!" They are tempted to refuse to float to unfamiliar settings. These nurses are faced with a moral and professional dilemma. Recall that the nurse has obligations to ensure both the welfare of the patient and meet the needs of the institution. In either case—in assigning a nurse to float or in accepting the assignment—one must be guided by the principles of nonmaleficence and beneficence: the actions that the nurse is expected to perform must be relatively certain to do good and do no harm. In that regard, neither the nurse, the patient, nor the institution will benefit from requiring a nurse to perform tasks for which there is no preparation. To do so would be unethical. When faced with situations of this sort, we should look to our codes of ethics for help. Regarding this particular situation, for example, the ICN *Code of Ethics for Nurses* (2000) is very specific about the nurse's duty: "The nurse uses judgment regarding individual competence when accepting and delegating responsibility." The Canadian Nurses Association *Code of Ethics for Registered Nurses* (2008) also addresses this type of situation: "Nurses practice within the limits of their competence. When aspects of care are beyond their level of competence, they seek additional information of knowledge, seek help from their supervisor or a competent practitioner and/or request a different work assignment. In the meantime, nurses remain with the person receiving care until another nurse is available." Similarly, the ANA *Code of Ethics for Nurses* (2001) states, "As the scope of nursing practice changes, the nurse must exercise judgment in accepting responsibilities, seeking consultation, and assigning activities to others who carry out nursing care."

Nevertheless, it could also be said that to refuse an assignment is unethical on a number of levels. As the CNA *Code of Ethics for Registered Nurses* (2008) states, we must not abandon patients in need of care. If there is no one else available to care for the patient, we are obligated to give care, albeit only the type of care for which we are prepared and competent. For example, nurses temporarily assigned to specialty units can be asked to give basic, supportive nursing care, but should not be asked to perform technical tasks for which they are unprepared. To do so is ethically wrong. In the same regard, we should not attempt tasks for which we are not prepared: to do so will compromise fidelity. We should not, however, refuse to accept float assignments simply because we fear the unknown, because familiarity is comfortable, or for other self-interested reasons.

CASE PRESENTATION

Facing a Dilemma in the Newborn Nursery

Maggie is a nurse employed in the newborn nursery of a small hospital. She is working toward completing her Master's degree and has an important seminar she must attend at 4:30 P.M. Though she is scheduled to leave work at 3:00 P.M., by 4:00 P.M. the nurse from the next shift has not yet arrived. There is an LPN who is capable of caring for the newborns, but hospital policy requires the presence of an RN in the unit at all times. The supervisor is unable to give her any assistance. All the babies are quiet; she expects the evening shift RN to arrive soon and feels the LPN can handle the nursery for a short time. Maggie is torn between honouring her duty to patients versus leaving to attend the seminar.

Think About It

What Should the Nurse Do?

- Is this a practical or an ethical dilemma? What factors make this either a practical or an ethical dilemma?
- Do you think Maggie's duty to stay outweighs her obligation to attend the seminar?
- What is the harm that could occur if she leaves before the evening shift RN arrives?
- What is the harm that could occur if she stays and misses her seminar?

The situation in the above case presentation regarding the newborn nursery constitutes a practical dilemma. Moral and nonmoral claims are in conflict. Based upon the principles of beneficence, nonmaleficence, and fidelity, Maggie has a moral obligation to the patients committed to her and to the institution. On the other hand, her obligation to attend class is a matter of self-interest and is not based upon moral principle per se. There is the potential for harm to the newborns if she leaves the unit inappropriately staffed. An emergency could arise for which the LPN is not prepared. Possibly the evening shift RN will not arrive at all. If Maggie utilizes Kant's moral imperative—one should do only that which could become a rule for all people—a decision to leave the unit unattended by an RN would be untenable. By leaving, she would create a situation that should not become a rule for all nurses in all situations. A rule suggesting that all nurses should leave patients improperly attended could harm many patients in the future and as a result could also harm society's faith in the profession of nursing. Based upon a comparison of moral versus practical considerations and the potential harm that could result if Maggie left the unit improperly attended, it seems clear that she should not leave. This is not meant to imply that nurses should always subjugate personal needs to patient or institutional ones. Staying at work later than scheduled as a result of an occasional, unpredictable circumstance is one thing; being required to stay repeatedly is something entirely different. If nurses find that they are being asked to stay late time and time again, they should approach the manager and nursing administration to ensure that there are adequate staffing plans and coverage in place across shifts and units. Coverage and staffing are essential parts of providing safe and quality nursing care to patients. Often, if the practice of staying late goes on consistently and nothing is said, it is understandable why nothing might be done about it by managers or administrators, as long as no negative events occur and no one speaks out. However, clearly, this is not a practice in the best interests of patients or nurses. It also might contribute to low morale and a difficult working environment. Supporting all nurses in being able to provide safe, quality care and not feel forced to subjugate personal needs to institutional ones is a key role of nursing leaders.

NURSES' RELATIONSHIPS WITH INSTITUTIONS

We enter the workforce with very different perceptions than our employing institutions. Having learned that autonomy and accountability are valuable components of the nursing role, we believe we have an overarching fiduciary duty to our patients. We also expect that our beliefs will be honoured and that our opinions and knowledge will be respected. Hospitals and other health care institutions, on the other hand, tend to be sharply hierarchical and bureaucratic institutions that expect nurses' and other subordinates' primary loyalty to be toward the institution (Jameton, 1984). Institutions expect nurses' actions to be directed toward attaining the goals of the system: goals that may focus strongly upon ensuring the well-being of the institution itself and sustaining patterns of power and control with secondary goals as "quality" patient care, defined usually by the institutions and not by individual providers. Difficulties arise when there is conflict between the goals of nurses and patients and those of the institution.

Problems arise, in part, because the institution's demands for loyalty are often inequitable (Jameton, 1984). Though requiring employees to accede to certain requests, institutions rarely reciprocate with similar loyalty to nurses. For example, due to budget constraints, most institutions are fairly rigid about nurses' work hours.

We are expected to arrive ready to begin and complete work according to a set schedule. We are sometimes directed to complete more work than can reasonably be done. Nurses, loyal to the institution and to the duty that they feel toward the patients in their care, are often willing to skip meals and breaks and complete work after "clocking out." In essence these practices, though very stressful for nurses, are financially appealing to institutions and often overlooked by nurse managers and unit administrators, also under pressure to adhere to budgetary constraints.

We need to balance professional obligation and the ideal of compassionate service with basic personal commitments. Most nursing organizations and regulatory bodies support the notion of professional development, which may include, at times, attending lectures, seminars, or other learning activities on your own time, with personal sacrifice, such as free time away from work, your lunch hour, or time with family and friends. Sometimes a patient situation or unit issue may require that an individual nurse or group of nurses stay after a shift or at times outside their required working hours, to discuss the situation or attend a meeting. Furthermore, most specialty units, such as coronary care, intensive care units, or operating rooms require nurses to have additional training and usually will provide financial reimbursement for such. The courses, however, are intense and difficult to fit into a full-time work schedule. These are the kinds of sacrifices and hardships that come along with being a professional and maintaining currency with one's profession. However, consistently repeated, self-sacrificing, altruistic behaviour on the part of nurses is self-defeating, and does not establish conditions of employment conducive to high-quality nursing care. It tends to support and perpetuate a flawed system; as long as nurses continue to work selflessly, the system (rather than the patient) benefits. Nurses willing to work in this way devalue the work of nurses and perpetuate the expectation that this type of one-sided self-sacrifice will continue. Of course, on rare occasions this sort of problem can occur in any institution, but when we repeatedly accept workloads that are unreasonable, we become complicit in continuing the wrongs. Although working extra appears to fulfill both professional obligations and the ideal of compassionate service, it "may only superficially meet obligations to clients and may actually lead to a less desirable state of affairs not only for nursing colleagues and the nursing profession, but ultimately for clients" (Benjamin & Curtis, 1986, p. 137). In the long run, this type of behaviour is harmful to both patients and nurses. Jameton says:

> A basic choice is forced on those who work in hospitals by the existence of prevalent and systematic problems in health care. If one fails to resist exploitation, incompetence, and corrupt practices, one becomes responsible for them. If one resists them, one enters into conflict with conventional conceptions of behavior for employees and thereby risks reprisals. One has to choose between complicity and self-sacrifice. . . . (1984, p. 289)

Jameton's term *self-sacrifice* is related to the willingness of some nurses to risk reprisals for resisting exploitation in the health care system. He does not suggest that nurses sacrifice all issues of self-interest in favour of institutional interests. Moreover, it is important to be clear that our fiduciary duty does not imply that we should sacrifice our well-being on a consistent basis, in order to protect and further the best interests of our patients. Certainly, if that is the case, it is highly indicative of an unhealthy and problematic work environment and one in which there are significant issues of organizational ethics.

In some instances, we base the motivation for altruism on misguided beliefs about duty. Some believe that altruism is necessary to fulfill their duty to patients. Though many philosophers consider altruism and sacrifice a virtue, Ayn Rand (1996) suggested that altruism has a dehumanizing effect. Rand believed that those who are altruistic have a nightmare view of existence—believing that people are trapped in a malevolent universe. Using the term *self-sacrifice* in a fashion nearly opposite that of Jameton, Rand viewed a persistent willingness to sacrifice as flowing from poor self-esteem and inappropriate priority setting. Moreover, she believed that those with poor self-esteem have difficulty valuing others. Because genuine regard is partially a product of sympathy (imagining oneself in the situation of another), one must value oneself in order to value others. Additionally, nurses who repeatedly sacrifice for the good of an institutional system fail to assume the power to change the wrongs that are committed.

CASE PRESENTATION

When Patients Suffer from Lack of Nursing Care

Tim, an RN, works weekends on the skilled nursing unit of a small rural hospital that recently underwent significant financial hardship. Forced to amalgamate with a much larger urban centre, the hospital then dismissed nearly one-third of the staff of the skilled nursing unit. Lately, when Tim comes to work, he feels totally overwhelmed. Although he always considered himself efficient, Tim is distressed because he rarely has enough time to complete his work. He knows that many of the patients suffer because of lack of attention. Those who are bedridden are not turned on a regular schedule, they often wait for assistance with eating until their food is cold, and medications are rarely given on time. Suffering from expressive aphasia and hemiplegia secondary to a CVA, Mrs. Wallace was admitted to the skilled nursing unit after two weeks in the intensive care unit. Mrs. Wallace has been on the skilled nursing unit for three weeks when her daughter, Nina, notices a large reddened area surrounding a small gray ulcer over her mother's coccyx. Concerned, Nina asks Tim what caused this problem. Even though Mrs. Wallace's nursing care plan calls for attention to activity including frequent turning and sitting in a chair twice daily, Tim suspects that this was not consistently done the previous week. He recognizes that the reddened area is the beginning of a large pressure ulcer, a problem that might have been prevented with proper attention to activity and good nutrition. Tim hesitates to tell Nina that the problem is a potentially serious one that might have been prevented by good nursing care measures. He believes she has a right to know but is hesitant to implicate himself or the other nurses, and he is afraid that he will lose his job if he complains.

Think About It

How Do Nurses Make Decisions When Loyalties Conflict?

- What are the ethical principles implicit in this situation?
- What are Tim's conflicting loyalties?
- The remaining staff on the unit is efficient and hard working—skipping lunch and staying overtime to complete their work. Do you believe the staff is responsible for the apparently poor nursing care that Mrs. Wallace is getting?
- Do you believe Tim should tell Nina the truth about the pressure sore?
- Should Tim risk losing his job by whistleblowing?
- Is this an ethical or practical dilemma?
- What harm can result from either option?
- What would you do?

The previous case presentation is another example of a practical dilemma. The conflict that Tim is experiencing is between the principle of beneficence (the desire to do good for the patient) and a sense of loyalty to the institution or the other nurses with whom he works. There may also be an element of self-interest—Tim may not want to be implicated in the harm that the patients are experiencing as a result of the staff cutbacks. Tim's fiduciary duty is owed to the patients—Mrs. Wallace, other patients suffering from the shortage of staff, and future patients who could be harmed by perpetuation of the problem. Keeping in mind that the notion of a fiduciary duty implies putting aside one's own interests or agendas, there are strong arguments that he should act to correct the situation. He may choose to take any number of actions: he can work through the administrative hierarchy to improve staffing; he can answer Nina's questions honestly; though his job will certainly be jeopardized, he can inform the media of the problems that were created by the drastic staffing shortages. In any case, if Tim fails to act to solve the problem, he will be complicit in its perpetuation and the subsequent harm to patients.

Another example related to institutions' inequitable demands for loyalty is seen in the customary practice of requiring nurses to complete incident reports. Institutions may discourage nurses from talking to patients about mistakes that have been made. They much prefer that nurses file incident reports. These documents, geared toward institutional goals, are filed and kept for use in the event the hospital needs a legal defence, in firing or disciplining workers, or in reorganizing services to prevent future incidents (Jameton, 1984). Thus, patient-centred goals based upon the principles of autonomy, fidelity, veracity, and respect for persons are subordinated to institutional subgoals of employee control and risk management.

Nurses' loyalty to the institution is an important mode of control. Without loyalty, administrators cannot manage institutions (Jameton, 1984). For this reason supervisors and administrators sometimes react negatively when nurses support and cooperate with each other to make changes. The ensuing perception of nonsupportive supervisors is a contributing factor for job stress and dissatisfaction (Moore, Kuhrik, Kuhrik, & Katz, 1996). In the end, this can be harmful to nurses and patients alike. Jameton says, "Where institutions as a whole fail to serve patients well, this demand for loyalty can interfere with the nurses' expressions of loyalty to nurses and patients" (1984, p. 121).

NURSES' RELATIONSHIPS WITH OTHER NURSES

Nurses work together in close proximity day in and day out. No other profession is so intimately connected with issues of life, death, and personal care. The knowledge gained from the intimate experiences of birth, illness, life, and death are powerful. Nurses are connected to each other and set apart from others: connected by common experience, language, and knowledge, and set apart through a perceived professional mystique. Nurses work together closely, identify with each other, and supervise or are supervised by other nurses. The practice of one affects that of others.

Loyalty is a natural product of long-term acquaintance and close working relationships. Some view loyalty among members as a distinguishing characteristic of a profession. Jameton defines loyalty as:

> showing sympathy, care, and reciprocity to those with whom we appropriately identify; working closely with others toward shared goals; keeping promises; making mutual concerns a priority; sacrificing personal interests to the relationship; and giving attention to these over a substantial period of time. It supports showing respect for persons. And it resolves potential conflicts in autonomy by making values and goals that I see as my own more like values and goals of those who work with me. (1984, p. 118)

Promoting faithfulness and commitment, loyalty is very limited and exclusive in its scope. Though normally viewed as admirable, loyalty is seldom regarded as a cardinal virtue because of the potential for fanaticism and blind injustice (Honderich, 1995).

In practical matters, loyalty is a productive virtue. It enhances unity, strength, and power. Facing bureaucratic, economic, and political forces, our loyalty to each other and to the profession adds strength to our call for improved patient care, public welfare, nursing autonomy, and optimum employment conditions.

While having the potential to strengthen the profession of nursing and improve the welfare of patients, loyalty among nurses can result in negative outcomes, when not prioritized alongside other loyalties and obligations. Though our primary obligation is to patients, those of us who are overly loyal to other nurses might act in ways that are harmful to patients' health status. For example, a nurse having blind loyalty to another might cover up a coworker's incompetent practice, illegal drug use, or other actions that have the potential to harm present or future patients. For this reason, we must be careful to maintain objectivity in balancing loyalty to nurses and the profession against the obligation owed to patients. Part of being a self-regulating profession means monitoring incidents of professional misconduct. Legal definitions of professional misconduct are complex and vary between provinces with different legislation ruling the regulatory practice of nursing. However, one principle is clear. Failure to report unethical or unsafe practice of another member of the profession is clearly misconduct. As a licensed professional, you have an ethical and professional responsibility (and in some case, a legal one as well) to report incidents of unsafe, harmful, or unethical behaviour of another licensed professional nurse. The method by which it is reported or addressed should be thoughtful, maintain confidentiality, and be directed toward the appropriate person, agency, or regulatory body (College of Nurses of Ontario, 2000).

NURSES' RELATIONSHIPS WITH PHYSICIANS

Nurses' relationships with physicians are an important factor in the quality of patient care. Ideally, the work of nurses and physicians should be complementary and synergistic. Because both professions hold claim to the primary goal of patient health, one would expect a sense of collegiality and collaboration between nurses and physicians. When this type of relationship exists, it is rewarding and productive. When there is conflict between nurses and physicians, the relationship is stressful and damaging to nurses, physicians, and patients alike. Because nurses and physicians work in close proximity, conflict that occurs between them is a strong contributor to the lack of job satisfaction for nurses.

Nurse–physician relationships have generally reflected the prevailing gender roles in society. These roles were well defined for centuries. The traditional nurse was expected to obey the physician, much as the wife was expected to obey her husband. Physicians demanded obedience, and nurses hesitated to disagree with physicians, even if there was good reason to do so. Unfortunately, these "time-worn attitudes" linger in both professions (Benjamin & Curtis, 1986, p. 86).

Given the bureaucratic nature of most health care institutions, particularly hospitals, the relationship between physicians and nurses is complex and peculiar. Generally, nurses are employees of the institutions, while physicians are independent practitioners who have the privilege of institutional practice. Physicians, who may not be employees of the institutions, have no formal chain-of-command relationship with the nurses who care for their patients. Curtin and Flaherty (1982) write, "This tradition of self-employed 'guest practitioners' in health care institutions having so much power over the large groups of 'full-time employees' of the institutions defies explanation, but it is a fact of life in health care" (p. 144). Though they issue orders to nurses directly, physicians are not employed by, subordinate to, or even responsible to the institutional administration. These dual lines of authority are confusing, and have the potential to severely limit the autonomous decision-making role of the nurse (Benjamin & Curtis, 1986, p. 82). Because most nurses are employees with either expressed or implied contracts with institutions, they have an obligation to perform the tasks required by the institutions. One of the major tasks that most institutions require of nurses is the implementation of physicians' orders. When nurses question or disagree with physicians, they may feel distressed, believing they are being disloyal to both the physician and the institution.

Another contributor to conflict in the nurse–physician relationship is the rapid advent of advanced practice nursing. Having an expanded knowledge base and a scope of practice that includes many functions that were once the sole domain of physicians, advanced practice nursing can contribute to the tensions that exist between nurses and physicians. The outmoded tradition of the nurse who obeys the physician is in direct conflict with the autonomous nurse who thinks independently, makes nursing diagnoses, and implements independent nursing actions (Benjamin & Curtis, 1986).

What actions should be taken by the nurse who questions or disagrees with an order or action of a physician? The nurse must remember that the primary obligation is owed the patient, not the physician. Nurses are autonomous practitioners. They have the knowledge and experience, and the legal and ethical responsibility, to make independent judgments even when carrying out physicians' orders. As a nurse is also responsible for patient care, carrying out orders that may be incorrect or unsafe may well constitute an ethical and legal issue for the nurse as well as the physician. When deciding what course to take in situations in which nurses disagree with physicians' orders, Benjamin and Curtis (1986) suggest that nurses apply the test of the **spectrum of urgency.** At one end of this spectrum are problems that are minor and may be solved at a leisurely pace. At the other end are urgent problems that require quick solutions and immediate actions. The low-urgency end of the spectrum includes situations in which there is little risk of serious harm, or there is significant time available to examine all aspects of the situation. The high-urgency end of the spectrum consists of emergencies in which lifesaving actions must be carried out at once. Nurses may have time to discuss and negotiate satisfactory solutions to problems at the low-urgency end of the spectrum, but problems at the high-urgency end of the spectrum require efficient and timely action.

CASE PRESENTATION

Making a Decision in an Urgent Situation

Marta is night-shift charge nurse in the emergency department of a small but busy hospital. She has advanced certification and twenty-five years of experience. Marta works well with the other members of the emergency room staff, and is comfortable and efficient in situations of extreme urgency. The emergency department is usually staffed by emergency physicians. Because one of the regular physicians recently moved away, there has been a series of physicians with various degrees of preparation and ability moonlighting in the department, particularly on night shift. During an unusually busy shift, an ambulance arrives with a middle-aged man having severe chest pain and dyspnea. His condition quickly deteriorates, and after a few minutes he experiences cardiac and respiratory arrest. The physician on duty, Dr. Andrews, is a family practice physician moonlighting after his regular shift at a local community health centre. Marta perceives Dr. Andrews as nervous and hesitant. During the first phase of the "code," Dr. Andrews seems uncertain of every detail. As the nurse in charge, Marta begins instituting a seldom-used protocol that was developed for use in the event that the nurses are faced with a cardiac arrest when no physician is present. All the nurses are trained in intubation techniques, but hospital policy prohibits them from performing that particular procedure. Marta suggests to Dr. Andrews that he intubate the patient.

After several clumsy attempts, Dr. Andrews angrily orders Marta to call an anesthesiologist at home to come and intubate the patient. Marta realizes that the patient's chances of survival are best if he is intubated quickly. She asks the unit clerk to call the anesthesiologist. Over his angry objections, Marta removes the laryngoscope and endotracheal tube from Dr. Andrews's trembling hands and proceeds to intubate the patient quickly and successfully. The patient responds to resuscitation attempts and is discharged five days later.

Think About It

Was Marta's Decision Correct?

- What is your immediate response to the situation in which Marta finds herself?
- Where would you place this situation on the "spectrum of urgency"?
- What are the arguments in favour of Marta's actions?
- What are the arguments in favour of Marta's following Dr. Andrews's orders?
- Do you consider Marta's actions to be based upon ethical principle?
- Did Marta place herself at risk of reprisal, legal action, or professional discliplinary action?
- What would you have done?

Nurses are charged with making thoughtful, fair, and knowledgeable decisions in relation to questioning physicians' orders, while also being careful to consider the overall harm that can result from any given action. Recognizing that the physician's goal, like that of the nurse, is the welfare of the patient, we must be mature and objective when questioning orders. Nurses have an ethical obligation to protect the patient from medical incompetence. Nevertheless, we must be careful in this regard, keeping in mind the overall harm that can result from the practice of constantly and inappropriately questioning insignificant aspects of physicians' orders.

WORKING AS PART OF A TEAM

While maintaining an awareness of the primary obligation owed to patients, nurses must be sensitive to those who work beside them. Each person is a moral agent and must be recognized as worthy of dignity and respect. As the coordinator of patient care, the professional nurse is accountable for the quality of nursing care rendered to patients. This accountability includes supervision, delegation of nursing care functions, and disciplining of other health care providers. The inherent practical, moral, and legal implications of these functions are facets of the role of professional nurse that must be undertaken with sensitivity and respect.

The structure of health care delivery in some institutional settings makes the professional nurse responsible for delegating a number of nursing functions to staff members, such as licensed practical nurses, personal support workers, personal care providers, and nursing students. As the coordinator of patient care, the registered nurse is accountable for all nursing care that patients receive, whether from the nurse directly or other members of the nursing care team, including nursing students.

Registered nurses have a twofold responsibility. Their primary duty is to the patient, to ensure that the care provided is appropriate, high-quality and individualized. However an ethical duty also exists to those with whom we work as a team. The Canadian Nurses Association notes in its *Code of Ethics* that, as part of being accountable, "Nurses share their knowledge and provide feedback, mentorship and guidance for the professional development of nursing students, novice nurses and other health-care team members" (CNA, 2008, p. 18). Furthermore, the code goes on to note that "Nurses treat each other, colleagues, students and other health-care workers in a respectful manner, recognizing the power differentials among those in formal leadership positions, staff and students. They work with others to resolve differences in a constructive way" (CNA, 2008, p. 49).

One discouraging phenomenon is poor treatment of and lack of mentorship for nursing students. Many students enter their clinical practice with high expectations and an overly idealistic outlook. While it is important to acclimatize them to the realities and challenges of the health care system, demoralizing them by belittling their abilities or acting in an intimidating manner serves no constructive purpose and furthers the image of nurses "eating their young." This expression has been reiterated over the years to describe the phenomenon of "being hard" on those who are up and coming, in order to teach them the realities of the roles which they are aiming to fulfill one day. It also refers to the practice of not supporting nursing students and novice nurses, by challenging them, leaving them on their own without adequate knowledge or resources, being unfriendly or unapproachable, or representing professional work and skills behind a veil of mystique, inaccessible to those novices or students not "in the know." These types of practices are counterproductive to quality patient care and sustainability of the profession. They are also unethical and highly unprofessional, even worthy of being labelled as professional misconduct, if serious enough.

In addition to delegation, the supervisory role of professional nurses occasionally includes disciplining of others. Disciplining is a difficult task that must be done with insight, respect, compassion, and logic. The nurse must be keenly aware of the effect of disciplinary action upon others and must focus on the intended goal. The traditional methods of discipline, such as punishment and chastisement, are damaging to the spirit and counterproductive in practice.

Nurse managers' method of disciplining may set the tone for the entire nursing unit. Discussing poor leadership, Dilley says, "Nurse managers from hell can be easily identified. They use coercion—as in, 'do as I say or you'll find yourself on the night shift.' They belittle their employees in front of patients or other staff. They communicate by memo rather than face-to-face. They change policies without input from others. They are rude and thoughtless" (2000, p. 9).

A good nurse manager may also set the tone of the unit through the style of discipline. Quoting the great teacher Maria Montessori, Leah Curtin (1996) writes, "'Our aim is to discipline for activity, for work, for good; not for immobility, not for passivity, not for obedience'" (p. 51). Curtin suggests that the most meaningful method is self-discipline, which corrects the problem, strengthens the character of the worker, and improves performance. She defines self-discipline as a process by which the rules are internalized and become a part of the individual's personality. This process is possible only if the person knows the rules, understands their purpose, and agrees that they deserve compliance. To achieve this result, the nurse must model the expected standard daily and have few rules—all of which are applied consistently, change infrequently, and apply to all personnel equally. The nurse has a moral obligation, to both patients and personnel, to uphold rules that protect the health or safety of patients, other employees, the institution, and oneself as leader (Curtin, 1996, p. 51).

WORKPLACE HARASSMENT

Harassment in the workplace is not a new problem. However, it is a poorly defined and a much too infrequently discussed problem. The Canadian Human Rights Commission (2006) defines "harassment" and "personal harassment" as follows:

> Harassment is any behaviour that demeans, humiliates or embarrasses a person, and that a reasonable person should have known would be unwelcome. It includes actions (e.g., touching, pushing), comments (e.g., jokes, name-calling), or displays (e.g., posters, cartoons). The *Canadian Human Rights Act* prohibits harassment related to race, national or ethnic origin, colour, religion, age, sex, marital status, family status, disability, pardoned conviction, or sexual orientation.
>
> Disrespectful behaviour, commonly known as "personal" harassment is not covered by human rights legislation. While it also involves unwelcome behaviour that demeans or embarrasses an employee, the behaviour is not based on one of the prohibited grounds named above. Nevertheless, some employers choose to include personal harassment in their anti-harassment policies. (p. 3)

Under Canada's *Labour Code,* all employers are required to design their own policies and guidelines for workplace harassment. However many institutions and employers do not have clear harassment policies and, if they do, many workers are unaware that such policies exist or that they have specific rights in regard to how they are treated by colleagues and supervisors.

In nursing, the issue of workplace harassment is often discussed as "bullying" in nursing (Randle, 2003). Bullying is defined as consistent behaviours that demean and degrade others (Adams, 1997). Randle's 2003 landmark article in the *Journal of Advanced Nursing* describes the experience of nursing students, who describe bullying behaviours from supervising nurses as "distressing" (p. 397). This phenomenon has been referred to colloquially in nursing, as *eating your young* (Truman, 2004), an expression that refers to, at best, the inability to nurture those who are younger or less experienced than you and, at worst, the practice of cutting down, demeaning, or demoralizing those who are younger. This practice, according to Truman and others who have also discussed this phenomenon (Pugh, 2005; Randle, 2003) contributes to low rates of job satisfaction, poor self-esteem, and low retention rates for nursing. Each of these, in turn, contributes to poor patient care, and in some cases, may lead to further and continued demeaning treatment to patients and other nurses in turn. In fact, Pugh (2005) and Randle (2003) both emphasize that bullying nursing students leads to those same students bullying others, patients, and younger nursing students. In other words, without attention and dialogue about this pervasive problem, it will continue in a cyclical fashion, with victims becoming perpetrators.

Does bullying and demeaning of younger workers occur only in nursing? Certainly not. It occurs across professions, genders, and environments (Pugh, 2005). It may be more visible in nursing because of the expectation that nurses will always display only nurturing and caring behaviours to all around them. It also may be more visible as the work of nursing is done in the public eye. Nursing stations are out in the open with conversations and activities visible to all who may walk by. Nursing care is often carried out in corridors and shared rooms. Medication rooms, utility rooms, and kitchens in hospitals are shared by a variety of allied health professionals as well as patients and family members. According to Pugh, who calls bullying between nurses lateral violence, the vulnerability of nurses to this phenomenon may be due to two things. First, it may be due to the tremendous workload that most nurses deal with on a daily basis. The stress and fatigue that go alongside this degree and intensity of work may contribute to the displacement of stress and anxiety on other nurses. With increasing technology, an aging workforce, and shortages in the profession in Canada, workload will continue to be an issue. The second factor to which Pugh refers is the fact that many nurses are, in fact, excluded from the power structure of their workplace and have limited input into decision making that affects their own professional lives. This lack of power can contribute to lateral violence, as is commonly seen in other kinds of social groups who are oppressed and lack power in their daily lives.

Many nurses who experience harassment or bullying, according to Pugh, leave the profession instead of seeking help or advice with the problem.

What options are available to nurses who experience harassment or bullying? First, most institutions now have policies regarding harassment or even officers or employees designated to deal with harassment and discrimination issues. Most universities have harassment and discrimination offices, which take complaints from students and faculty members and conduct investigations. Making managers and nurse leaders aware of these kinds of problems can help. Programs and support can be put in place to address issues like these and create initiatives and simple solutions for addressing these kinds of behaviours, making the workplace an easier and more positive environment, and increasing satisfaction, self-esteem, and retention.

SUMMARY

In the professional realm, nurses are faced with the dichotomy of striving to meet their primary obligation to patients while dealing with problems among providers and within the institutional system. Nurses must be prepared to examine personal beliefs, prioritize obligations, and devise morally sound solutions to problems. Solutions must reflect an overall respect for persons and recognize the moral agency of individuals. Nurses are guided in this endeavour by personal values and beliefs and by professional codes of ethics.

CHAPTER HIGHLIGHTS

- As a moral agent, each person has the duty to pursue solutions to moral problems.
- Solutions to practical and ethical problems in the professional realm must be sensitive to personal values and beliefs.
- Nurses must be able to identify and prioritize conflicting obligations.
- It is important for nurses to determine the nature of conflicts in the professional realm.
- Problem resolution requires thoughtful consideration and weighing of alternative solutions.
- In solving problems, nurses must recognize that each person is an autonomous being, worthy of respect.
- Nurses must seek solutions to moral problems related to conflicting role expectations in the institutional setting.
- Nurses must seek solutions to moral and practical problems related to relationships among nurses, physicians, and subordinates.

DISCUSSION QUESTIONS AND ACTIVITIES

1. Describe potential problems in the professional realm that fall into each of the following categories:
    - Conflicts of obligation
    - Conflicts of principle
    - Practical dilemmas
    - Conflicts of loyalty

2. Discuss with your classmates situations that could reasonably occur in the work setting that would constitute an appeal to conscience.

3. Interview nurses who have been in practice one year or less. Ask them to compare their expectations of the work environment with the reality that they faced upon graduation.

4. Discuss the conflict that results as shrinking institutional budgets require cutbacks in nursing staff.

5. List the positive and negative aspects of loyalty. Do you feel loyalty is a virtue?

6. Describe the ideal professional relationships that can occur between nurses and physicians.

7. Role-play a situation in which a nurse is sensitive and respectful in disciplining a subordinate, focusing on the goal of improving performance rather than punishing.

REFERENCES

Adams, A. (1997). *Bullying at work—How to confront and overcome it*. Virago Press: London.

American Nurses Association (2001). *Code of ethics for nurses*. Washington, DC: Author.

Benjamin, M., & Curtis, J. (1986). *Ethics in nursing* (2nd ed.). New York: Oxford University Press.

Canadian Human Rights Commission. (2006). *Anti-harassment policies for the workplace: An employer's guide*. Ottawa: Canadian Human Rights Commission. Retrieved January 29, 2009, from http://www.chrc-ccdp.ca/publications/anti_harassment_toc-en.asp#12.

Canadian Nurses Association (2008). *Code of ethics for registered nurses*. Author.

Childress, J. (1978). Appeals to conscience. *Ethics, 89*, 316–321.

College of Nurses of Ontario. (2000). Accountability means taking action. *Communiqué, 25*(4). Retrieved August 19, 2008, from http://www.cno.org/pubs/mag/cmqVol25no4.pdf.

Curtin, L. (1996). Ethics, discipline and discharge. *Nursing Management, 27*(3), 51–52.

Curtin, L., & Flaherty, M. J. (1982). *Nursing ethics: Theories and pragmatics*. Bowie, MD: Brady.

Department of Justice Canada. (1985). *Canada Labour Code*. Ottawa: Department of Justice. Retrieved January 29, 2009, from http://laws.justice.gc.ca/en/L-2/.

Dilley, K. B. (2000). Out from under their thumbs. *American Journal of Nursing, 100*(5), 9.

Gadow, S. (1980). Existential advocacy: Philosophical foundation of nursing. In S. F. Spicker and S. Gadow, eds., *Nursing: Images and ideals, opening dialogue with the humanities* (pp. 90–91). New York: Springer.

Honderich, T., ed. (1995). *The Oxford companion to philosophy*. New York: Oxford University Press.

International Council of Nurses (2000). *The ICN code of ethics for nurses*. International Council of Nurses, Geneva, Switzerland. Retrieved January 23, 2001 from http://icn.ch/index.html.

Jameton, A. (1984). *Nursing practice: The ethical issues*. Englewood Cliffs, NJ: Prentice-Hall.

Moore, S., Kuhrik, M., Kuhrik, N., & Katz, B. (1996). Coping with downsizing: Stress, self-esteem and social intimacy. *Nursing Management, 27*(3), 28–30.

Pugh, A. (2005). Bullying in nursing: Building a culture of respect combats lateral violence. *Cross Currents* (Winter) (n.p.).

Rand, A. (1996). The ethics of emergencies. In J. Feinberg, ed., *Reason and responsibility: Readings in some basic problems of philosophy* (9th ed., pp. 541–545). Belmont, CA: Wadsworth.

Randle, J. (2003). Bullying in the nursing profession. *Journal of Advanced Nursing. 43*(4), 395–401.

Truman, K. M. (2004). Education enhances recruitment and retention in the emergency department. Don't eat your young, nurse them. *Nursing Management, 35*(7), pp. 45–48.

CHAPTER 10

Practice Issues Related to Technology

OBJECTIVES

After completing this chapter, the reader should be able to:

1. Discuss the impact of technology on nursing and health care.
2. Apply beneficence and nonmaleficence to decisions about technology.
3. Discuss issues and dilemmas related to current technology and to life-sustaining interventions.
4. Relate the concept of medical futility to health care decisions.
5. Relate economics to decisions regarding health technology.

6. Discuss considerations in decisions about cardiopulmonary resuscitation and artificial sources of nutrition for patients.

7. Describe legal issues associated with health care technology.

8. Discuss issues and dilemmas associated with technologies affecting reproduction, genetics, and organ transplantation.

9. Describe nursing considerations for patient care in the midst of technology.

INTRODUCTION

Nursing care is inextricably intertwined with ever-expanding advances of scientific knowledge and technology. Few would deny the benefits of medical advances, often referred to in terms such as *wonders* or *miracles*. However, the many benefits brought to the health care arena by technology are often accompanied by serious dilemmas for both practitioners and patients. Technology brings to the fore many questions related to issues of living and dying, and the changing definitions of both that are brought on by scientific advances. Dilemmas include availability of and accessibility to technologies, what patient situations warrant the use of available technologies, and who decides when to initiate and when to withdraw particular interventions. The rising cost of providing accessible technological advances also raises issues in the realms of priority setting and distributive justice. Additionally, nurses must be concerned about the amount of nursing energy and attention that technology requires. As much as we say that nursing focuses on holistic caring for the patient, nurses are faced with increasing demands to focus attention on technology rather than on their patients.

This chapter focuses on common issues related to technology encountered in today's health care settings. Issues of technology, patient self-determination, and feasibility are intertwined. Nurses who are directly involved in dilemmas, as well as those who are more on the periphery, must be aware of considerations regarding the effect of technology on patient care. These considerations include values, attitudes, communication, and attention to the humanistic caring role. The term *technology* includes the vast range of scientific advances that affect health and health care. Changing technologies bring with them the challenge of dealing with new issues, and nurses need to be prepared to face this challenge.

BENEFITS AND CHALLENGES OF TECHNOLOGY

Scientific advances in the past one hundred years have been phenomenal. They include medications, surgical techniques, machines and equipment, diagnostic procedures, specialized treatments, expanded understanding of the causes of and progression of disease, gene diagnosis and therapy, and greater insight into what is required for people to stay healthy. New interventions have saved lives, improved quality of life, alleviated suffering, and significantly decreased the incidence of some diseases.

Before the advent of many modern health-related technologies, people experienced illness and death as an inevitable part of the cycle of their lives. Although death was not necessarily welcomed, it was expected as the natural outcome when the body could no longer ward off the effects of certain diseases or injuries. If someone was born with, or developed, a deformity, it may have been seen as a curse, but was also considered part of who the person was. Life began when the infant started breathing, and life ended when the heart and breathing stopped.

Current technology makes it possible to restart arrested hearts, use machines to breathe for people, correct deformities, assist the body in dealing with disease through use of medications and other interventions, eliminate diseased parts through surgery, and even to replace malfunctioning or diseased vital organs. The ability to prolong life, or at least to extend the functioning of the physical being, has prompted the necessity of dealing with some very important issues. One dilemma relates to questions of quality of life, and whether physical existence is synonymous with living. Another issue relates to whether the availability of certain technologies means they should always be used. Many issues relate to decisions about how and for whom technologies will be used.

Quality of Life

The ability to keep people alive and physically functioning through use of technology has led to much reflection and discussion about what constitutes life and living. Some people believe that biological life must be preserved, regardless of the effect on the person whose body is being kept alive. This belief is sometimes referred to as the "sanctity of life" position. A frequently asked question is whether a person is truly alive in situations where there is merely physiological functioning, without awareness of oneself or others. Others suggest that living implies a quality that goes beyond physical existence. **Quality of life,** a subjective appraisal of factors that make life worth living and contribute to a positive experience of living, means different things to different people. It is difficult to find a clear and concise definition of quality of life, because of the multidisciplinary usage and variable cultural understandings, making it a very subjective notion. Farquhar (1995) points out that definitions of quality of life derive from both lay and "expert" sources and range from global understandings of the concept, such as satisfaction with life, to focused definitions used for research; for example, health or functional ability. Ideas incorporated in understandings of the concept include fulfillment, satisfaction/dissatisfaction, conditions of life, happiness/ unhappiness, experiences of life, and factors such as comfort, functional status, socioeconomic status, independence, and conditions in one's environment.

Farquhar (1995) suggests that deciding what weight to give different dimensions of the concept presents problems in defining quality of life. For instance, when evaluating personal quality of life, which does a person rank as more important, happiness, or functional status, such as the ability to get around and care for oneself? Nurses need to understand patient perspectives of what constitutes quality in their lives in order to incorporate these factors into goal setting and care planning.

Quality of life is a personal perspective that is determined by each individual. Recognizing this, we should not judge the quality of another's life based on our own values. If judgments are made about a person's worth and quality of life based on factors such as contributions to society, age, mental capacity, or ability to function, discrimination against those who are judged to have a lesser quality of life may easily follow. Perceptions of quality of life often change with age and life experiences. For example, persons with debilitating health concerns may rate the quality of their lives quite positively, although others might feel that they could never live with such limitations. When patients and families are confronted with technological options, nurses need to help them clarify their perceptions regarding quality of life, and discuss not only how life might be extended, but also how quality of life may be affected by various options.

Principles of Beneficence and Nonmaleficence

When dealing with issues of technology, the principles of **beneficence** and **nonmaleficence** may be in conflict. A particular technology, which may be implemented with the intention of *doing good* (beneficence), may result in much suffering for the patient. Inducing such suffering is counter to the maxim of *do no harm* (nonmaleficence). In some circumstances this is accepted as part of the treatment process, such as pain associated with surgery or side effects of chemotherapy. We are willing to endure the discomfort because there is an expectation of recovery, that we will ultimately be or feel more healthy. In circumstances in which there is little or no expectation of recovery or improved functioning, the essential question is whether the harm imposed by technology outweighs the good intended by its use. Suffering associated with technology may include physical, spiritual, and emotional elements for both patient and family. Making decisions regarding use of technology may cause pain, and there is suffering in living with unknown results of these ongoing decisions. Relief of suffering, a goal of healing from its earliest days, needs to be addressed in all patient encounters.

CURRENT TECHNOLOGY: ISSUES AND DILEMMAS

Current technologies related to organ and tissue transplantation, genetic engineering, reproduction, and sustaining life have profound potential for affecting our lives and health in positive ways. Their use also presents dilemmas for patients, families, professionals, and society. Nurses generally do not make the decisions regarding implementing or withdrawing particular technologies (except perhaps in situations like initiating cardiopulmonary recuscitation following specific protocols), yet we are involved as the caregivers of those receiving interventions and in many levels of patient care that involve technology. In most health care environments, nurses function as part of an interprofessional team, providing key information for, and contributing to, decisions regarding patient care and the use of technology. One of nursing's primary responsibilities is to help patients and families deal with the purposes, benefits, and limitations of the specific technologies. This section focuses primarily on the issue of withdrawing or withholding treatment as a prime example of a dilemma related to technology. Other issues related to technology are discussed briefly, and the reader is encouraged to further explore particular areas as the need or interest arises.

Treating Patients: When to Intervene and to What End

One of the most controversial bioethical topics of recent years centres around withholding or withdrawing life-sustaining treatments when they are deemed to have poor outcomes or offer no benefit. Decisions about withholding or withdrawing medical treatment are generally made by physicians in consultation with patients and family members. Approaches to dealing with these decisions reflect varying attitudes and concerns and may be confusing for all involved. A brief look at history sheds light on current attitudes regarding dealing with contemporary medical treatment. Questions related to the ethical limitations of medical care date back to the time of Hippocrates, when physicians were taught that the goal of medicine was to relieve suffering and reduce the effects of disease by lending support to natural processes. Medicine was not intended for situations in which the body was overpowered by disease, since interventions might merely prolong the suffering. The accepted ethical stance recognized the limitations of medicine, and withheld treatments that held little potential for healing (Jecker, 1995).

The scientific era that began emerging in the seventeenth century fostered a change in this ethical stance. Rather than revering and working with natural processes, conquering and dominating nature became the goal of science. In the nineteenth century, as medicine began to align more with science and biologic causes for diseases were discovered, the goal of medicine became the conquest of disease by exercising power over nature. Jecker notes that ethical problems involving aggressive medical treatments where there is little likelihood of success or poor quality of expected outcomes "are the outgrowth of a scientific tradition whose mission is to control and dominate, whose proving ground is nature, and whose means is an unfailing faith in the scientific method" (1995, p. 144). Within this narrow focus of curing disease, ethical issues of personal quality of life and dimensions of suffering are often unrecognized and neglected. With their attention to healing and caring, nurses play an important role in calling attention to concerns that go beyond the narrow focus of curing.

Issues of Life, Death, and Dying

Ethical dilemmas faced in health care settings often relate to issues of and attitudes toward living and dying. Important questions that are deliberated by those involved include "When does life begin?," "When does life end?," "How can we be sure that someone has died?," and "Who decides?" Technology has stretched the boundaries and clouded the waters surrounding life's beginning and ending. Perspectives vary from the belief that life begins at conception to the view that it begins when an infant can survive outside the womb. Technology makes this discussion even more complex and raises questions such as "What happens when conception cannot occur 'naturally' and artificial processes are employed either in vivo or in vitro?" and "Is the laboratory embryo a life?"

Today, many low-birth-weight infants and those with certain birth defects, who would not have survived in prior eras, survive with the support of machines, medications, and surgical procedures. In the process, however, some babies are kept alive only to die after months of invasive and burdensome treatment. Others survive to face chronic health problems, with their associated financial, emotional, and physical strains on families and the health care system. There is no definitive way to predict which infants will have problems as they grow and develop. Dilemmas arise regarding how much effort to invest in "saving" a few infants who have a high probability of living only a short time or with significant health problems.

Ask Yourself

When Does Life Begin?

- What are your beliefs about when life begins? What shaped these beliefs?
- How should decisions regarding situations such as extremely low birth weight infants or infants born with serious intractable conditions, be made?
- Who should have a say in these kinds of decisions?
- How should diverse values be considered? Whose opinion counts? Who has the responsibility for the final decision, and why?
- If an infant will die without technology and the technology is withdrawn, do you consider that a natural or unnatural end of life? Why?

In our society, death has become an unnatural event, frequently associated with hospitals and other institutions, surrounded by tubes, machinery, and what are often labelled as heroic efforts. Determining when life ends has become a critical issue related to use of technology, prompting the involvement of courts in decision making. The general attitude, especially among health care providers, is that death is the enemy to be overcome or kept at bay for as long as possible, regardless of the age or health condition of the person. Thus death is often viewed as a failure on the part of the health care provider. It is understandable, therefore, that many health care providers have difficulty dealing with death as a possible outcome for patients, and find it a difficult topic to discuss. Another reason that the topic of death may be avoided is that discussing death requires us to face issues of meaning in life and anxieties and fears regarding our own mortality. However, lack of discussion of death as a possible outcome may lead families and patients to have unreasonable expectations and false hopes of what the system can offer. Demands for inappropriate interventions, or accusations that not enough was done, may arise from such situations. Patients and families need support in recognizing and honouring their responses, beliefs, and fears regarding death. By facing our own issues about death, we are better able to facilitate this process with patients and their families.

In many cultures, death is viewed as part of our life cycle that comes in its own time. Health care focused on curing is provided when there is reasonable hope of benefit, but people recognize when it is time for care to mean letting go and facilitating the transition through the dying process. In such cultures, dying often occurs at home, surrounded by family and friends.

Ask Yourself

What Are Your Views of Death and Dying?

What many people fear most regarding death is suffering and dying alone.

- How does technology contribute to this concern or attitude?
- What has your experience been related to death, what has shaped your attitudes regarding death, and what are your fears related to death?
- How can nurses minimize or deal with the effects of technology on patients in the dying process?
- How can nurses support patients and families in recognizing and honouring their own responses and beliefs regarding death?
- If machines and medication are keeping a body functioning, even if the person is apparently unaware, is that person still alive? Discuss your response.
- Do you think that brain wave activity in the midst of severe deterioration of major systems constitutes living? Discuss your response.

Personal attitudes prompt different expectations and scenarios when we are faced with decisions about heroic efforts and life-sustaining technologies. We must be aware of our own attitudes concerning living and dying, as well as the beliefs and expectations of patients, families, and other health care providers. Such awareness alerts us to situations in which there are differing attitudes among the parties involved, and provides an opportunity for opening lines of communication before a serious dilemma arises. Consider, for example, the patient who tells the nurse that he feels that his body is just giving up in spite of all the medications and treatments he is receiving, and he would like to go home to die peacefully, yet the physician is considering another surgery that is helpful about 30 percent of the time. In such a situation it would be important for the nurse to explore this area further with the patient, and either communicate his wishes to the physician or facilitate the patient's talking with the physician about his wishes.

CASE PRESENTATION

A Child with Leukemia

Lucia, a twelve-year-old child with leukemia, has relapsed in spite of routine chemotherapeutic interventions. This child has suffered the side effects of the treatment, including nausea, hair loss, and frequent hospitalizations with infections, and is deteriorating physically. She says she feels as if she is being tortured with all the needles, spinal taps, and bone marrow samples; that she has no friends; and that this kind of life is not worth living. A bone marrow transplant (the only hope for a cure at this point) would mean subjecting her to intensive chemotherapy, total body irradiation, and weeks in isolation following the transplant. The family is told that there is a forty percent chance that the transplant will be effective.

? Think About It

Factors Influencing Choices Regarding Medical Technology

- What factors do you think need to be considered in making the decision about having the bone marrow transplant?
- How do percentages of risk and benefit affect your decision making?
- In this situation, do you think a forty percent chance of success is enough to go ahead with the transplant? What if it were sixty percent? What about twenty percent?
- Consider a similar situation, but in the case of an elderly patient. Would you then think a forty percent chance is worth it? Why or why not? What has changed in your contemplation of the case?
- How can you help patients and families use statistical information in deliberating their decisions? What other factors would you help them to consider?
- Who should be involved in making this decision?

We must remember that dying is more than a medical occurrence; it is a spiritual process touching the individual, family, and community. Although medical interventions can assist and support those in the dying process, current technologies can prolong suffering by prolonging the dying process, and separate people from their families by actual physical barriers and institutionalization. Relieving suffering and supporting a dignified death are important elements of the nursing role. Nurses also can be instrumental in helping negotiate different views on what constitutes quality of life, and dignity in death, for individuals, families, and the medical and multidisciplinary team. Certainly, nurses play a significant role in helping patients and families understand the impact of technology on life and death as patients make decisions in a very difficult time.

Medical Futility

Ethical and legal arguments for initiating or discontinuing life-sustaining treatments are based primarily on the relative benefits and burdens for the patient. "Although many health care professionals feel reluctant to discontinue life-sustaining treatments, most philosophical and legal commentators find no important ethical or legal distinction between not instituting a treatment and discontinuing treatment already initiated" (Rushton, 1994, p. 517). Withholding or removing life-sustaining treatments in situations in which the burden or harm has been determined to outweigh the benefits is, in essence, allowing the person to die as a result of the natural progression of the illness process. This is different from **euthanasia**, which is causing the painless death of a person in order to end or prevent suffering. Curtin (1996) suggests that it is not reasonable to say that removal of artificial interventions cause death; rather, it is the condition (such as disease or accident), in response to which artificial interventions were initiated, that causes death.

In deliberations regarding withholding, initiating, or withdrawing life-sustaining interventions, **medical futility** related to the patient's situation has been discussed as a major factor. Medical futility refers to situations in which interventions are judged to have no medical benefit, or in which the chance for success is low. The Canadian Nurses Association defines futility as "a medical treatment that is seen to be non-beneficial because it is believed to offer no reasonable hope of recovery or improvement of the patient's condition" (Canadian Nurses Association, 2001, p. 1). Traditional views of medical futility have considered only the perspective of the physician in determining what constitutes a futile measure. Others have challenged or broadened this view by offering that the physician alone should not be the only one who can define an intervention, treatment, or outcome as futile or not (Somerville, 2000; Taylor, 1995, Wiejer, 1998). Taylor (1995, p. 301) suggests that futility can be considered in four different ways:

1. Not futile; beneficial to both physical and overall well-being;
2. Futile; non-beneficial to both physical and overall well-being;
3. Futile from the patient's perspective; medically indicated but not valued by the patient;
4. Futile from the clinician's perspective; valued by the patient but not medically indicated.

The fourth category, according to the Canadian Nurses Association, has sparked the most debate. Treatments and requests for treatments that fall into this category are those that are most difficult to negotiate and rationalize, when requested by the patient or family of the medical team. Understandably, a physician may be reticent to agree to provide treatment that is, from her or his perspective, futile. Lo (1995) suggests that there are strict definitions of futility that would justify unilateral decisions by physicians to withhold or withdraw interventions, and *loose,* value-laden definitions of the concept that would not justify such unilateral decisions.

Loose definitions of futility include situations that prompt variable interpretations and thus are more confusing—for example, situations in which the likelihood of success is very small; no worthwhile goals of care can be achieved; patient quality of life is unacceptable; and prospective benefit is not worth the resources required. In these situations, the meaning of futility must consider perceptions of the patient and family and judgments of the health care team. In the absence of clear external guidelines, these less clear situations require more skillful nursing care, as persons draw on their own understandings and resources shaped by personal beliefs and cultural values.

Somerville (2000) and others might respond to Lo's claim, stating that there should never be a situation in which a health care professional alone makes a decision regarding futility without consideration of the views of those mostly closely involved, the contexts of the situation, and the values and beliefs of the patient and family or support network. Making difficult decisions regarding the futility or utility of proposed or available medical treatments in complex health care situations requires that there is significant discussion and negotiation, with an emphasis on articulation of values and beliefs and negotiation of diversity.

In its 1999 publication, *The Joint Statement on Preventing and Resolving Conflicts Involving Health Care Providers and Persons Receiving Care,* the Canadian Nurses Association acknowledged the challenges of such negotiations, as well as the key advocacy and educational role that nurses play in such processes.

Futility is often discussed in relation to cardiopulmonary resuscitation (CPR), but it relates as well to interventions that preserve patients in persistent vegetative states or dependent on the technology of tertiary care settings. One difficulty associated with medical futility is that there is no set definition of the concept, only suggested parameters that vary greatly in guiding health care providers.

Ask Yourself

What Constitutes Medical Futility?

- Discuss what you consider to be the main ethical dilemmas involving the notion of futility.
- Would you consider an expensive treatment that works 20 percent of the time to be futile? What if it works only 5 percent of the time? Explain.
- Should medical futility be an issue when treatments are not expensive? Explain. If so, then is the issue really one of simply expense?
- Do you think a decision about futile treatment should be different with children and younger adults than with the elderly? Discuss your response. Consider the values and beliefs you may hold about age and quantity or quality of life.

Because personal values come into play, health care providers, patients, and families may have differing views of what is a benefit or burden. Because of the difficulty in defining and developing clear guidelines for medical futility, recent literature focuses less on the concept of futility, and more on the process of working with the patient and family to explain fully the medical circumstances, and negotiate care that is in the best interest of the patient. *The Joint Statement on Preventing and Resolving Conflicts Involving Health Care Providers and Persons Receiving Care* focuses on this very important process, emphasizing the roles that nurses can play (Canadian Nurses Association, 1999). For example, a patient or family may find hope and be willing to consider a treatment that has a 5 percent likelihood of success, while the health care providers see this as a futile effort. When considering quality of life, the perspective of the patient and family is essential in any determination of futility. Deciding when it is not worth continuing life-sustaining treatment is another circumstance in which the views of the parties involved may differ.

CASE PRESENTATION

Mr. Mason and His Son

Mr. Mason is a seventy-eight-year-old retired, widowed ironworker. He has been estranged from his adult son, an only child, for many years. He was recently diagnosed with advanced lung cancer. He recognized that he needed to make some plans for his immediate future, so he contacted his son and has appointed him power of attorney for personal care/substitute decision maker. Mr. Mason has now been admitted to your unit in severe pain. He is somewhat confused, and you are unable to elicit information from him about his wishes regarding life-sustaining measures. You note that his most recent chart entry indicates that he does not have a written advance directive or a "living will" prepared. You carefully begin discussing this difficult subject with his son, as it is your hospital's policy that everyone admitted to your oncology unit be informed about advance directives. Following are three possible twists this case could take, each of which is based on a real-life situation.

Ending 1. Mr. Mason's son begins to sob uncontrollably, saying, "I was never a very good son. I left home when I was barely nineteen and didn't even write or call for many years. I am just getting to know my dad, and now this happens. I want as much time with him as possible. He told me a few days ago that he was ready to die and didn't want to be kept alive on machines. But it is so unfair to me. I want him alive and more time with him. Please, do everything you can to keep him alive. I need some more time with him. I need for him to forgive me."

Ending 2. Mr. Mason's son seems impatient, continually looking at his watch as you talk to him. Finally, seeming exasperated, he says, "Look, I know he's going to die. I've worked through it already. I know he wouldn't want to suffer, but that's about it. After all, I don't think anyone in their right mind would choose to suffer, would they? Listen, I don't mean to sound cold, but we haven't been close over the years and I can't pretend to be upset. It isn't fair to me or to him. We've talked a bit about the financials and I am in the process of selling his house so I'll make sure his wishes about his money are respected. I've told my kids that basically, he's gone and I have no intention of bringing them in to see him. Anyways, he can't talk to anyone in this state. I'd like to just clean this up today, let him go in peace, and move on."

Ending 3. The son quickly acknowledges that he understands the question. Without hesitation he says, "Look I know you don't need to hear all this but we have been estranged for many years, mainly because of how horrible he was to my mother and me. He was barely around during my childhood and when he was, he was a tyrant. He's never apologized, never even tried to make it up. So I'm not sure why, now, I should be asked to be merciful to him. He has never showed us an ounce of mercy. So keep him alive. I'd like to give him some time to suffer and think about the things he has done."

Think About It

Family Reactions to Medically Futile Situations

- What would be your response to the son's statement in each of these scenarios? Include both your thinking response and your feeling response.
- How would your feelings lead you to advise one option over another?
- How do you think the nurse should react to each response?
- What values and dilemmas are evident in each scenario?
- Identify your personal and professional values related to each scenario.
- Who should make the decision? Do you feel conflicting loyalties?
- How would you respond to the son's decision and offer him additional support?

Economics and Medical Futility.   The cost of health care, particularly in relation to technology, has brought economic factors into discussions of futility. Some suggest that the principle of justice indicates that if a particular intervention is judged to be of limited or no benefit for one person, it should be discontinued so it is available for another patient who can make better use of the scarce resource. Lantos (1994) notes that political and economic developments in medicine in recent years, particularly in models such as the American medical system, have prompted physicians and hospitals to look more closely at futile treatments. With decreasing health care transfer payments from the federal government to each province and territory, institutions are forced to allocate resources and set priorities in all areas. Lantos suggests that it is ethical and justifiable for physicians to limit access to treatments that are expensive while offering limited benefits, and that, given limited health care resources, such decisions are socially responsible. Such an argument is consistent with utilitarian ethics, a perspective often used by government agencies when deciding about distribution of goods and services.

Ask Yourself

How Are Economics and Decisions About Medical Futility Related?

- Under what circumstances do you believe physicians or institutions should be able to limit a patient's access to expensive treatments?
- How do you think economics affects decisions about medical futility?
- How might patient care be affected by these decisions?

Do Not Resuscitate Orders

Cardiopulmonary resuscitation (CPR) is an area in which nurses have an active role in initiating or withholding life-sustaining treatment. Considering whether to initiate CPR with a patient requires attention to professional, ethical, legal, and institutional considerations. Principles utilized to justify decisions regarding resuscitation include autonomy, self-determination, nonmaleficence, and respect for persons.

The general practice regarding CPR is that it must be initiated unless (1) it would clearly be futile to do so, or (2) the practitioner has specific instructions not to do so. The legal definition of do not recuscitate (DNR) is not to initiate CPR in the event of a cardiac or pulmonary arrest. DNR orders are written directives placed in a patient's medical record indicating that the use of cardiopulmonary resuscitation is to be avoided. *The Joint Statement on Resuscitative Interventions* (1995, p. 1) states that "unless a specific order to the contrary (do not resuscitate [DNR] has been recorded on the person's health record by the responsible physician [CPR] has come to be used as a standard intervention in virtually all cases of sudden cardiac or respiratory arrest, whether unexpected or not." DNR orders should be documented immediately in a patient's health care record, noting the reason the order was written, who gave consent and who was involved in the discussion, whether the patient was competent to give consent or who was authorized to do so, and the time frame for the DNR order (Thibault-Prevost, Jensen, & Hodgins, 2000). In situations of the strict definitions of medical futility noted above, Lo (1995) suggests that decisions to withhold or stop CPR are appropriately made by physicians and that, in such situations, resuscitation need not be offered as an option for patients. Some suggest that nurses are as well qualified as physicians to write DNR orders. Because nurses are the professionals who are in close and continuous contact with patients, they are perhaps better able to help patients and families articulate their views regarding end-of-life care and concerns as well as negotiate terms of care with the multidisciplinary team. (Canadian Nurses Association, 2008; Martin & Redland, 1988; American Nurses' Association, 1992a; Thibault-Prevost, Jensen, & Hodgins, 2000). DNR decisions require open communication among the patient or surrogate, the family, and the health care team. This communication needs to include explicit discussion of the efficacy and desirability of CPR, balanced with the potential harm and suffering it may cause the patient. In addition to clear communication with the health care team and an understanding of the risks and benefits of CPR, patients must be attuned to their own values around resuscitation, and be aware of or inquire about existing institutional policies regarding CPR as well as their right to refuse such interventions. Their health care team must be clear about the fact that refusing CPR does not mean that other treatments, including palliative care, will be withdrawn or not available. These other treatments must be discussed, offered, and negotiated with patients, as they decision make about CPR and/or DNR orders (Canadian Nurses Association, 2008). People often overestimate the effectiveness of CPR, and do not understand that CPR is not always medically indicated. Many people derive their concept of CPR from what they see in the media. In their study of how CPR is portrayed on television, Diem, Lantos, and Tulsky (1996) discovered that rates of survival after CPR in television dramas were much higher than the most optimistic survival rates in the medical literature. In order to make informed decisions regarding CPR, patients and families need to understand their clinical condition and prognosis. People rarely appreciate that CPR is a harsh and traumatic procedure, and that patients with multiple, severe, chronic health problems who receive CPR rarely survive to discharge (Quill, 2000; Moss, 2001).

Tomlinson and Brody (1988) note that the relevance of considering the patient's or family's values in justifying DNR orders may vary, depending on the rationale given for the decision. In situations in which there would be no medical benefits, patient autonomy and consent may be considered less relevant. However, when rationale for the decision is based on the patient's quality of life, either after or before CPR, determination of whether the benefit of continued life outweighs the risk of harmful consequences, such as debility or suffering, must flow from the values of the patient or patient's proxy or substitute decision maker (SDM). Competent patients have the right to refuse CPR and may request DNR orders after they have been informed of the risks and benefits involved. Good communication is the most critical key factor in assuring that any DNR decision is acceptable to all parties involved.

CASE PRESENTATION

Mistaken Resuscitation

Jacob has had a chronic lung condition for the past ten of his thirty-two years. The condition causes some restrictions on his life, but he has kept up with a regular job and is very involved in his church. He is currently hospitalized with a severe respiratory infection. Although his condition did not seem to be that serious, when he was admitted he made sure that there was a DNR order in his chart. Because of a staff shortage, Lashanda, a registered nurse who usually works on another unit, has been assigned to Jacob's unit. Although she has been working on the other side of the unit, she is currently covering the whole unit while other staff are at lunch. As she answers a call light from Jacob's roommate, she notices that Jacob is not breathing and has no pulse. Since she is unfamiliar with Jacob's DNR request, she immediately calls a "code" and initiates CPR, figuring that there would be no question that this would be the appropriate action for someone of this age. Although Jacob is successfully resuscitated with no serious sequelae, he is intensely angry, saying that resuscitation, while successful, violated his rights.

Think About It

Decisions Regarding Resuscitation

- What do you think about Jacob's request for a DNR order? What ethical principles are involved in his choice?
- What do you think about Lashanda's response in the situation? Do you think she acted appropriately under the circumstances? What principles may have guided her actions?
- How do you think you might respond in a similar situation? What principles would guide your actions?
- Imagine yourself in Jacob's situation. How would you feel and why?
- What other strategies might a hospital unit use, in cases like these, in order to ensure patient's wishes are always followed?

DNR orders apply only to resuscitation. The fact that CPR might be considered futile does not necessarily imply that other life-sustaining interventions are futile or that other treatments will not be used. Health care providers often fail to make this distinction explicitly, thus causing confusion for patients as well. Many institutions require more specific instructions regarding what is and is not to be done for a patient. These interventions might include treatment of physiological abnormalities like fever or cardiac arrhythmias, nutrition, and hydration, provision of antibiotics, or use of mechanical ventilation. Plans for and parameters of DNR orders need to be discussed with all members of the health care team so that the goal of care and the patient's wishes are clear. The presence of DNR orders requires nurses to become even more focused on providing supportive and comfort interventions, and to ensure that there is no reduction in the level of care for the patient and family. A DNR order means only that, in the event of cardiac or respiratory arrest, there are to be no attempts to resuscitate. Presuming no arrest occurs, the patient may recover from the problem necessitating hospitalization and return home.

At a more philosophical level, Scofield suggests that decisions to not resuscitate ask us "individually and collectively, to arrive at a consensus on how to integrate death and decisions about it into the legitimating values of our moral universe. Deciding what kind of life we want involves deciding what kind of death we can face" (1995, p. 184). He notes that death, which was once considered fate, is now often a matter of a choice that we do not want to have to make. This is the dilemma that faces those involved in DNR decisions.

Nursing Considerations Related to DNR Orders. Although it is generally considered the domain of the physician to write a DNR order, nurses need to be aware of parameters surrounding such orders. Nurses need to know which patients under their care have DNR orders, and these orders need to be documented clearly in a patient's chart, and perhaps at the bedside, and reviewed periodically as the patient's condition changes and in adherence with institutional policies. If a patient or appropriate proxy or SDM indicates to the nurse the desire not to be resuscitated and there is no order in the chart, the nurse should document the request in the patient's chart and bring this to the immediate attention of the health care team. The nurse may wish to explore the request with the patient or proxy, and may need to facilitate discussion of the issue between patient and other members of the health care team. Orders should specify which interventions are to be withheld, and considerations regarding circumstances in which they are to be withheld. All persons involved in the care of the patient need to know about the orders. Since attitudes affect one's approach to others, nurses need to reflect on their own attitudes toward decisions regarding withholding of interventions, both in general and in particular patient situations, remembering that their priority should be to advocate for the patient's best interests.

Artificial Sources of Nutrition

Maintaining nutrition is a natural life-sustaining measure and a common part of the nursing role. Once a person has difficulty with functions associated with nutrition, such as chewing or swallowing, or is not conscious enough to participate in these activities, decisions about artificial sources of nutrition must be made. Ethical dilemmas arise concerning whether to classify such interventions as feeding or as medical treatments, as ordinary or extraordinary measures.

Utilizing artificial sources of nutrition may present dilemmas in situations involving persons in persistent vegetative states or end-stage dying processes for whom this intervention is maintaining physical life. We know that withholding food will eventually lead to starvation and death and, under most circumstances, is not considered an ethical action. However, it is considered appropriate to withhold or discontinue life-sustaining medical interventions when they are not benefiting the patient or are contrary to the patient's wishes. There are fewer complexities surrounding decisions to withhold artificial sources of nutrition than there are regarding decisions to withdraw medical interventions. However, as nutrition and hydration are considered by many people to constitute basic needs, and are considered in a highly emotional and value-based way, these kinds of decisions can be especially difficult for patients, families, and SDMs.

As with any such decision, we must consider the wishes of the patient or surrogate. Quality of life is an important factor, and if interventions contribute to, more than relieve, a patient's suffering, the principle of nonmaleficence may sway one toward a decision of not implementing or of discontinuing such therapies. Evidence suggests that tube feeding does not improve outcomes, and has substantial risks in some patients, particularly those with dementia or multisystem illness (Finucane, Christmas, & Travis, 1999; McCann, 1999; Moss, 2001). Curtin reflects that if a person is willing and able to eat and drink, even when death is imminent and the patient is suffering, attempts to quicken death by withholding ordinary nourishment is morally repugnant. However, "in situations in which death is inevitable and the conditions of living intolerable (involve extensive technological isolation from human touch, futile pain and pointless extensions of dying), highly sophisticated means of feeding are not in a patient's best interests and may be withheld or withdrawn" (1996, p. 82). Once artificial measures have been implemented, it is psychologically more difficult to decide on their removal. Curtin suggests that, unless a rational adult refuses them, such measures should be continued as long as sentient life is a reasonable expectation, but that they may be terminated when there is a reliable prediction of permanent unconsciousness. With any technological intervention we must consider whether its use is prolonging living or prolonging dying. When competent patients refuse food or fluid, respect for persons directs nurses to honour this refusal. Nurses need to help family and other caretakers understand that people who are dying often have a decline in appetite, and that the care of keeping the person comfortable does not need to include efforts to maintain nutrition. Involved parties may view the use of such interventions from different perspectives.

Legal Issues Related to Technology

As noted in Chapter 7, what is considered an ethical decision by some may not be upheld as a legal action. In the area of health care technology, the courts have intervened in some decisions related to withholding or withdrawing life-sustaining treatments when there has been disagreement among the involved parties. Legal precedents regarding issues such as what constitutes clear evidence of a person's wishes related to these treatments and what is considered standard practice have been set in the process. Examples of two such cases are presented here. When one looks at dilemmas faced by families, health care providers, institutions, and the legal system in situations such as these, the importance of having advance directives becomes evident. **Advance directives** are instructions indicating one's wishes regarding health care interventions or designating someone to act as a surrogate in making such decisions in the event that one loses decision-making capacity. The Canadian Nurses Association defines an advanced directive as "a document prepared by a competent person intended to direct the kind of treatment that a person will receive if he or she later becomes incompetent. The two basic forms of advance directives include instructional directives about particular treatments and directives that name a substitute decision maker" (Canadian Nurses Association, 2000, p. 3). Based on a respect for the autonomy of individuals, and the acknowledgment that individuals have the right to consent, an advance directive allows for persons to have their authentic and autonomous wishes known, even if they cannot articulate them (Canadian Nurses Association, 1994). Advance directives, when contained in a comprehensive document such as a living will, can provide health care teams with clear directions as well as ensure that family members are not conflicted over not having a clear idea of the patient's authentic wishes at the end of life (Singer, 1994, 2002). These directives are discussed further in Chapter 11.

Although the following two cases took place in the United States, they remain fundamental "benchmark" cases for discussions of the notion of advance directives. Note the use of the term "guardian *ad litem*." This term refers to a person who is appointed by a court to protect the best interests of another, in a very specific context only. In these two cases: a guardian *ad litem* acted to speak for these two women's best interests related to health care decision making.

CASE PRESENTATION

Karen Quinlan

The well known case of Karen Quinlan (Devettere, 1995; Pence, 1995) is a story of a twenty-one-year-old woman who, in 1975, was found to have suffered cardiopulmonary arrest at home alone after having been drinking at a local bar. After the ambulance crew restored heartbeat through CPR, she was admitted to the local hospital and placed on a ventilator. Within a few days she was transferred to a larger hospital where she was kept alive with the assistance of a respirator and feeding tube. Over months she lost weight, developed contractures, and was given no hope of regaining awareness. After much deliberation, the family asked that the respirator be discontinued, but the hospital indicated that it could not grant the request unless the father was named as her guardian. When the father asked the court to appoint him guardian with authority to make decisions to discontinue extraordinary interventions, the court appointed him guardian of her property, but not of her person, and appointed a **guardian *ad litem*** to represent Karen. The guardian *ad litem* felt responsible for preserving Karen's life, and opposed removing the respirator. The physician's lawyer argued that removing a respirator from a living person was not standard medical procedure, and the judge sided with this view. When the family appealed the ruling to the New Jersey Supreme Court, the decision of the lower court was reversed and the father was appointed as her guardian. When the father requested that the respirator be removed, the physicians initiated a process of weaning her from it, resulting in her being able to breathe without the machine. Totally unconscious with severe contractures, she was transferred to a nursing home, where she died ten years later.

CASE PRESENTATION

Nancy Cruzan

In another well known case, Nancy Cruzan (Angell, 1990; Annas, 1990; Pence, 1995) was found unconscious and not breathing after her car went into a ditch in the winter of 1983. Although emergency personnel restored her breathing, she never regained consciousness. After a year of being sustained through the use of a gastrostomy tube for artificial nutrition, it was determined that she was in a persistent vegetative state. When her parents, acting as her guardians, asked that the artificial feeding be discontinued because she had indicated previously that she would not want to be kept alive in this condition, the physicians and hospital refused. When the case went to court, the evidence supporting discontinuing the feeding was based primarily on a statement she had made to a roommate that she would not want to live if she were a vegetable. The judge ruled that the medical nutrition could be removed, but that decision was appealed to the Missouri State Supreme Court by a **guardian *ad litem***. The Missouri court reversed the previous

(Continued)

decision, claiming that there was no clear and convincing evidence that this would be her wish, that she was not terminally ill or suffering, and that there was no reason to act contrary to the state's interest in preserving life, regardless of how minimal that life had become. An appeal to the United States Supreme Court upheld the decision that medical nutrition could not be withdrawn because of the lack of clear and convincing evidence. In 1990, almost eight years after her accident, Nancy's parents appealed again to the local court with the evidence of three of her friends who stated that she had told them that she would not want to live in a vegetative state. At that time, the physician agreed that it was no longer in her best interests to be medically nourished, and the judge agreed that there was now clear and convincing evidence indicating that it was in her best interests to terminate artificial nutrition. Almost seven years after her automobile accident, Nancy Cruzan's artificial nutrition was discontinued in December 1990, and she died later that month.

Think About It

When the Courts Intervene

- As you reflect on these two cases, which position do you support, that of the family or that of the guardian *ad litem*?

- Which court decisions do you think are more valid? Defend your position.

- Describe ethical dilemmas and principles involved in these situations.

- If one of your family members was in a similar situation, how do you think you would respond? Would you expect solidarity or disagreement with this position from other members of your family?

- Consider that you are a nurse caring for Karen or Nancy at various stages in her situation. How would you respond to the various parties involved as decisions about her care are being discussed?

- What do you think about the role of the legal system in decisions regarding use of technology?

Palliative Care

Two primary obligations that we have to people who are dying are comfort and company (Moss, 2001). When life-sustaining interventions are no longer of benefit or are not desired by the patient, the focus of care becomes palliative, that is, directed toward comfort and support. **Palliative care** is comprehensive, interdisciplinary, and total care, focusing primarily on comfort and support of patients and families who face illness that is chronic or not responsive to curative treatment (Critchley et al., 1999; Billings, 2000; Moss, 2001). Palliative care focuses on the best quality of life for patient and family through meticulous control of pain and other symptoms, a personalized plan to optimize quality of life as defined by patient and family, and spiritual and psychosocial care. Palliative care requires delivery of coordinated and continuous services in home, hospice, skilled nursing facilities, or hospital, and includes support in bereavement. Members of the palliative care team include nurses, physicians, spiritual support persons, pharmacists, social services, mental health services, and pain services.

The backbone of palliative care is good nursing care that continues to support the dignity and self-respect of patient and family. In addition to providing care to the patient and the family, nurses often coordinate palliative care teams. When families are in disagreement about when it is time to stop other interventions and focus on palliative care, the nurse's ability to communicate effectively with and facilitate communication among those involved is crucial. Families often need time to see what we see regarding the patient's condition and expected outcomes of various interventions. We have to be willing to take as much time as necessary and as often as needed to explain and negotiate care decisions. Robin Shirley (personal communication, January 18, 2001) shares the following process that she uses in her role of palliative care nurse.

Palliative Care Conference

- Have a holistic view of the patient, including present health status, prognosis, significant relationships, living situation, family dynamics, decision-making capacity, advance directives or surrogate, and spiritual support.

- If the patient does not have decision-making capacity and there is no surrogate, seek to have a surrogate named.

- Prior to scheduling the conference, inform the surrogate that the purpose of the meeting is to determine the best way to provide quality end-of-life care to the patient and family, and stress the need for all family and significant persons, including spiritual support persons, to participate. The conference is set at a time when most people can be there. Primary nurse, physician, and other involved health care team members should be included.

- In opening the meeting, the palliative care nurse describes the process that will be followed in order to allow everyone an opportunity to speak and ask questions, and to arrive at a consensus regarding what is truly best for the patient.

- The meeting is opened by introducing everyone present and their role or relationship with the patient. In order to prevent disorder that can occur with the high emotions of the circumstances, those present are then asked one by one to name things that the patient enjoyed in life. This process also helps the physician and other care providers to step back from the clinical picture and see the patient as a person with individual values and meaning. Next, the physician is asked to discuss current status and prognosis, allowing an opportunity for family to ask any questions. The primary nurse is then asked to discuss daily care and interactions with the patient, and to respond to any questions. Through this process the family is often able to acknowledge that their loved one will not return to the state they once enjoyed, which leads to the beginning of acceptance and consideration of what is truly best for the patient at this time.

- Everyone in turn is then asked what they know or believe to be the desires of their loved one regarding end-of-life care. This includes the values of the patient, and what family members consider to be in the best interest. This process often prompts tears and reminiscing. Spiritual support persons may comment about the patient's spiritual values and considerations, or intervene as needed to support those participating.

- Throughout this process the palliative care nurse periodically restates what the general consensus of the group seems to be. This helps to clarify what is being said, and provides those not in agreement an opportunity to bring up concerns or issues. The meeting generally concludes with consensus regarding what is best for their loved one and discussion regarding comfort measures desired by the family and that the care providers feel will best suit the patient. (In some situations more than one meeting may be needed before consensus is reached.)

- All involved frequently join around the patient's bedside following the meeting for reminiscing. The family usually has open visitation, and are involved as much as they wish in care for the patient.

- Documentation of the process, participants, content, and outcomes is completed in the patient's record and ongoing follow-up is initiated.

Examples of Potential Dilemmas with Other Technology

In addition to life-sustaining interventions, advances in technology affect nursing and health care in other arenas as well. Examples of a few such technologies are briefly presented here. Nurses who work with patients whose care involves such technologies need to be aware of potential ethical issues associated with their use, as well as the benefits of such interventions. The intention here is to alert the student to some of the questions and dilemmas that may be associated with these technologies. The student is encouraged to explore these areas further, reflecting on personal values related to each technology.

Reproductive Technology.   Because the inability to conceive and bear children can be a very distressing experience for a couple, any technology that can facilitate the process may well be viewed as a life-affirming gift for those who have a strong desire to bear children, but cannot. Such technologies include artificial insemination by donor, in vitro fertilization, and surrogate embryo transfer. While scientists develop and refine these technologies to benefit people, ethicists and others raise questions related to moral implications of their use. Some questions focus on the potential for changing society's concept of family and parenthood. For example, in the case of surrogacy, is the mother of the baby the woman whose ovum is joined with her partner's sperm, or the woman who donates her body for the baby's development and birth? We must consider whether the use of such technologies might relegate childbearing into little more than the production of a product. Yet, we must also consider that the product, a viable pregnancy and child, is often welcomed by many who have few options available to them. Other ethical questions arise regarding who has custody of frozen embryos, and whether these embryos have rights. These considerations relate to ideas, values, and beliefs that individuals hold regarding the beginning of life. While these values and beliefs are often deeply held, they vary significantly between individuals and groups. This accounts for much of the heated debates around these issues, at individual, community, and government levels. A related consideration is the potential that women may become more exploited than liberated by the use of these technologies. The issue of stem cell research is a hot topic of debate. Until 1992, there were no overarching policies regulating stem cell research in Canada. In 2002, the Canadian Institutes of Health Research (CIHR) published guidelines for human pluripotent stem cell research. Pluripotent stem cells refer to cells that are capable of giving rise to most other cell types or tissues of the human body. The Institutes also integrated guiding principles into the ***Tri-Council Policy Statement on Ethical Conduct for Research Involving Humans***. This document makes up the federal guidelines for the conduct of research in Canada.

Genetic Diagnosis, Engineering, and Screening.   Advances in molecular biology, new reproductive technologies, and the Human Genome Project have prompted rapid breakthroughs in genetic research. This research has advanced our knowledge of the use of genetic interventions as possible remedies for diseases caused by genetic disorders. The possibilities of these interventions, however, raise ethical as well as legal and social justice questions (Frankel & Chapman, 2000). **Genetic diagnosis,** which is usually done within an in vitro fertilization program, involves a process of biopsy of embryos to determine the presence of genetic flaws and gender prior to implantation. At present, such diagnosis is aimed at couples who have a high risk of conceiving a child with a serious genetic disorder, with the intent that only embryos that are free of genetic flaws would be implanted. **Genetic engineering** is the ability to alter organisms genetically for a variety of purposes, such as developing more disease-resistant fruits and vegetables, or eventually being able to alter embryos genetically so that the fetus and baby will be healthier. Through **genetic screening** it is possible to determine if persons are predisposed to certain diseases, and whether couples have the possibility of giving birth to a genetically impaired infant. The implications of having such technologies available include the potential for correcting some genetic defects in embryo, eliminating some very serious genetic diseases, and producing food that is more nourishing and resilient. Frankel and Chapman (2000) make a distinction between the therapeutic use of these interventions, and the possibility that these interventions may be used to modify human characteristics beyond those that are needed to sustain or restore health. The possibility of their use to enhance certain human characteristics has significant social implications. For example, such interventions could offer control over the genetic inheritance, including the biological properties and personality traits of our children. They suggest that the ability to discard "undesirable" traits and improve those that are "desirable" may lead to a form of **eugenics**, meaning "good birth." The eugenics movement of the early twentieth century sought to promote traits that proponents felt were desirable for society, while weeding out what they considered undesirable. Around the world, eugenics led to efforts to discourage procreation among people deemed to be "socially inferior" through compulsory sterilization of many people, particularly those who were poor, in prison, or in mental institutions. Another concern that these authors raise is that these technologies may lead to the imposition of a skewed or harmful definition of what is normal regarding human traits, and what is considered abnormal or undesirable. Because individuals and societies tend to impose their values and standards on others, this could lead to serious transcultural implications.

Concerns related to these technologies are as varied as their potential benefits, particularly the recognition that relaxing criteria related to a person's value or rights in one arena may lead to abuses or exploitation in other circumstances. Ethicists often speak of these concerns in terms of a *slippery slope* where, for example, one decision based on relaxing criteria supporting the value of human life makes it easy to slide into acceptance of lower standards as ethical guides. For example, one concern is that genetic engineering might produce organisms that could be harmful to humans; another is that employers or insurers might use information gained from genetic screening to exclude people with particular traits from certain jobs or from being insured. Might genetic screening and diagnosis lead to abuses, such as forbidding people with certain traits to have children, insurers refusing to cover expenses if insured mothers give birth to genetically impaired infants, or prohibiting the birth of babies with particular genetic features deemed undesirable by those in power in a society? These areas include other broad societal implications, such as who pays for the procedures, who determines guidelines for their use, and to whom they are made available.

Organ and Tissue Procurement and Transplantation. Organ transplantation is no longer considered as extraordinary or uncommon a health care event as it was in the not too distant past. As techniques become more refined, the possibility of a transplant becomes a hope for more and more people afflicted with the failure of a vital organ. Because the demand for organs is great and the supply limited, dilemmas related to allocation of scarce resources emerge. Questions arise regarding eligibility of recipients for organ transplant. Should these determinations be made based on a potential recipient's expectation of survival posttransplant, or power and prestige, or some combination of these and other factors? Transplantation may involve organs from dead or living human donors, animals, or artificial appliances, and there are dilemmas associated with each. Our discussion focuses on human donor issues.

Because transplantation requires well-nourished organs, procurement must occur as soon after death as possible. Thus, having criteria for determining when death occurs is imperative. Irreversible cessation of cardiopulmonary functioning is one such criterion. If a person has been maintained on life support technology, brain death is the most likely criteria to be used, which leads to issues regarding what constitutes brain death. Some suggest that current criteria for brain death which indicate that all functions of the entire brain must cease are more stringent than necessary, and that irreversible cessation of higher brain functions would be sufficient criteria. Additionally, adherence to a strict brain-death-only donation criteria has often been blamed for the lack of available organs for donation. Currently, the percentage of hospital deaths resulting from brain death are estimated at one to three percent. Using other criteria, such as cardiac death, has been a subject of much debate in Canada. After the criteria for brain death was published in 1968, (Ad Hoc Committee of the Harvard Medical School to Examine the Definition of Brain Death), all organ donations in Canada were from persons who met this criteria. However in 2006, the Ottawa Hospital announced that it had carried out an organ donation from a patient following cardiac death, or donation after cardiac death (DCD), formerly known as non-heart-beating organ donations (NHBD). This is, as Doig (2006) notes, "a major change in end-of-life practice and poses significant ethical problems for end-of-life decision-making in intensive care units (ICUs)" (p. 206). Worries over the lack of definitive criteria for cardiac death and the notion of reversibility of cardiac death have fuelled the debate and the reluctance of some provinces and institutions to carry out DCD.

The topic of DCD has been debated actively at a number of forums, sponsored by the Canadian Council for Donation and Transplantation, which has publicly noted that the option of DCD should move forward, in particular contexts with significant ethical guidance and intensive education (2005).

The scarcity of available organs and the long waiting lists of potential recipients raise the possibility that people may be declared dead prematurely in cases of both DBD and DCD. This scarcity of organs also affects organ procurement from living human beings. With living donors, issues related to voluntary informed consent and the buying and selling of organs are of concern. There are places in the world where organs are taken from people who are living in extreme poverty or from prisoners, without their knowledge or against their will, and sold to procurement centres in more affluent countries. Desperate straits have prompted some individuals to sell an organ to raise money for personal or family needs, raising a question about whether there can be true voluntary informed consent under such circumstances.

In cases of sudden accidental death, family members may be asked to consider donation of viable organs. Consider whether there can be true voluntary consent when the family is in the midst of crisis and shock. With the urgency for a decision due to time factors for harvesting organs, coercion could be a factor. In many settings, nurses function as transplant coordinators and are asked to approach patients or families about considering organ donation. In such situations these nurses are often trained to be clear about their own feelings regarding organ procurement and transplantation, and to attend to the needs of the families while also considering the constraints of organ harvesting.

NURSING PRACTICE IN THE MIDST OF TECHNOLOGY

Nursing practice continues to evolve with expanding knowledge and scientific advances in many arenas. As technology has been developed and refined, related nursing responsibilities have expanded. In the midst of these changes, the essence of nursing remains the human focus of caring for patients and families—being attentive to the needs of persons whose lives are affected by the technology. Integrating caring and technology and juggling the demands of each present challenges for nurses in any area of practice. As new technologies become available, they will bring with them associated issues of concern. Regardless of the technology, important considerations for nursing relate to attitudes and values, communication, and maintaining the human focus of care.

Attitudes and Values

The importance of self-awareness related to values, beliefs, and reactions is especially significant when dealing with issues related to technology. The process of being more attentive to personal perspectives regarding such issues as quality of life, living, dying, medical futility, and allocation of scarce resources may be facilitated by pondering questions such as those posed throughout this chapter. Such awareness enables the nurse to differentiate personal values from those of patients and others involved in the situation. Principles of self-determination and autonomy counsel the nurse to understand that individuals may judge benefits of an intervention from varying perspectives. Recognizing where personal values may be different enables nurses to be more attentive to fostering good communication, encouraging others to make their own decisions, avoiding judgment about the rightness or wrongness of the decision based on personal values, and accepting those decisions if they are different from what the nurse would do.

As the various examples presented in this chapter suggest, many dilemmas that emerge surrounding technology relate to differing values among the parties involved. Facilitating discussion of values among patients and families may help them to clarify their own perspectives. Nurses also need to be alert to situations in which there may be differences in values among the patient, family physician, or other health care team member. Encouraging timely communication may avert a major dilemma, or facilitate more effective resolution of the concern. Nurses who cannot reconcile their values with a particular situation need to take the necessary steps to remove themselves from that situation so as to not compromise patient care or personal integrity. In so doing, it is essential to avoid abandoning the patient by ensuring that there are others who will provide the needed care for the patient.

The Importance of Communication: Who Decides?

As has been noted, there are many factors involved in making decisions about withholding or withdrawing life-sustaining treatments and utilizing other technologies. Nurses need to determine who is involved in making the decision, and how the nurse fits into the scenario. Utilizing the decision-making process described in Chapter 6 may assist in this process. Nurses need to be aware of institutional policies and protocols regarding various technologies. Such policies should include approaches to reaching decisions about particular patients; ways of dealing with conflicts that may arise; protection of patient rights; description of roles of those involved in the decision-making process; and directions for documenting the decision in the patient's chart. In most situations, the patient or the patient's SDM has the ultimate authority to decide which interventions to use or withhold.

Because nurses are in close and continual contact with patients, they are often perceived as more available and more approachable than physicians. Patients or family members may discuss their concerns about interventions more readily with the nurse, seeking information or advice. It is important to know what they have been told by the physician, determine the patient's and family's level of understanding about the situation, and whether they have the necessary information to make an informed decision. If information is needed in such areas as risks, discomforts, side effects, potential benefits, likelihood of success, or treatment alternatives, advocating for the patient in this regard is an expected nursing response. Nurses are in a key position to utilize conversations with patients and families to discover areas of confusion and to elicit information about the patient's wishes regarding interventions.

Sometimes people just need to talk out their concerns and sort through sometimes conflicting messages. Providing a listening presence can help people vent emotions, speak their fears, and clarify their concerns. At times the concern may be such that the nurse must advocate for the patient by facilitating communication with the physician or other support persons, such as family members, a patient representative, or a member of the ethics committee. Collaboration among all involved is important to ensure an informed choice. Effective communication can be facilitated by providing an environment that is not rushed; using terms and language that are understood by the other person and avoiding "medical-ese"; allowing time for and encouraging questions; practising attentive listening; and offering a caring presence.

Caring: The Human Focus

In the context of expanding scientific and technological knowledge, nurses have the responsibility for helping patients and families benefit from what technology offers, while always remembering the human focus of care. Davis (1991) suggests that when medical treatment is deemed futile, nursing care in its fullest meaning is most essential. This is evident especially in nursing's role in palliative care. However alert, and in whatever stage of living and dying, an individual has a life story that continues to unfold, a story that continues to intertwine with lives of others. In the midst of the technology, nurses can encourage family and loved ones to talk with, touch, and be in touch with the patient. In this way nurses acknowledge the primary importance of relationships, even in a health care setting filled with machines, noises, and other evidences of advanced technology.

Attention to the human focus includes helping patients and families become more comfortable with the sometimes formidable array of machines and equipment, and make sense of the large amounts of clinical data that are generated. Incorporating family members in caring for the patient provides time for connecting and observing the patient in both good and bad moments, and engenders a more realistic view of the patient's condition. Rather than engendering anxiety and mistrust by shutting the family out of the patient's life and experiences at critical moments, nurses should encourage them to share directly in the patient's journey. This provides families more experiences upon which to base hard decisions.

The nursing role of providing care and comfort is paramount in any health care setting, and has many facets. It may take the shape of explaining, as often as necessary, the purpose and problems related to interventions. Caring requires that the nurse see the experience from another's point of view, so that questions, fears, concerns, and frustrations may be addressed appropriately. Providing care and comfort also requires that the nurse support and encourage behaviours that enable patients and families to choose in accordance with their own beliefs and values. Being proficient in technical skills with the intent of doing what is best for the patient is part of human care, as is the ability to be with and wait with persons as they struggle through difficult situations.

SUMMARY

Many of the major ethical dilemmas encountered by nurses and other health care providers today are associated with advances in scientific knowledge and technology. In order to recognize and to deal with such dilemmas, nurses need to clarify their own values, and to appreciate differences in values among the various people involved in making patient care decisions. The potential of technology has raised very deep questions about life and death that must be addressed on individual, professional, and societal levels. Issues of quality of life, relief of suffering, and futility of interventions are some facets of these questions. Decisions about when to intervene and reasonable goals of interventions are made more difficult because of varying perceptions of the value of such interventions, nondefinitive outcomes, and issues related to availability of interventions. Principles of beneficence, nonmaleficence, justice, and autonomy provide the basis for arguments on different sides of issues related to technology. Nurses must take into account their responsibilities to patients and the profession, as well as personal integrity, when dealing with ethical dilemmas engendered by technology. Nurses must remember that, in the midst of the technology with its associated dilemmas, there are persons who need the human focus of care that is basic to nursing practice.

CHAPTER HIGHLIGHTS

- The use of technology in health care has prompted the need to address important ethical questions regarding life, death, and allocation of resources.

- Utilization of health care technology may give rise to conflicts between the principles of beneficence and nonmaleficence.

- Appropriate utilization of health care technologies requires that health care providers, patients, and families understand the purposes, benefits, and limitations of specific technologies.

- Attitudes and beliefs concerning life and death affect how health care providers, patients, families, and the legal system approach issues related to health care technology. Ethical dilemmas may arise when there are differing opinions related to the use of technology among the parties involved.

- Determination of medical futility is an important consideration in decisions to withhold or withdraw life-sustaining interventions. Ethical decisions regarding these measures require consideration of whether they are prolonging living, or prolonging dying.

- Economics may factor into decisions related to medical futility, availability of technology, and accessibility to many interventions.

- Withholding or withdrawing life-sustaining treatments in situations in which the burden or harm has been determined to outweigh the benefits constitutes allowing a person to die, and is not euthanasia. Dilemmas may arise regarding whether to classify the use of specific interventions as ordinary or extraordinary measures. The courts have sometimes been involved in making this determination.

- Patient self-determination and distributive justice must be considered in decisions regarding technology. Vigilance is required to ensure that people are not harmed, exploited, controlled, discriminated against, or excluded from care by the use of health care technologies.

- Nurses are in a key position to help patients and families articulate their preferences regarding technological interventions, and to facilitate communication with other health team members in this regard. This role requires familiarity with patient and family decisions and institutional policies regarding life-sustaining interventions, and awareness that when medical care is deemed futile, nursing care in its fullest meaning is most essential.

DISCUSSION QUESTIONS AND ACTIVITIES

1. Develop advance directives for yourself, considering interventions you would choose and parameters regarding these choices. Discuss and compare your directives with classmates.

2. Go on-line and download a living will from the Joint Centre for Bioethics at the University of Toronto (www.jointcentreforbioethics.ca/tools/livingwill.shtml). Critically examine the document to see if it addresses all your wishes and choices, were you completing it.

3. Discuss your beliefs regarding determinants of the beginning and end of life.

4. Describe quality of life as it relates to health care decisions.

5. Discuss potential *slippery slope* elements related to reproductive and genetic technologies, and organ procurement and transplantation.

6. Plan and engage in a debate in your class focused on economic and justice issues related to health care technologies.

7. Observe several patients who are receiving technological interventions, and note how the technology is affecting them and their families; issues surrounding its use; the focus of nursing care; and your reaction to the situation. Describe strengths of the nursing care you observe, and aspects that you might do differently if you were providing care. Talk to nurses and patients regarding the impact of technology on their health and care.

8. Discuss your view about nurses writing DNR orders.

9. How would you handle a situation where you feel the physician's decision regarding life-sustaining interventions is inappropriate for your patient?

10. Choose one of the topics discussed in this chapter and explore the websites of the CNA, and the ICN regarding policies or positions statements on this issue. You may include information from other disciplines as well. Compare and contrast positions of the various organizations. Discuss your views about this issue, and how they compare with the positions of the professional organizations.

    CNA—http://www.cna-nurses.ca

    ICN—http://www.icn.ch

11. Role-play a palliative care conference with students in the class, using a real or hypothetical patient case situation.

REFERENCES

Ad Hoc Committee of the Harvard Medical School to Examine the Definition of Brain Death. (1968). A definition of irreversible coma. *Journal of the American Medical Association,* 205: 337–40.

American Nurses' Association (1992a, April 2). Position statement: Nursing care and do-not-resuscitate decisions. Author. Retrieved January 7, 2001, from http://www.nursingworld.org/readroom/position/ethics/etdnr.htm.

American Nurses' Association (1992b, April 2). Position statement: Forgoing nutrition and hydration. Author. Retrieved January 7, 2001, from http://www.nursingworld.org/readroom/position/ethicsetnutr.htm.

Angell, M. (1990). Prisoners of technology: The case of Nancy Cruzan. *New England Journal of Medicine, 322*, 1226–1228.

Annas, G. J. (1990). Nancy Cruzan and the right to die. *New England Journal of Medicine, 323*, 670–672.

Billings, J. A. (2000). Palliative care: Recent advances. *British Medical Journal, 321*, 555–558.

Canadian Nurses Association. (1994). Joint statement on advance directives. Retrieved January 2, 2009, from http://www.cna-aiic.ca/CNA/documents/pdf/publications/PS20_Advance_Directives_Sept_1994_e.pdf.

Canadian Nurses Association. (1995). *Joint statement on resuscitative interventions.* Approved by the Canadian Healthcare Association, the Canadian Medical Association, the Canadian Nurses' Association, the Catholic Health Association of Canada, and in collaboration with the Canadian Bar Association. Ottawa: Authors.

Canadian Nurses Association. (1999). Joint statement on preventing and resolving conflicts involving health care providers and persons receiving care. Ottawa: Author.

Canadian Nurses Association. (2000). End-of-life issues. Retrieved January 2, 2009, from http://www.cna-aiic.ca/CNA/documents/pdf/publications/PS43_End_of_Life_Issues_Nov_2000_e.pdf.

Canadian Nurses Association. (2001). *Futility presents many challenges for nurses.* Ethics in Practice series paper. Ottawa: Author.

Canadian Nurses Association. (2008). *Standards and best practices: CPR.* Retrieved January 2, 2009, from http://www.cna-aiic.ca/CNA/practice/standards/cpr/default_e.aspx.

Critchley, P., Jadad, A. R., Taniguchi, A., Woods, A., Stevens, R., Reyno, L., & Whelan, T. J. (1999). Are some palliative care delivery systems more effective and efficient than others? A systematic review of comparative studies. *Journal of Palliative Care, 15*(4), 40–47.

Curtin, L. (1996). *Nursing: Into the 21st century.* Springhouse, PA: Springhouse.

Davis, A. J. (1991). Ethical issues in nursing research: My own experience. *Western Journal of Nursing Research, 13*, 414–415.

Devettere, R. J. (1995). *Practical decision making in health care ethics: Cases and concepts.* Washington, DC: Georgetown University Press.

Diem, S. J., Lantos, J. D., & Tulsky, J. A. (1996). Cardiopulmonary resuscitation on television. *New England Journal of Medicine, 334*(24), 1579–1582.

Doig, C. J. (2006). Is the Canadian health care system ready for donation after cardiac death? A note of caution. *Canadian Medical Association Journal, 175*(8), 905–906.

Farquhar, M. (1995). Definitions of quality of life: A taxonomy. *Journal of Advanced Nursing, 22*, 502–508.

Finucane, T. E., Christmas, C., & Travis, K. (1999). Tube feeding in patients with advanced dementia. *Journal of the American Medical Association, 282*(14), 1365–1370.

Frankel, M. S., & Chapman, A. R. (2000). *Human inheritable genetic modifications: Assessing scientific, ethical, religious, and policy issues.* Washington, DC: The American Association for the Advancement of Science.

Jecker, N. S. (1995). Knowing when to stop: The limits of medicine. In J. H. Howell & W. F. Sale, eds., *Life choices: A Hastings Center introduction to bioethics* (pp. 139–148). Washington, DC: Georgetown University Press.

Lantos, J. D. (1994). Futility assessments and the doctor-patient relationship. *JAGS, 42*, 868–870.

Lo, B. (1995). *Resolving ethical dilemmas: A guide for clinicians*. Baltimore: Williams & Wilkins.

McCann, R. (1999). Lack of evidence about tube feeding: Food for thought. *Journal of the American Medical Association, 282*(14), 1381.

Martin, D. A., & Redland, A. R. (1988). Legal and ethical issues in resuscitation and withholding of treatment. *Critical Care Nurse, 10*, 1–8.

Moss, A. H. (2001). What's new? Progress in palliative care, CPR, and advance directives. Seminar at Raleigh General Hospital, Beckley, WV. January 18, 2001.

Pence, G. E. (1995). *Classic cases in medical ethics*. New York: McGraw-Hill.

Quill, T. E. (2000). Initiating end-of-life discussions about seriously ill patients: Addressing the "elephant in the room." *Journal of the American Medical Association, 284*(19), 2502–2507.

Roberts, D. (2000). Race, gender, justice, and reproductive health policy. Presentation at *New century, new challenges: Intensive bioethics course XXVI*, Kennedy Institute of Ethics, Georgetown University, Washington, DC, June 9, 2000.

Rushton, C. H. (1994). Guidelines on forgoing life-sustaining medical treatment. *Pediatric Nursing, 20*, 517–521.

Scofield, G. R. (1995). Is consent useful when resuscitation isn't? In J. H. Howell & W. F. Sale, eds., *Life choices: A Hastings Center introduction to bioethics* (pp. 172–187). Washington, DC: Georgetown University Press.

Singer, P. A. (1994). Advance directives in palliative care. *Journal of Palliative Care, 10*(3), 111–116.

Singer, P. A. (2002). *Living will*. Toronto: University of Toronto Joint Centre for Bioethics.

Somerville, M. A. (2000). *The ethical canary science, society and the human spirit*. Toronto: Viking.

Taylor, C. (1995). Medical futility and nursing. *Image: Journal of Nursing Scholarship, 27*(4): 301–306.

Thibault-Provost, J., Jensen, L. A., & Hodgins, M. (2000). Critical care nurses' perceptions of DNR orders. *Journal of Nursing Scholarship, 32*(3), 259–265.

Tomlinson, T., & Brody, H. (1988). Ethics and communication in do-not-resuscitate orders. *New England Journal of Medicine, 318*, 43–46.

Weijer, C. (1998). Cardio pulmonary resuscitation for patients in a persistent vegetative state: Futile or acceptable. *Canadian Medical Association Journal, 158*(4), 491–493.

SUGGESTED READINGS

Devettere, R. J. (1995). *Practical decision making in health care ethics: Cases and concepts*. Washington, DC: Georgetown University Press.

Howell, J. H., & Sale, W. F., eds. (1995). *Life choices: A Hastings Center introduction to bioethics*. Washington, DC: Georgetown University Press.

Jonsen, A. R., Veach, R. M., & Walters, L., eds. (1998). *Source book in bioethics: A documentary history*. Washington, DC: Georgetown University Press.

Pence, G. E. (1995). *Classic cases in medical ethics*. New York: McGraw-Hill.

CHAPTER 11

Practice Issues Related to Patient Self-Determination

OBJECTIVES

After completing this chapter, the reader should be able to:

1. Discuss autonomy and paternalism as they relate to patient self-determination.

2. Describe factors that may threaten autonomy in health care settings and situations in which autonomy may be limited.

3. Examine the interaction of justice and autonomy.

4. Discuss informed consent as it relates to patient self-determination.

5. Examine legal and ethical elements of informed consent.

6. Describe the nursing role and responsibilities related to informed consent.

7. Discuss the place of advance directives in health care decisions.

8. Discuss patient autonomy related to choices for life and health.

9. Describe the nursing role and responsibilities related to patient lifestyle and health choices.

10. Describe confidentiality in relation to health care choices.

INTRODUCTION

The role of the patient and that of the health care practitioner, and the implied responsibilities of each, have varied throughout history and in different cultures. In some cultures, decisions regarding "what is best" for the patient are deferred to the health care practitioner, who is presumed to know what will bring about healing. Indeed, until recent years, the physician was often viewed in this light. Such paternalism, even well meaning, has been challenged in recent years, and greater emphasis has been placed on the role and rights of patients in making health care decisions. This chapter focuses on practice issues related to patient self-determination. Discussion of these issues includes both ethical and legal components, and is intertwined with issues of technology and economics.

AUTONOMY AND PATERNALISM

Self-determination derives from the principle of autonomy. **Autonomy**, which is discussed in detail in Chapter 3, denotes having the freedom to make choices about issues that affect our life and to make decisions about personal goals. Autonomy, which means self-governing, implies respect for persons, the ability to determine personal goals and decide on a plan of action, and the freedom to act on the choices made. The value placed on the primacy of the individual implicit in autonomy is primarily a westernized concept, and may not be fully accepted in other, less liberal, cultures. Sherwin (1992) suggests that the notion of autonomy is more than a sense of an isolated self, and must include an appreciation for the self in relation to others, recognizing that choices are made in the context of community. Implications of this view for autonomy within the context of health care include viewing patients as members of a social world, in which health care decisions affect others and are made in conjunction with trusted persons.

Factors that may threaten autonomy in health care settings include a prevailing paternalistic attitude that promotes the dependent role of the patient; assumptions that a patient's values and thought processes are the same as those of the health care provider; failure to appreciate a difference in knowledge level regarding health matters; and a focus on technology rather than caring. Persisting paternalistic attitudes have contributed to increased numbers of patients and families struggling with health care providers over control of health care decisions. **Paternalism** "derives from the privileges associated with the patriarchal family, where fathers are granted the right and responsibility to use their supposedly superior knowledge and judgment to make decisions on behalf of other family members" (Sherwin, 1992, p. 138). Paternalism implies well-intended actions of benevolent decision making, leadership, protection, and discipline. In the health care arena paternalism manifests in the making of decisions on behalf of patients without their full consent or knowledge. Although the principle of beneficence suggests that decisions are focused on the patient's well-being, the power inherent in such a hierarchical arrangement can be abused, and decisions made may reflect the interests of those other than the patient. Consider, for example, many elderly patients in nursing homes who are routinely sedated "for their own protection" because of "agitation and confusion." It is worth pondering whether medication used in this way is for the benefit of the patient, or to make life easier for the staff.

CASE PRESENTATION

Who Should Decide What Is Best?

Maureen is a thirty-eight-year-old woman with a diagnosis of multiple sclerosis (MS). She has had MS since her early twenties and has managed her life with the progressive disease, getting married, having a child, and establishing herself in a career as a counsellor at a local youth shelter. She is also actively involved in her local MS Society and is a strong advocate for living independently with the disease.

Over the past two years, her condition has markedly worsened. She can no longer carry out her activities of daily living nor can she drive or work. She has a daily caregiver in her home to assist her with self-care as well as the care of her four-year-old child. Her mother also helps out a great deal, but finds that it is difficult as she is seventy-two and has advanced arthritis herself. Maureen's husband, a financial planner, works long hours and is feeling the strain of caring for her when her respite worker is not present. In the past two weeks, she has had episodes of forgetfulness and has had one serious fall. She has had to call her husband to come home early from evening meetings to help her with the care of their daughter. The caregiver has told Maureen's husband that she no longer considers the situation to be a safe one, either for Maureen or her daughter.

Maureen's neurologist has informed her that the disease is especially aggressive in her case and that she is no longer eligible, because of the progression, for a new experimental drug, which she was hoping she could try as part of a clinical trial, which offers a great deal of potential hope for those with MS.

Her husband, John, and Maureen's mother, approach her along with her neurologist to discuss the option of being in a residence. They assure her that it would be better for her, her daughter, and her husband. He would not be worried about her when he was at work. Her daughter would be cared for by a nanny, her grandmother, and her father, and would be brought frequently to visit with Maureen. The residence that they have researched caters to younger clients and is close to home. They could decorate the unit to Maureen's taste and they emphasize, she would be able to receive twenty-four-hour care there.

Maureen is very upset when they discuss this with her. She accuses them of "conspiring" against her and tells them that she is "not dead yet" nor is she "unable to make her own decisions." She adamantly refuses to consider this option, stating that she wishes to be home with her daughter and that there is nothing wrong with the current situation, with a few adaptations. She states that it appears that they have not considered other options. She is also angry that her physician is part of the discussion and appears to have already discussed it with her husband and mother, out of her presence.

Think About It

- Are John and Maureen's mother being paternalistic? Why or why not?
- Is Maureen's neurologist being paternalistic? What are the implications for his involvement in the discussion, from an ethical perspective?
- What ethical issues are evident in this case?
- What ethical issues do you think are relevant to the discussion of this case?
- Are there any other options that might be possible in this case?
- What do you think should happen next?
- What kinds of things should be considered in the discussion of Maureen's immediate future?

Inherent in the authoritarian medical model is the "belief that neither patients nor health care professionals other than physicians possess the appropriate skills and capacities to exercise decision-making power. In particular, patients (and their guardians) are thought to be too uneducated, too emotionally distraught, or too stupid to make adequate decisions in the face of illness" (Sherwin, 1992, p. 145). What this attitude does not address, however, is that decisions about health require more than scientific expertise. Such decisions must take into account factors such as the patient's values, culture, spiritual and other beliefs; evaluation of risks, benefits, and economic considerations; and effects on lifestyle and role. All the factors need to be considered within the context of the patient's life. For this to occur, patients must be engaged in the decision-making process as autonomous agents in relationship with others who can facilitate the decision-making processes.

How Far Does Autonomy Go?

Although the principle of autonomy has become a key consideration in health care ethics, it does have limits. Practitioners are not obligated to honour requests from patients or families for interventions that, in the best judgment of the practitioner, are outside accepted standards of care or that are contrary to the practitioner's own ethical views. Autonomy may also be limited by availability of resources and economic circumstances.

In discussions of patient self-determination, the principle of justice needs to be considered along with that of autonomy. **Justice** implies fair, equitable, and appropriate treatment in light of what is due or owed to persons, recognizing that giving to some may deny receipt to others who might otherwise have received these things. In determining who deserves what portion of finite health care resources, autonomy and justice may conflict where needs or demands for health care by autonomous patients outweigh available resources. Having finite resources implies necessarily that the rights of family members and of society must be considered in relation to the needs of individuals. Hardwig (1995) suggests that the medical and nonmedical impact of treatment decisions on both the patient and the family needs to be considered. He reflects that patient autonomy implies the responsible use of freedom, which means considering the needs of family and society as well as our own desires. The limited availability and expense of many medical interventions bring such questions to the fore. Since people can be maintained on highly technological treatments (which are costly to the health care system) for prolonged periods of time, justice requires us to ask not only who deserves an intervention, but also who will gain the most benefit from it. Justice also requires that we are clear and explicit about the criteria we consider when making such decisions. Although the moral relevance of considering the interests of the family and society at large is not well addressed in current ethical theory, dilemmas faced by patients, families, and practitioners include these issues, and it is well worth pondering their implications.

Ask Yourself

Should There Be Limits to Patient Autonomy?

- How would you describe nursing's role regarding patient autonomy?
- How have you experienced paternalism in nursing?
- How do you feel about the suggestion that the physician is most qualified to make health care decisions? What have you experienced in this regard?

INFORMED CONSENT

Informed consent provides protection of a patient's right to personal autonomy. The concept of informed consent is one that has come to mean that patients are given the opportunity to autonomously choose a course of action in regard to plans for health care. The choice includes the right to refuse interventions or recommendations about care, and to choose from available therapeutic alternatives. This is usually discussed in relation to surgery and complex medical procedures, but also includes consent to more common interventions that may have undesirable side effects, such as immunizations and contraceptives. Even in a simple intervention such as the provision of a bed bath or insertion of an intravenous line, the consent of the patient must always be sought. Exceptions to informed consent include emergencies in which there is no time to disclose the information, situations in which a person is deemed not competent to provide an informed consent, and waivers by patients who do not want to know their prognosis or risks of treatment. Consent is considered to be informed if information is given to the person that any reasonable person might wish in the circumstances, in order to make such a decision, and the person also received answers to any questions or concerns that he or she may have (Ontario College of Nurses, 2005). We will discuss in greater detail the necessary elements of an informed consent process below.

The emergence of informed consent as we know it has been affected by several factors. One factor has been the institutionalization of health care in hospitals, with their associated technologies and life-prolonging techniques over which people are often assumed to have little control and limited understanding. However, with the availability of sophisticated medical information as easy to access as the Internet, patients often do have knowledge about technology, treatments, and techniques. When health providers visited in the home, informed consent was not as necessary, because people had more control and better understanding of traditional remedies (Devettere, 1995). The courts, however, have exerted the most significant influence on shaping the doctrine of informed consent.

The history of the concept dates back to at least three landmark legal cases. In *Slater v. Baker & Stapleton* (1767), a decision was made that prohibited "unauthorized touching." This decision held that a person has a right to know what is to be done to his or her body. It did not require any participation in the decision-making process. In the 1905 case of *Mobe v. Williams* (Husted & Husted, 1995, p. 61) and the case of *Schloendorff v. The Society of New York Hospital* (1914), separate rulings established the patient's right to know what was to be done, and also the right to give or withhold consent. These decisions did not address the patient's right to be informed about risks of treatment or nontreatment or about the existence of alternative therapies. In the case of *Salgo v. Leland Stanford, Jr.* (1957), the California Supreme Court ruled in favour of a patient who had not been informed of the risks of aortography and subsequently became paralyzed. This ruling established a patient's right to be advised of the risks involved in any proposed treatment (Husted & Husted, 1995).

Ethical and Legal Elements of Informed Consent

We must remember that, although the informed consent doctrine has foundations in law, it is essentially an ethical imperative. According to Williams (2008), "the notion of consent is grounded in the fundamental mental ethical principles of patient autonomy and respect for persons. Autonomy refers to the patient's right to make free decisions about his or her healthcare. Respect for persons requires that healthcare professionals foster patients' control over their own lives and refrain from carrying out unwanted interventions." (p. 12)

Information. The information component of informed consent includes both disclosure and understanding of the essential information. Figure 11–1 lists the information that must be included in an informed consent. People need access to sufficient information to help them understand their health concerns and make decisions regarding treatment. The information provided need not be "textbook" detail, but does need

Figure 11–1 **Elements of an Informed Consent**

- A description of the health concern, diagnosis, and prognosis.
- Details about the consequences/prognosis associated with each option for treatment/intervention as well as with no treatment.
- A description of the treatment or intervention.
- Details about potential risks for harm (physical, emotional, psychological, social, financial, etc.)
- Details about strategies in place to ameliorate potential risks for harm.
- Information about potential benefits, both to the individual, and in the case of consent for participation in research, information to society.
- Information about the voluntary nature of consent.
- For research participation, information about the voluntary nature of participation and the right to withdraw.
- For research participation, information on how confidentiality and privacy will be maintained.
- Consent information should be provided at a level of understanding appropriate to the patient with limited use of medical or legal terms and full explanation, in lay language, of any such term.
- Consent processes should not be rushed or hurried (except for cases of urgent or emergent health situations). Patients should be given time to reflect on the available options and discuss the decision with their support network and significant others.
- For consent to participate in research projects, the consent process should be clearly separated from both the recruitment phases and the intervention phases, to allow optimal time for reflection and informed decision making and decrease feelings of pressure or coercion to participate.

to offer enough explanation for the person to have a clear picture of the situation, what is being offered, and the alternatives and their risks, benefits, and consequences. Determining the adequacy of information disclosed in an informed consent is based on one or more standards: (1) *the professional practice standard*—the disclosure is consistent with the standards of the profession; (2) the *reasonable person standard*—the disclosure is what a reasonable person in similar circumstances would need in order to make an informed decision; and (3) the *subjective standard*—the disclosure is what the particular person wants or needs to know. Again, the challenge is to provide accurate and clear information in keeping with the standards, which, when considered separately, imply very different obligations of disclosure. Informed consent implies that the person has received the information and understands what is provided. Verification of understanding can be accomplished through discussion, in which patients have an opportunity to ask questions and are asked to describe their understanding of the nature of the intervention, alternatives, risks, and benefits. Although many people associate the informed consent process with a consent form, such a form is simply a representation that a clear, informed discussion took place and that the patient had an opportunity to hear, understand, and reflect upon the options available and the full information that needs to be provided in such a process. The most important part of the process is not the form per se, but the actual discussion that must take place, in a timely, unhurried, and thoughtful manner.

"Free and informed consent lies at the heart of ethical research involving human subjects. It encompasses a process that begins with the initial contact and carries through to the end of the involvement of research subjects in the project. . . . the process of free and informed consent refers to the dialogue, information sharing and general process through which prospective subjects choose to participate in research involving themselves" (TCPS, Article 2.1[d], 2005).

Consent. Consent to something implies the freedom to accept or reject it. This means that consent to health care interventions must be voluntary, without coercion, force, or manipulation from health care providers or family. Force entails making someone do something against his or her will. Coercion and manipulation may be overt or subtle, and may include threats, rewards, deception, or inducing excessive fear. The voluntary nature of consent does not prohibit health care providers from making recommendations or attempting to persuade patients to accept their suggestions. However, we must be alert to situations in which persuasion takes on qualities of coercion or manipulation.

CASE PRESENTATION

Language and Informed Consent

Christopher is a sixty-seven-year-old deaf man who was admitted to the hospital with atrial fibrillation. The nurse notes that he is alert, apparently oriented, and able to follow simple directions that she acts out, although he does look apprehensive as she cares for him. Christopher's social history indicates that he was brought into the hospital by a community worker who looks in on him because he is deaf and illiterate and has no family in the area. She had indicated that he came to the area as a new immigrant a number of years ago, along with a brother who died the previous year. She had also noted that two of his five siblings were also deaf, and they had developed a type of sign language that was understood only by family members. At the interdisciplinary care conference, the medical resident who is in charge of his case voices frustration because of the need to get the patient's permission to do a stress test and to talk to him about medications and risk for stroke. He suggests that they should just get the patient to make an X on the form so they can go ahead with the treatment protocol because it is in the patient's best interest to do so. The social worker suggests that they get an interpreter for the deaf to come in and try to talk to him through sign language, although she is not sure he will understand.

❓ Think About It

Obtaining Informed Consent When There Is No Common Language

- What ethical dilemmas are evident in this case?
- What do you think about Christopher decision-making capacity?
- Do you think it is possible to obtain an informed consent from Christopher? Support your position with discussion of elements of informed consent and decision-making capacity.
- In a situation such as this, it is evident that the patient has capacity for language, and comprehension although it is not understood by the health care providers, and that he has been able to care for himself with some assistance. How would these factors enter into determination of his decision-making capacity?
- How does the inability of the health care provider to communicate with a patient affect determination of the patient's decision-making capacity?
- What are the implications of denying Christopher important services because of lack of common language and subsequent inability to ensure informed consent?

Nursing Role and Responsibilities: Informed Consent

While the practice of documenting informed consent for a procedure usually ends with the signing of a consent form, the process is much more complex. Following the rules laid out previously, informed consent must include explicit verification that the patient is aware of all options, the possible outcomes of each option, and the likely outcome with nontreatment. The patient must also recognize the implications that each option will have upon his or her lifestyle. The nurse must be sensitive to the fact that the very act of asking a patient to sign a form giving permission for a particular treatment may constitute a form of coercion. It is the nurse's responsibility as advocate for the patient to ensure that all criteria for autonomous decision making are met. If the nurse believes that the patient does not understand the implications of any part of the process, including nontreatment and alternative options, or that the patient is unable to deliberate and to reason on the various choices, a nurse is ethically obligated to intervene or speak up on a patient's behalf. The nurse must act if it becomes apparent that the patient is not informed. Actions may include notifying the physician and requesting further information for the patient, or stopping the process until it is ensured that the decision can be made autonomously. Although the mechanics of the process usually require the nurse to obtain the patient's signature on a consent form, the primary concern of the nurse is to ensure that all criteria for autonomous decision making are met.

Remember, a consent form is a representation of a process, in which a patient is fully informed and volitionally able to decision make, autonomously.

Witnessing a patient's signature on a consent form implies accountability on the part of the nurse. Sullivan (1998) notes that the nurse's signature attests that the patient is giving consent willingly, is competent in that moment to give consent, and that the patient's signature is authentic. She cautions nurses who are not present when the treatment is explained to the patient to verify the patient's understanding of the procedure, inquire if there are any questions that need to be discussed with the physician, and to not let a patient sign a consent form if there is any indication of coercion. She also stresses the importance of nurses documenting their communication with the patient and with the physician regarding any questions, concerns, or teaching related to the informed consent. Any special circumstances, such as the patient's inability to read or write, or the use of an interpreter if the patient speaks a different language, should also be documented.

ADVANCE DIRECTIVES

Given the dilemmas that can arise regarding the use of technology, we must encourage and assist people to make their wishes known concerning the use of such interventions. For those who are mentally alert and capable of making decisions, informed consent is needed prior to initiating any life-sustaining interventions. To ensure that our wishes regarding treatment are followed in the event that we have lost decision-making capacity, advance directives are needed. **Advance directives** are instructions that indicate health care interventions to initiate or withhold, or that designate someone who will act as a surrogate or proxy in making such decisions in the event that we lose decision-making capacity. Such directives can be considered as a kind of informed consent for future interventions. Advance directives support people in making decisions on their own behalf, and help to ensure that patients have the kind of end-of-life care they want. In order to help patients be as clear as possible about their choices, the various life-sustaining measures that may be considered in end-of-life care should be discussed openly and clearly. Patients should be encouraged to express verbally, or in writing, their wishes about specific interventions such as tube feedings, breathing machines, cardiopulmonary resuscitation, antibiotics, withdrawal of food and/or fluids, and dialysis. Consideration of interventions should include how long they might want to stay on an intervention if it is initiated and their condition continues to decline or is not improving. In addition to enabling people to have choices in their dying process, the presence of clearly understood advance directives can alleviate stress on family and clinicians when dealing with end-of-life concerns.

Perhaps the most important factor in decision making regarding end-of-life care is clear and open communication between the patient or the surrogate/proxy and health care providers. We need to do more than merely seek to know which potential life-sustaining technology a person does or does not want. We need to see and get to know the person who is making these decisions along with the values and beliefs that clearly underlie the more pragmatic decisions. Eliciting a clear statement of personal values is basic to this process. What does the person value in life? What constitutes quality of life for the person? What are his or her personal beliefs and concerns about dying? We must recognize the influence of cultural, societal, spiritual, and family norms and perspectives on personal values. For example, in some cultures, speaking of death and dying is believed to bring bad luck. Family wishes may influence personal choices, and in some cultures the patient may defer decisions about end-of-life care to the family. When discussing different interventions, we need to ensure that patients understand what the procedure is and what it involves. They also need to appreciate that risks and benefits of life-sustaining interventions vary with age, health condition, and circumstances that prompt the consideration of the intervention. For example, the literature shows no evidence that tube feedings prolong life or improve quality of life for patients with dementia or multisystem illness (Finucane, Christmas, & Travis, 1999; McCann, 1999; Moss, 2001). We need to understand why the patient or family wants a particular intervention, and what it is that they think it will do for them.

Advance directives include living wills and durable powers of attorney. **Living wills** are legal documents giving directions to health care providers related to withholding or withdrawing life support if certain conditions exist. Statutes regulating living wills vary from province to province, so nurses must be familiar with their own provincial laws and statutes. Additionally, nomenclature varies between provinces. Living wills guide decisions by indicating a person's desires regarding life-sustaining interventions; however, they also raise issues of concern. Directives in living wills may be vague, and may address only the interventions a person does not want. Ideally, a living will should achieve two ends. First, it should articulate the patient's clear wishes regarding specific health care interventions and decision-making processes, based on authentic values. Second, it should clearly identify a proxy or substitute decision maker who will communicate and enact the patient's wishes, if she or he is unable to do so.

Part of an advance directive is indicating who it is you want to be your proxy or Substitute decision-maker (SDM), in the case that you are unable to make your own decisions. This person, in his or her role as proxy, would be responsible for ensuring that your wishes about health and personal care, as articulated in a living will or proxy directive, are carried out in the event of your incapacity. As noted, in different provinces, this role is called something different. The term "attorney for personal care" is used in Ontario, while other provinces such as Nova Scotia, New Brunswick, Manitoba, and Alberta use the term "proxy" and in Quebec, this role is called a "mandatary." No matter what the label, the fundamental roles and responsibilities are the same—to make decisions on another person's behalf in keeping with their wishes, values, and beliefs, who can no longer do so autonomously. In effect, an advance directive and identification of an SDM essentially extends one's autonomy when one can no longer do so.

An important part of identifying a proxy decision maker is to ensure that there is a thoughtful and thorough discussion between the two parties, about values, beliefs, and wishes regarding health, illness, and personal care. While it isn't necessary to have values completely aligned, it is key to ensure that the proxy decision maker has both an understanding of the values of the person creating an advance directive as well as the motivation and will to keep the best interests of that person in mind.

Decision-Making Capacity

Conscious adults are presumed to have decision-making capacity, unless there is evidence to the contrary. **Decision-making capacity** is a medical determination relating only to the issue at hand, as people may have the ability to make decisions about some areas and not others. For example, a person may be able to make decisions about health, while unable to make reasonable decisions about household or financial matters. Persons may have decision-making capacity at some times and not others, and in each specific situation, there must be a determination that they have, or do not have, the capacity. The fact that a person makes a decision that seems unreasonable to the health care provider does not necessarily mean a lack of decision-making capacity; it may merely reflect a difference in values. If the decision seems unreasonable, or not in keeping with the patient's previously stated authentic values and beliefs, however, it is wise to explore the patient's rationales and/or capacity regarding decision making.

Elements of Decision-Making Capacity. When evaluating a patient or surrogate decision maker (SDM) for decision-making capacity, several elements must be present. These are listed in Figure 11-2. First, the patient must be able to understand all relevant information, including the nature of the health care problem, the prognosis, treatment options and recommendations, and the risks, benefits, and consequences of each. Second, the patient must be able to communicate this understanding and her or his choices. Third, the patient must possess a set of values and goals that enable evaluation regarding whether this health care decision will be of benefit in terms of personal goals. Fourth, the patient must have the ability to reason and to deliberate about available choices, which includes the ability to grasp notions such as risk and percentage, cause and effect, and chance and probability. Although it is not unreasonable to see some indecision, or even a change of mind once a choice has been made, a great deal of vacillation between choices may suggest the need to re-evaluate decision-making capacity. It may also indicate a lack of understanding necessitating education or intervention by the nurse. Nurses are in a key position to observe patients and families for the presence of these elements of decision-making capacity. As patient advocates, nurses need to assess, document, and communicate to appropriate members of the health care team any concerns in this regard.

Figure 11-2 **Elements of Decision-Making Capacity**

The patient must:
- have the ability to understand all information.
- have the ability to communicate understanding and choices.
- have personal values and goals that guide the decision.
- have the ability to reason and deliberate.

Physicians usually have legal authority and responsibility to determine decision-making capacity. Determining incapacity is best done in consultation with family or others who have the patient's best interest in mind. We must make a distinction between decision-making capacity and competence. Decisions about **competence,** which is the ability to make meaningful life decisions, require a legal action and always require more than simply one person to evaluate and assess competence. Legally, persons are considered competent unless there is a ruling by a judge that they cannot make meaningful life decisions.

When a patient lacks decision-making capacity, someone else must be identified as an SDM to make decisions for the patient. In the case of children, the surrogate is usually a parent or legal guardian. With adults, the SDM may be a spouse, parent, adult children, other relatives, or other person named as SDM in the patient's advance directives. In situations in where a patient has no advance directives, or has not named a surrogate to make decisions in the event of incapacity, health care providers should work with family and others to identify an SDM. The legal process for choosing an SDM varies from province to province and you need to be familiar with the process in your province. The person chosen as SDM should be someone willing to serve in this role and who can make health care decisions in accordance with the patient's wishes, or that are consistent with the patient's best interest if these wishes are not known or cannot be reasonably discerned. Whenever possible, the SDM should demonstrate care and concern for, and have regular contact with, the patient. In addition, the surrogate should be willing and able to participate fully in the decision-making process, and engage in face-to-face contact and communication with caregivers. Close family members such as parents, adult children, adult siblings, and adult grandchildren are often considered first if the patient has not designated an SDM. However, close friends or neighbours may at times be better qualified to make these decisions. The decisions made by the SDM should reflect the patient's values, including cultural and spiritual perspective, to the extent that these are reasonably known.

As noted earlier in the chapter, in different provinces, surrogate or substitute decision makers are referred to by a variety of labels and names (Singer, 2002). Furthermore, in each province, the roles are articulated and enacted somewhat differently. It is up to the nurse in each jurisdiction to have a working knowledge of the law as it pertains to advance care planning.

Nursing Role and Responsibilities: Advance Care Planning

Advance care planning refers to a communication process that may involve the creation of a living will along with identification of a person to make health care or personal care decisions for you, if you are incapacitated and unable to advocate for yourself. The goals of such a process are to ensure that your authentic choices, thoughtfully made while competent, can be carried out in the case that you are unable to articulate such wishes. Writing a living will allows you to maintain your autonomy, even when unable to directly enact choices or articulate preferences.

A living will is a document that allows you to clearly articulate advance directives. These are instructions, made in advance, that instruct others on how to provide your health care or personal care, or make choices for you and in your best interest. Best interests, in the case of a living will, means maintaining integrity of the choices made by the person.

There are two parts to an advance directive: an instruction directive and a proxy directive. A proxy directive identifies a person whom you wish to make decisions on your behalf when you are no longer able to do so. A proxy must be carefully chosen, and should have a clear idea of your authentic choices, wishes, values, and beliefs. Together, you should have thorough discussions of your wishes and values as you construct your living will.

An instruction directive is a set of instructions for the proxy to carry out. These instructions may pertain to health care decisions such as treatment, diagnostic care, or interventions, or they may be related to personal care decisions involving hygiene, nutrition, and hydration. Again, clearly, the values and beliefs that underlie such decisions should be articulated in such a document, to further guide decision making (Singer, 2002).

Living wills are legal documents and should be respected as such by health care teams and family members. In different provinces, however, they do have different roles and vocabulary along with different understanding of how advanced directives can be carried out, under varying provincial legislation regarding the use of living wills. Most provinces have legalized the use of living wills. The Canadian Medical Association has a policy clearly endorsing the use of living wills and the Canadian Nurses Association's *Code of Ethics* for Registered Nurses identifies "promoting and respecting informed decision making" as an ethical principle (Canadian Nurses Association, 2008, p. 11). The Code of Ethics states that nurses have a responsibility to "consider and respect the best interests of the person receiving care and any previously known wishes or advance directives that apply . . ." (Canadian Nurses Association, 2002, p. 12). Additionally, the Canadian Nurses Association, published a Joint Statement on Advance Directives in 1994, outlining the responsibilities of health care practitioners and agencies to facilitate the use of advance directives, and underpinned by principles of autonomy, self-determination, and rights (Canadian Nurses Association, 1994).

What is the nursing role and responsibility regarding advance directives? Whatever the work setting, nurses have a key role and responsibility in ensuring that patients have an opportunity to complete advance directives, and in interpreting and following through with patients' wishes as expressed through these directives. As nurses, we need to be aware of legislation and institutional policies that guide and govern advance directives. We also need to be aware of the policies and procedures regarding advance directives where we work. Tilden (2000) urges us to complete our own advance directives. Doing so helps us to reflect on our own values, beliefs, and concerns associated with end-of-life issues, to learn more about the specific forms and processes involved, and ultimately to have more empathy with patients going through this process. Information concerning advance directives is often provided to patients on admission to a facility by a clerical worker; however, in many cases, a nurse completing an initial assessment, upon admission, should be asking about advance directives, living wills, and substitute decision makers. Nurses can use this as an opportunity to stress the importance of having such directives, and to advocate for patients who may need assistance in developing advance directives. This is also a beginning opportunity for us to help patients explore personal values, their understanding of themselves in the context of their current situation, and significant cultural or other issues that may influence decision making. The one realistic constraint on having this kind of thorough and thoughtful discussion is lack of time. Nurses often cite heavy patient loads, limited time to conduct thorough assessments, and multiple competing priorities as preventing them from having meaningful discussion with patients about issues such as these. As nurses, we need to be familiar with our patients' directives for care, and ensure that care is consistent with the patient's wishes as expressed in the advance directives. We also need to ensure that we make the time to promote meaningful discussions on advance directives, or at the very least, direct interested patients toward helpful resources on creating advance directives. Nursing's advocacy role includes informing other health team members of the presence and content of advance directives, alerting appropriate team members to changes in patient wishes or to evidence of changes in the patient's decision-making capacity, and intervening on behalf of the patient when wishes expressed in advance directives are not being followed. As nurses, we have an important role in increasing public awareness about advance directives through patient and community education, through research, and through education of nurses and other health care providers. It remains, arguably, that one of the most important parts of increasing awareness is to begin by creating your own living will and assisting your family and friends to do so, as well. Encouraging patients to create an advance directive and emphasizing the importance of having a clear articulation of your wishes in place is much more effective if you have also done so. Having the experience of thinking through your own wishes, values and beliefs about health, illness, and personal care, as you create your own advance directive and include those around you in the discussion, also helps to increase your own comfort with discussing similar kinds of issues in an open way, with patients, who may feel uncomfortable, ill at ease, or frightened by the idea of discussing or creating an advance directive.

CASE PRESENTATION

The Absence of Advance Directives

Ninety-year-old Mr. Moshe did not have advance directives when he was admitted to the hospital with Alzheimer's disease and renal failure. Although he was coherent at times and could converse with caregivers, the doctor determined Mr. Moshe did not have decision-making capacity and named his daughter Zelda, with whom he had been residing, as his SDM. The nursing staff questioned this choice because of their concerns about the quality of care Mr. Moshe had been receiving from Zelda and her husband Josh. As Mr. Moshe's health began to deteriorate rapidly, the nurses inquired about his DNR status. Josh replied he wanted Mr. Moshe kept alive, and that this was what Mr. Moshe would have also wanted. Zelda concurred with this. Although Zelda's four siblings called frequently inquiring about their father, Zelda would not inform them about their father's condition nor allow them access to him. Because of this conflict and their concerns regarding the motives for his DNR status, the nurses notified the physician about the family issues and requested an ethics committee consultation to determine the best interests of the patient. The ethics committee representative convened a family meeting that included all five siblings, the physician, Mr. Moshe's primary nurse, and two members of the multidisciplinary team providing care to Mr. Moshe. After explaining that the purpose of the meeting was to discuss the type of care that would be in the best interests of their father, not to resolve family issues, the physician was asked to discuss Mr. Moshe's current health status and prognosis. Each of the children were given the opportunity to ask questions of the physician and primary nurse. Then each family member was asked to voice what their father valued in life, and what they believed to be his wishes regarding end-of-life care. Even though some of the siblings had not spoken to each other for nearly ten years, they each stated the same thing, that their father had told them he would never want to be on life support. Zelda, who was asked to speak last, agreed, much to the dismay of her husband, that her father would not want to be placed on life support. The siblings also requested that they be allowed to visit their father and to call and check on him. When they were informed that there currently was no legal SDM for their father, they all agreed to have Zelda continue in that role, providing she allow them access to him. They stated that even though they were upset with her, they believed she loved him and provided good care for him. To close the meeting all family members were invited to go join together at their father's bedside where they shared prayer and family stories. Mr. Moshe died that night.

? Think About It

Considering the Patient's Best Interests

- Because Mr. Moshe was coherent at times, do you think the health care team should have asked him what he would want regarding life support?
- What do you think of the choice of a surrogate for Mr. Moshe? What factors do you think were considered in appointing Zelda as surrogate? Are there factors you think should have been considered that were not?
- As the nurse caring for Mr. Moshe, what would be your concerns regarding his situation? How do you think you would have responded in this situation?
- How did the process of the family meeting address the communication that is needed for making end-of-life decisions?
- Reflecting on this case, think about your own choice of a proxy decision maker. What factors did you consider in your choice and why?

CHOICES CONCERNING LIFE AND HEALTH

Although discussion of patient autonomy frequently centres around issues of informed consent and end-of-life decisions, issues related to self-determination can arise in any area of nursing practice. In every area of practice nurses must deal with the effects of lifestyle choices on patients' health and healing. Many people who come into our care are suffering from ill effects of such things as overeating; tobacco, drug, or alcohol use; risky or unprotected sexual activity; or work-related stress. These factors are considered by many to be lifestyle "choices." By virtue of this label, the implication is that some people make good choices while others do not. Our job is to deal with the present health concern while encouraging change toward healthier living. However, patients are often not willing or able to follow the treatment plan and make the changes needed for healthier living. Dealing with patients whose health problems are clearly related to lifestyle choices, yet who are not willing or able to change their behaviours, may present ethical or moral dilemmas for nurses. Although nurses may acknowledge that the autonomous person has the right to choose healthy or unhealthy behaviours, it may be difficult to be as caring toward those who are perceived to have brought problems on themselves.

This is another area where the principle of justice may temper the bounds of autonomy. In situations where resources are limited, questions arise regarding whether it is ethical to put resources into treatments for people whose health problems are brought on by unhealthy life choices. This is countered by the question of whether it is ethical to refuse treatment or provide a lesser level of care to someone because the provider does not agree with the lifestyle choices. It can also be countered by the argument that for some, what may appear to be "poor choices" are not in fact, choices at all. Consider the example of a woman who drinks excessive amounts of alcohol. There may be multiple factors that have an effect upon whether or not this behaviour is truly a choice: her genetic predisposition, her past experiences and support, her level of education, and her ability to enact choices in other areas of her life. As another example, think of the mother who makes very poor nutritional choices for her children. She chooses food that is quick, highly processed, and easy instead of nutritional, complex, and vitamin rich. At first glance, she may appear to be making poor choices. But if we care to look deeper, we may see that she is a single mother, working two jobs, and unable to spend time preparing food. She also has never had any education on nutrition and making healthy food choices. Furthermore, she feels tremendous guilt at not being home enough for her children and finds that giving in to their wishes for junk food is one way she can demonstrate her love. Finally, think of the patient who has an ongoing peptic ulcer related to extreme stress at work and home. While some of us may think that the obvious choice is to change jobs or leave the current job, it may not be a choice that is easy for that patient to make. He may be the sole supporter of a family. Others may voice trite solutions to stress at home such as "Make time for yourself" to the patient. It is likely far more helpful to discuss the patient's family situation and see if there are available resources that might offer the patient assistance, such as counselling or respite care for elderly parents or children with disabilities.

So while we might view "poor" health and lifestyle choices as in fact, choices, it is important to look more deeply into the contextual situations of persons in an attempt to discover why they are making these choices before judging harshly or assuming that they have no interest in making healthier or different choices.

Choices Regarding Recommended Treatment

What are nurses to do when patients are well informed and apparently able to follow plans of care, yet do not? Certainly one hears of physicians who refuse to continue to care for patients who do not comply with instructions—smoking cessation, for example. In a climate of limited resources this is a question worthy of contemplation.

Ask Yourself

How Should We Think About Lifestyle Choices When Making Allocation Decisions?

Autonomy implies that persons have the right to make choices about things that affect their lives, whether these choices have a positive or negative effect, unless these choices impinge on the rights of others. There is an argument that the societal and financial burden of resultant health problems by those persons who make "poor" lifestyle choices (such as smoking, overeating, or taking illegal drugs) may in fact infringe upon the rights of others.

To make the point more clear, let's consider an example. Queues exist for access to particular diagnostic or therapeutic interventions, such as CT or MRI scans. Some might feel that those who have a problem related to a genetic or acquired problem should be in the queue ahead of those who have a problem related to a lifestyle "choice."

This is commonly and quite dangerously implied in many discussions of those who are diagnosed with HIV and AIDS. Many feel that those who may have contracted the virus through blood transfusions should be considered or treated differently than those who contracted it through unprotected sexual contact. The implication, of course, is that those who contracted HIV through a blood transfusion were not making a choice and are "innocent victims" while the concomitant assumption is that unprotected sexual activity is always an informed choice.

Other places in which these kinds of discussions surface is in the area of organ transplantation and eligibility for surgery. Consider the decision of the health care team who must choose between two clearly viable candidates for a liver transplant: one of whom has a congenital or acquired liver disease, such as primary biliary cirrhosis and the other who is a self-identified lapsed alcoholic. While many believe that factors such as these should not play a part in the decision as to "who may receive the liver" or "who may receive the liver first," it is clear that they can and do play a part in such assessments and decisions.

While these decisions may be framed as purely "clinical" decisions, they often do, realistically, include judgment, by clinicians, about the "goodness" or "badness" of a patient's decision to smoke, drink alcohol, take illegal drugs, overeat, or engage in risky sexual behaviour (Walton et al., 2007).

(Continued)

- What factors do you think should be considered when organizing patients into a queue, say, for hip replacement surgery or cardiac surgery?

- What factors should not be part of the decision and why?

- Is it fair that taxes are paid by all persons to support health care services that are used more often by those who might be overweight, smokers, or sedentary individuals? Why or why not?

- What kinds of personal values, beliefs, or biases are you identifying as you think about these questions?

- If you were making choices about allocation of health care resources, how would you consider, if at all, factors we consider to be *lifestyle choices* (smoking, overeating, drinking alcohol, exposure to stress, or drug use, etc.)?

- What kind of consequences, for patients, do you foresee if they know that they are being "judged" by health care professionals to whom they turn for advocacy, support, and holistic care?

- Have you encountered a patient who has disclosed what you consider to be a "poor" lifestyle choice? How did you feel toward the patient? Did it change your approach to her or him?

- Reflect on your own lifestyle choices. Are there any that others might think are "unhealthy" or a "poor" choice? How does that make you feel? What if you had to disclose this to a health professional? Would you feel hesitant to do so?

In the most recent iteration of its *Code of Ethics for Registered Nurses,* the Canadian Nurses Association states that, as part of promoting and respecting informed decision making, "Nurses respect the informed decision-making capability of capable persons, including choices of lifestyles or treatment not conducive to good health" (Canadian Nurses Association, 2008, p. 12). Further, quality of nursing care must not be affected by the patients' individual differences in background, customs, attitudes, and beliefs. Health care practices are an integral part of patients' backgrounds, customs, and beliefs. Therefore, it is clear that refusal to participate in a plan of care, regardless of the outcome, is the prerogative of the patient, and must not affect the caring attitude of the nurse. Unhealthy life practices are part of the whole person, and should be taken into consideration when revising plans of care.

Ultimately, choices about health care practices belong to patients. If allowed to choose, patients should not be labelled in a negative way for choices with which nurses do not agree. It is not appropriate for professionals who express the belief that all competent patients have the right to autonomous choice to then make value

CASE PRESENTATION

A Challenging Patient

Rochelle, a thirty-six-year-old woman who is a known cocaine addict, presented to the emergency room (ER) with severe left leg pain and swelling. The triage nurse reviewed her chart and presenting problem, noting that she had been seen two days prior for chest pain and left leg pain. Assuming these complaints were evaluated then, the nurse sent her to the "fast track" area to be seen by the nurse practitioner (NP). The NP noted that her chart was flagged regarding her cocaine addiction and that the physician who had seen her at the previous visit, after doing an EKG, CBC, electrolytes (which were normal), and a urine drug screen (which was positive for cocaine), discharged her with diagnoses of atypical chest pain and drug use. The NP's assessment revealed no shortness of breath, cough, or chest pain; severe swelling and skin tightness of the left leg, with exquisite tenderness and positive Homan's sign, were suggestive of deep vein thrombosis. When the NP went to the ER physician saying that the patient needed to be evaluated by him, she was told to keep the patient over there and do the workup because he had a patient with a "more serious" problem in the ER.

When the ultrasound confirmed extensive deep vein thrombosis, the NP told the patient the situation and that she needed to be hospitalized. The patient immediately said that she could not stay because she had no one to watch her nine-year-old-daughter, and she began to put on her shoes to leave. The NP told her that she could choose to leave but that the reason for the insistence on her staying was that this was a very serious problem from which she could die. Rochelle's response was to start crying, saying that she thought she would go home anyway because she had nothing to live for since her husband had died, so she would go home to die. When the NP called Rochelle's primary physician to alert him to the situation, he responded that he would come in to see her only if Rochelle agreed to stay; otherwise, it would be a waste of his time. After considerable effort, the NP contacted Rochelle's mother, who reluctantly agreed to keep her granddaughter when the NP explained the situation, and Rochelle agreed to stay.

Think About It

Dealing with Patients Who Make Apparently Unhealthy Choices

- What issues of patient self-determination are evident in this case?
- How do you see lifestyle choices affecting Rochelle's care? What ethical issues must be considered here?
- Take an honest look at how you think you might react to Rochelle, knowing that she frequently shows up in the ER and is a cocaine addict.

(Continued)

- As the nurse in this situation, how would you deal with the patient's saying she could not stay? What do you think of the way the NP handled it?
- Evaluate ethical issues involved in the responses of the various health care practitioners in this case.

---

judgments about the choices made, and subsequently label patients as noncompliant, uncooperative, or difficult. In fact, it is worth pondering whether the term "noncompliant" even belongs in nursing vocabulary. The notion of compliance relates to a paternalistic view that health care providers know what is best for patients and that, providing patients follow these directions, they will get well. Nurses should speak more appropriately in terms of motivation to follow a mutually agreed upon plan of care that incorporates patient and family values and beliefs. We must remember that patients have a right to refuse interventions, and they have a right to seek therapies other than those offered by conventional western medicine.

Complementary Therapies.   Many people utilize therapies that may be termed complementary, alternative, or unconventional in regard to Western allopathic medicine (Eisenberg, Kessler, Foster, Norlock, Calkins, & Delbanco, 1993; Eisenberg, et al., 1998). Examples of **complementary therapies** include acupuncture, herbal and nutritional interventions, healing touch, massage, and guided imagery. Most people tend to use such therapies along with conventional modalities, but some will choose to use them in lieu of what is offered by medical practitioners. Many people do not inform their medical practitioner that they are using these therapies.

Several issues regarding the use of complementary therapies need to be considered. First, people have a right to use modalities other than Western medicine to address their health care needs. Second, nurses and other health care practitioners need to develop at least a talking knowledge, and better yet a working knowledge, of such therapies in order to be better able to discuss their use with patients. Many therapies work as an adjunct to medical interventions, some may interact in unhealthy ways, and the efficacy of many modalities is not yet known. Nurses need not be practitioners of other modalities in order to discuss them with patients any more than they need to be able to do surgery in order to discuss it. Nurses should create an atmosphere that encourages nonjudgmental discussion of all modalities being considered or employed, with a goal of using whatever is beneficial for the particular patient. Transcultural considerations (which are discussed in Chapter 18) may influence a person's choice of treatment modalities. Third, complementary modalities should not be discounted merely because they are not understood within the Western medical framework; however, it is also important to counsel patients to explore the validity of claims made about a particular therapy. Fourth, as research continues and expands in the area of complementary therapies, the question of whether informed consent will need to at least acknowledge these therapies as treatment options must be addressed. Fifth, nurses who are skilled in complementary therapies need to be clear about what is within their scope of practice according to their provincial regulatory body. The ethical stance with complementary therapies, as with other interventions, requires offering an explanation of the intervention and receiving permission from the patient or family prior to initiating the therapy. Because these therapies can affect conventional interventions, practitioners should apprise other health team members of their use and document both treatments and their effects.

Controversial Choices

The value of patient self-determination is cited to support two decisions that have been the focus of much controversy in this country for many years: abortion and active euthanasia. Both of these choices are embedded in many people's fundamental values and beliefs regarding life and death. Abortion in particular is an example of an issue in which legal answers have been sought for ethical dilemmas. As well, the potential for transmission of HIV infections within health care settings raises controversial issues regarding testing and disclosure. This discussion presents some of the arguments on both sides of these three issues.

Nurses need to be very clear about their own values regarding each of these issues, and find a balance between personal values and professional obligations to patients and families. Nurses must sort out their own beliefs about what is right and wrong, so that they can differentiate between tasks and roles that are consistent with their ethical stance and those that are not, and make responsible practice decisions accordingly. Davis & Aroskar (1991) suggest that in the process of reasoning through dilemmas such as those involved with these issues, the least that can be expected is that the nurse not abandon the patient. In fact, it is ethically problematic to ever abandon a patient and in all cases, care must be in place and assured to all patients, regardless of choices or decisions. "The most that can be hoped is that each nurse regard the rights of others as precious, as she would want her own regarded, and that within this complex context she view her obligations to self, to the patient, to nursing, and to her place of employment" (p. 136).

Abortion. The abortion debate sparks passionate, emotion-laden arguments in political, social, legal, religious, and moral arenas. Issues of self-determination arise regarding the mother's right to control her body and her life (right to choose) in contrast to rights of the unborn fetus to a chance at life (right to life). Those in the right-to-life camp believe that abortion constitutes murder of an unborn person, suggesting that it is a legal as well as an ethical matter. This has raised questions about the role of government in dealing with this ethical concern. Those who hold to the right to choose maintain that the right to privacy regarding health care decisions includes a woman's reproductive choices, implying that governmental regulation is an infringement on this privacy.

Values in relation to life are fundamental considerations in regard to abortion. Such values include beliefs about when life begins, considerations regarding quality of life for children who are unwanted, and concerns about the mother's life and health. Some believe that life starts at conception, while others hold that life begins only when a fetus is viable outside the womb. Discussions regarding viability continue to change as technology enables the survival of babies of lower and lower birth weights, and results in saving some imperiled newborns of the same gestational age as some aborted fetuses.

Opponents of abortion hold the position that because a fetus possesses humanity and the potential for viable life, it must be accorded all human rights, including the right to life. Proponents of abortion argue that, based on autonomy, a woman has a right to her own body, and that no woman should be forced to bear a child that she does not want. Because abortion is a situation in which many feel that two lives are involved, dilemmas arise regarding who has rights, and whose rights take precedence.

> Some take the position that pregnant women, no matter what the circumstances of conception, have obligations toward the life and well-being of the fetus that overshadow any discussion of the woman's rights. . . . So we have a moral argument, where the stakes are high, in which some people support abortion on demand based on the woman's autonomy. At the same time we have people who oppose abortion perhaps except to save the life of the mother or not at all, based on the sanctity of life principle and the personhood of the fetus. To think in a simple way about this ethical dilemma, on the one hand the fetus is viewed as an object or thing while on the other, the woman is viewed as an object or thing. (Davis & Aroskar, 1991, pp. 130–131)

From either perspective, the consideration of abortion presents a dilemma for those involved.

There is no agreement about the morality of abortion in our society. It is a complex issue with many facets to consider. Although debate generally focuses on areas related to rights of the woman or the fetus, Mahowald (1995) suggests that it is also important to consider the morality of circumstances that provide fertile ground for abortion. She notes that immoral conditions that sometimes occasion abortion include: poverty, lack of social and medical supports for pregnancy and parenthood, stereotypic views of sex roles and biological parenthood, and a eugenic mentality that welcomes only "premium babies," those babies that meet the parents' desired specifications (p. 107). She stresses the need for society to direct more effort into rectifying these conditions.

Active Euthanasia.   As noted in Chapter 10, technology has caused death to become an unnatural event in the lives of many people. In Canada, active euthanasia and assisted suicide are both illegal and taking part in either of them is a criminal act, even if carried out with merciful intentions or the goal of relieving suffering. Section 14 of Canada's *Criminal Code* states "No person is entitled to consent to have death inflicted on him, and such consent does not affect the criminal responsibility of any person by whom death may be inflicted on the person by whom consent is given." Additionally, section 241 refers to suicidal behaviour indicating that "Everyone who counsels a person to commit suicide or aids or abets a person to commit suicide, whether suicide ensues or not, is guilty of an indictable offence and liable to imprisonment for a term not exceeding fourteen years." In Canada, euthanasia and assisted suicide are considered criminal conduct.

Because of the concern that health care providers will not adhere to personal wishes regarding end-of-life issues, fears about prolonged suffering resulting from prolongation of dying, and the lack of control that each of these engenders, many people consider the possibility of active euthanasia or assisted suicide. **Active voluntary euthanasia** is an act in which the physician both provides the means of death and administers it, such as a lethal dose of medication. With **assisted suicide** the patients receive the means of death from someone, such as a physician, but activate the process themselves. Justification offered by proponents of these acts include respect for the person's autonomy in choosing to end his or her life if it is deemed intolerable due to conditions of a lingering terminal illness, and compassion exhibited in relief of the patient's suffering. Opponents argue from a stance of the sanctity of life, saying that any such act violates the prohibition against killing human beings. They hold that suffering can almost always be relieved, and they voice concerns about potential abuses, such as **involuntary euthanasia** to contain health care costs, if such acts were permitted (Lo, 1995).

It is particularly important to consider the reason for a patient's request for assisted suicide or euthanasia. When the patient indicates that life has become intolerable, we must determine why this is so. Often, inadequate pain management and depression are factors that enter into this perception, which, when treated appropriately, may change the patient's perspective. This may not always be the case, however, and nurses need to be able to support patients and families as they struggle with questions regarding whether natural death is always the best and most loving choice (Hooks & Daly, 2000). Attending to the nature and cause of a person's suffering and providing comfort care throughout the dying process are important components of the nursing role that may influence choices regarding active voluntary euthanasia or assisted suicide.

Issues Related to HIV/AIDS. We know that human immunodeficiency virus and acquired immunodeficiency syndrome (HIV/AIDS) is a major worldwide health concern, and that the virus is generally contracted through unprotected sexual contact. The virus can also be spread through maternal–infant transmission and intravenous drug use.

Because of the risk of exposure to HIV in health care settings, questions arise regarding issues of autonomy and confidentiality in relation to HIV testing and status. One issue relates to whether patients can be required to submit to HIV testing in situations of potential or actual percutaneous exposure of health care workers to their blood. In order to protect persons from potential discrimination, confidentiality of HIV testing and status is generally assured by law; thus, it is generally illegal to perform HIV testing or for that matter, many other kinds of tests, without a person's clear written consent. "Ethically speaking, HIV testing over the patient's objections violates the patient's autonomy and privacy as well as the spirit of informed consent . . . consent for HIV testing is important because stigma and discrimination may occur if other people know that the patient is seropositive" (Lo, 1995, p. 332).

Because of concerns about potential stigma in work or home settings related to having a documented HIV test, regardless of its result, patients may refuse a test even if they are sure it will be negative. In order to ensure confidentiality and to encourage patient agreement to testing in the event of exposure of a health care worker to a patient's blood, Lo (1995) suggests an approach of anonymous testing of the patient. In this way the health care worker could know if he or she is at risk, while protecting the patient from potential stigma resulting from the test.

Another issue that has become a public concern relates to potential exposure of patients to the blood of a seropositive health care worker. Questions arise whether HIV testing among health care workers, or at least those involved in certain invasive procedures, should be mandatory; whether seropositive health care workers should have restrictions on their practice; and whether the HIV status of health care workers should be made known to patients. Some argue that if it becomes mandatory for health care workers to be tested, then it should be mandatory for all patients as well. Principles of autonomy, confidentiality, and nonmaleficence become part of this discussion. Health care workers, as well as patients, have a right to autonomy and confidentiality regarding health matters, particularly where discrimination could result from disclosure. At the same time, nonmaleficence directs them to do no harm to patients, and the doctrine of informed consent requires advising patients of potential risks related to interventions being considered. Economic factors enter into the discussion as well. At the present time, presuming health care workers follow universal infection control precautions, the risk of a patient contracting HIV from a seropositive health care worker is low, in contrast to the high cost of mandatory testing. Requiring such testing could well divert money from other, more effective areas of health promotion and protection. Resources may be better used and result in more sustainable changes, if they were directed toward ensuring that all health care professionals are practising universal precautions.

Current issues related to HIV/AIDS may become less of a concern as technology advances toward more effective prevention and treatment of the disease. However, ethical concerns surrounding these issues apply to other health problems of similar nature. Nurses and other health care workers must be aware of any factors in their own health that might put their patients at risk, and take necessary precautions to protect patients from harm. It is also essential that nurses follow universal precautions aimed at protecting themselves and others from harm. If behaviours on the part of health care workers are observed that might put patients at risk, the imperatives of beneficence and nonmaleficence direct nurses to do what is necessary to protect the patient. Actions may include approaching the person involved, reporting the situation to appropriate persons within the agency, and working with groups to institute changes to prevent similar situations from occurring.

Although cases of HIV/AIDS must be reported, as with other infectious diseases, caregivers cannot disclose a person's HIV status (or any kind of personal health information) without consent. The legal and ethical right to confidentiality regarding HIV/AIDS raises an ethical issue related to protection of others when the infected individual continues behaviours that may expose others to the infection. In some circumstances, physicians are allowed limited disclosure without consent, such as to the patient's spouse. In such situations the imperative of confidentiality must be weighed against the duty to warn others in order to protect them from potential harm. At the present time there are no clear directives in this area for health care providers.

Confidentiality

The imperative of **confidentiality** in health care, which is discussed in Chapter 3, can be traced at least as far back as the Hippocratic vow not to reveal secrets. In order to care for people with health concerns, nurses must be privy to very personal, and sometimes secret, information. Without assurance of confidentiality, many people would not disclose information that is important in diagnosis and treatment of, and caring for, health concerns. This is especially true in situations where there is stigma attached to, or other risks for social repercussions from, the information disclosed. Nurses need to remember that a patient's trust is sacred, and any breach of confidentiality, no matter how small it might seem to the nurse, is a violation of this trust. As with so many other areas, there are situations where other factors override confidentiality. In circumstances such as court cases, the law might require disclosure. In situations where secrets entrusted to the nurse suggest potential harm for the patient or others, the duty to warn may take precedence over confidentiality. For example, if a patient tells a nurse about suicide plans that the nurse believes are genuine, and the patient is not willing to be hospitalized, protection of the patient may require the nurse to initiate the process of involuntary hospitalization.

SUMMARY

This chapter discussed considerations for nursing practice related to patient self-determination. The concept of self-determination derives from the principle of autonomy, and denotes the right and freedom to make choices about issues that affect one's life. Principles of justice, beneficence, and nonmaleficence may temper the bounds of autonomy in some circumstances. The doctrine of informed consent is both a legal and ethical imperative for protecting a person's right to self-determination in health care decisions. Informed consent implies the right to accept or reject recommended treatment plans. As patient advocates, we need to be alert for situations in which patient autonomy may be limited, or in which there is a lack of sufficient information for the patient or family to make informed decisions. Nurses have a particular responsibility for facilitating informed decision making regarding patient choices for end-of-life care. Nursing's professional code directs nurses to provide services with respect for the rights and dignity of the patient regardless of a person's background or the nature of the health concern. If professional responsibilities expected of a nurse in a patient care situation are inconsistent with the nurse's ethical stance, integrity and accountability, she should remove herself from that situation after ensuring that there are others to assume care for the patient. A nurse's attention to the many-faceted issues surrounding patient self-determination may be the factor that ensures the patient's involvement in important health care decisions.

CHAPTER HIGHLIGHTS

- Self-determination derives from the principle of autonomy, and implies having freedom to make choices about issues affecting one's life, an ability to make decisions about personal goals, and an appreciation for self in relation to others.

- Autonomy may be threatened by factors such as paternalism; presumptions that a patient's values, knowledge level, and ways of dealing with issues are consistent with those of health care providers; and greater attention to technology than caring. In some situations, principles such as justice or nonmaleficence may temper the bounds of autonomy.

- Decisions about health care require attention to patient values, culture, and beliefs; effects of lifestyle and role; others who are affected by a patient's choices; and evaluation of risks, benefits, and economic considerations.

- Practitioners may not be required to honour requests for interventions that are outside accepted standards of care or contrary to the practitioner's ethical views. However, patients cannot be abandoned.

- Informed consent provides legal and ethical protection of a patient's right to personal autonomy regarding plans for health care, including the right to refuse interventions and to choose from available alternatives. Information necessary in an informed consent includes the nature of the concern and prognosis if nothing is done; description of treatment options; and benefits, risks, and consequences of treatment options or nonintervention.

- Decision-making capacity, which is a medical determination and essential for informed consent, includes evidence of the ability to understand information, to communicate understanding and choices, to evaluate decisions in relation to personal values and goals, and to reason and to deliberate. Conscious adults are presumed to have decision-making capacity, unless there is evidence to the contrary.

- Nursing responsibility regarding informed consent includes verifying that the patient is aware of options and the implications of each, and advocating for patients to ensure that criteria for autonomous decision making are met in situations where the physician has not attended to these criteria. Nurses in advanced practice must obtain informed consent for interventions that they initiate within their scope of practice.

- Advance directives, which include living wills and durable powers of attorney, provide instructions regarding health care interventions in the event that one loses decision-making capacity.

- In dealing with patient lifestyle choices, nurses must remember to provide quality nursing care with respect for human dignity and to avoid value judgments related to differences in background, customs, attitudes, and beliefs.

- Nurses need to be aware of their own values and beliefs regarding various lifestyle and health care choices, and know how these affect their care with patients.

- Nurses must recognize the patient's right to use complementary therapies, become more knowledgeable about other modalities, and create an atmosphere encouraging of nonjudgmental discussion of such interventions.
- Ethical codes direct nurses to maintain confidentiality regarding patient health status and choices, except in special circumstances in which the "secrets" revealed suggest potential harm for the patient or another.

DISCUSSION QUESTIONS AND ACTIVITIES

1. Discuss your understanding of patient self-determination, including its ethical and legal basis, and nursing practice considerations.

2. Describe dilemmas that nurses may face related to patient self-determination and suggest approaches for dealing with such dilemmas.

3. Explore how practising nurses in your institution perceive their role regarding informed consent. What dilemmas related to consent have they encountered and how did they deal with these issues?

4. Analyze your own values regarding abortion and active voluntary euthanasia. How would you respond to a patient under your care who was deliberating such a choice?

5. Explore your provincial legislation regarding advance directives, HIV testing and disclosure, euthanasia, assisted suicide, and abortion. What are the implications of these regulations for nursing practice in your province?

6. What are your views on mandatory HIV testing for health care professionals? What about limiting the practice of seropositive health care workers? Review current literature to determine recommendations by professional organizations concerning these issues.

7. What is the process for obtaining support and guidance for dealing with ethical concerns and dilemmas in your institution? If there is an ethics committee, how are referrals made? Who is on the committee, and how are members chosen? Talk with a member of an ethics committee, and discuss how she or he sees the role and the effectiveness of the committee.

8. Select a case situation in which there are ethical concerns that warrant referral to the ethics committee. With classmates, role-play the ethics committee discussion, decisions, and actions regarding the case. Explain why you take the position that you do, and how you feel about the outcome.

9. Choose one of the issues discussed in this chapter and explore the websites of the CNA, the ANA, and the ICN regarding policies or position statements on this issue. Compare and contrast positions of the various organizations. Discuss your views about this issue and how they compare with the positions of the professional organizations.

    CNA—http://www.cna-nurses.ca/cna

    ANA—http://www.nursingworld.org

    ICN—http://www.icn.ch

REFERENCES

Canadian Institutes of Health Research, Natural Sciences and Engineering Research Council of Canada, Social Sciences and Humanities Research Council of Canada. *The council policy statement: Ethical conduct for research involving humans, 1998* (with 2000, 2002, 2005, amendments).

Canadian Nurses Association. (1994). Joint statement on advance directives. Ottawa: Author. Retrieved January 2, 2009, from http://www.cna-aiic.ca/CNA/documents/pdf/publications/PS20_Advance_Directives_Sept_1994_e.pdf.

Canadian Nurses Association. (1998, May). Advance directives: the nurse's role. *Ethics in Practice*. Retrieved January 9, 2001 from http://www.cna-nurses.ca/pages/ethics_sec... cs%20in%20practice/advance_directives.htm.

Canadian Nurses Association. (2008). Code of ethics for registered nurses. Ottawa: Canadian Nurses Association. Retrieved January 2, 2009, from http://www.cna-nurses.ca/CNA/practice/ethics/code/default_e.aspx.

Curtin, L. (1982). Autonomy, accountability, and nursing practice. *Topics in Clinical Nursing, 4,* 7–14.

Davis, A. J., & Aroskar, M. A. (1991). *Ethical dilemmas and nursing practice* (3rd ed.). Norwalk, CT: Appleton & Lange.

Department of Justice, Government of Canada. (1985). *Criminal Code* (R.S., 1985, c. C-46).

Devettere, R. J. (1995). *Practical decision making in health care ethics: Cases and concepts.* Washington, DC: Georgetown University Press.

Eisenberg, D. M., Kessler, R. C., Foster, C., Norlock, F. E., Calkins, D. R., & Delbanco, T. L. (1993). Unconventional medicine in the United States. *New England Journal of Medicine, 328,* 246–252.

Eisenberg, D. M., Rogers, B. D., Ettner, S., Appel, S., Wilkey, S., Van Rompay, M., & Kessler, R. C. (1998). Trends in alternative medicine in the United States, 1990–1997. *Journal of the American Medical Association, 280*(18), 1569–1575.

Finucane, T. E., Christmas, C., & Travis, K. (1999). Tube feeding in patients with advanced dementia. *Journal of the American Medical Association, 282*(14), 1265–1370.

Hardwig, J. (1995). What about the family? In J. H. Howell & W. F. Sale, eds., *Life choices: A Hastings Center introduction to bioethics* (pp. 53–67). Washington, DC: Georgetown University Press.

Hooks, F. J., & Daly, B. J. (2000). Hastening death. *American Journal of Nursing, 100*(5), 56–63.

Husted, G., & Husted, J. (1995). *Ethical decision making in nursing* (2nd ed.). St. Louis, MO: Mosby.

Lo, B. (1995). *Resolving ethical dilemmas: A guide for clinicians.* Baltimore: Williams & Wilkins.

McCann, R. (1999). Lack of evidence about tube feeding: Food for thought. *Journal of the American Medical Association, 282*(14), 1381.

Mahowald, M. B. (1995). Is there life after *Roe v. Wade?* In J. H. Howell & W. F. Sale, eds., *Life choices: A Hastings Center introduction to bioethics* (pp. 96–110). Washington, DC: Georgetown University Press.

Moss, A. H. (2001). What's new? Progress in palliative care, CPR, and advance directives. Seminar at Raleigh General Hospital, Beckley, WV. January 18, 2001.

Ontario College of Nurses. (2005). *Practice guideline: Consent*. Toronto: Author. Retrieved January 2, 2009, from http://www.cno.org/docs/policy/41020_consent.pdf.

Salgo v. Leland Stanford Jr. (1957). 317 P. 2d 170 (Cal. Dis. Ct. App; 1951).

Schloendorff v. The Society of New York Hospital. (1914) 211 NY125, 105 N.E. 92 (1914).

Sherwin, W. (1992). Paternalism. In *No longer patient: Feminist ethics and health care* (pp. 137–157). Philadelphia: Temple University Press.

Singer, P. (2002). University of Toronto Joint Centre for Bioethics. *Living will*. Toronto: University of Toronto Joint Centre for Bioethics.

Slater v. Baker & Stapleton. (1767). High Court of Justice, King's Bench Division. English Reports, vol. 95, pp. 860–863.

Sullivan, G. H. (1998). Getting informed consent. *RN* (April), 59–62.

Tilden, V. P. (2000). Advance directives. *American Journal of Nursing, 100*(12), 49, 50.

Walton, N., Martin, D. K., Peter, E., Pringle, D., & Singer, P. A. (2007). Priority setting and cardiac surgery: A qualitative case study. *Health Policy, 80,* 444–458.

Williams, J. R. (2008). Consent. In P. A. Singer and A. M. Viens, eds., *The Cambridge textbook of bioethics*. Cambridge: Cambridge University Press.

CHAPTER 12

Scholarship Issues

OBJECTIVES

After completing this chapter, the reader should be able to:

1. Describe scholarship issues encountered by nurses in academic, clinical, and research settings.
2. Discuss principles basic to academic and research integrity.
3. Describe principles and standards underpinning the protection of human rights in research.

4. Explain why informed consent is mandated for research involving human participants, and describe the elements required for this consent.

5. Discuss the nursing role regarding protection of human rights in research.

6. Describe principles guiding personal response to dilemmas regarding nursing scholarship.

INTRODUCTION

Scholarship issues face students, teachers, researchers, and clinicians from the moment a person enters a nursing program and throughout that person's professional career. This chapter discusses principles that undergird ethical behaviour in academic matters, in conducting research, and in the treatment of data both during the research process and in presentations or publication. Respect for all persons, including ourselves, is basic to ethical behaviour regarding scholarship. Personal values affect how we approach situations that present ethical dilemmas. It is essential that nurses be knowledgeable about principles guiding ethical conduct, whether dealing with academic assignments, research data, or research with human participants.

ACADEMIC HONESTY

Integrity in upholding the principles of veracity and fidelity is expected of nurses in any setting and is at the core of academic honesty. Veracity refers to truth telling, which is an essential ingredient for trust among humans. Husted and Husted (1995) suggest that true interaction and communication cannot occur where there is no trust. These authors describe fidelity as promise keeping, suggesting that it is the form that truth takes in an agreement between persons such as nurse–patient, researcher–participant, or student–teacher. Integrity implies respect for self and others, and a personal commitment to principled behaviour over time in our personal and professional lives. When integrity is present, there is no need for monitoring a person's behaviour; rather, there is an implicit trust that we represent ourselves in a truthful way. Honesty and integrity are key considerations in both academic and clinical situations. Personal values such as honesty serve as the basis for professional integrity.

Students at all levels face many stresses in regard to academic performance, and nursing students are no exception. Pressures may come from many areas, such as family expectations, personal goals of being accepted into graduate school, needing a certain grade to receive tuition reimbursement, or self-expectations that say "I always get good grades." When pressures become intense, values such as honesty and integrity may become challenged.

Issues of academic integrity include plagiarism, cheating, misrepresentation of personal performance, and submission of false information. **Cheating** refers to dishonesty and deception, which may include the use of the work of others without authorization or without citation, the use of unauthorized information that is shared or received from others, and manipulating situations in which testing or evaluation is being carried out (Cizek, 1999; Cox, 2003).

Plagiarism exists when a person submits the work or part of the work of another and claims this work as his or her own (Simon Fraser University, 2000). **Misrepresentation of personal performance** includes submitting work that has been taken from another and represented as one's own, allowing someone else to write an exam using your name, or not being forthright with academic records or documents. Finally, **submission of false information** may include examples such as submitting a false statement such as a medical certificate to avoid completing an assignment or writing an exam, submitting false academic records, or altering official academic documents (Ryerson University, Office of Academic Integrity, 2005).

Ask Yourself

What Are Your Perspectives on Academic Honesty?

- One of your closest friends is in a different section of the same course, and his section meets two days after yours. You know he has been very stressed because of his mother's illness and that he needs good grades to keep his scholarship. You have just taken the mid-term exam, and he asks you to give him an idea of the topics covered so he can focus his studying. What would you do? How do you feel in this situation? What principles would guide your decisions?

- During an exam you notice two students passing what appear to be notes between them. You are fairly sure that the instructor has not seen this. How do you feel in response to this? What would you do, and why?

- You are struggling with an assignment that is due in just a few days. A classmate says she has a paper that her cousin did for this same course three years ago that she is using as a guide, changing the text so that it seems like her writing. She offers to let you see her cousin's paper to do the same. What do you think about her plan? How would you respond? What would guide your decision?

- You are studying for an important final exam. You note that the professor has indicated that, on her website, the teaching assistant has provided a set of practice questions to complete to prepare for the exam. You work through them carefully, as do your colleagues. While in the final exam, you notice that the exam questions are the same as the practice questions. Everyone around you notices the same thing, but no one tells the professor. What would you do? What principles would influence or guide your decision making?

- You are writing a long paper that you are finding particularly difficult. Remembering that you did a paper on a similar topic two years ago, you find it and decide that you will simply "cut and paste" sections from your previous paper into this paper. You are sure that this isn't plagiarism and that since the paper is your own work, you can do this without feeling uneasy about it. Is that true? Should you feel uneasy about this decision? If so, why?

- At the end of term, you have a number of important assignments due all at once. In addition, you have an on-line discussion in which you need to participate. When preparing for posting a response to the on-line discussion, for participation marks only, you research your topic on the Internet. You find a great deal of good non-scholarly, lay resources on the topic and decide that you will just cut the sections of text, paste them into the on-line discussion and change a few words. You do this, complete your on-line discussion quickly, and receive full participation marks. Since they weren't scholarly resources and the marks were simply for participation and not really for merit of work, you are fairly sure that this was acceptable. Later on, you are feeling that perhaps this wasn't the best way to approach the work. Why do you think you are uneasy? What would you do?

Implicit in academic honesty is a trust that work submitted by a student, whether papers, projects, or exams, is indeed the work of that student. When material from other sources is included in papers, students must utilize appropriate referencing so as to avoid plagiarizing. The breach of trust and potential consequences within a student–teacher relationship that academic dishonesty engenders are self-evident. Litigation is another potential consequence in severe situations. Because of the value of honesty, academic institutions frequently have written policies that may carry consequences as serious as the student's being suspended or expelled for dishonest practices.

CASE PRESENTATION

Suspicions of Dishonesty

Sabrina and Jude have been close friends and study partners throughout their nursing program. They discuss their readings and class notes and frequently choose the same topic, sharing articles between them when writing papers. After a recent submission of papers, the instructor called them in and noted that their papers were almost identical, including mistakes in grammar, and said that it appeared that one had copied the other's paper. They each denied copying from the other.

Think About It

Considering Consequences for Academic Dishonesty

- What ethical issues are involved in this situation?
- How do you feel about incidences of academic dishonesty?
- How do you think this situation should be handled? What consequences would you consider?
- In light of the standards that guide nursing practice, what is your position on allowing a student who has violated academic honesty through plagiarism, cheating, or forgery to continue in a nursing program?
- Should nursing students be held to a higher standard for academic honesty? Why or why not?

RESEARCH ISSUES AND ETHICS

Nurses must be accountable for the quality of care they deliver, and research is one way of documenting the efficacy of nursing practice as well as furthering the profession and dessiminating innovative approaches to practice. Both the art and science of nursing are expanded through research. Research is necessary for the ongoing development of the unique body of knowledge that undergirds the discipline of nursing, and provides an organizing framework for nursing practice. Research is an integral part of practice and education in nursing.

Participating in research can be exciting and encourage professional growth. It can also present some dilemmas for the nurse and nurse researcher in the academic and clinical realms. Seeking new knowledge and understanding is the expected motivation for conducting research. However, personal or institutional gains related to rewards like grant funds, prestige, the need to succeed, or promoting a product can be other motivating factors that may challenge principled behaviour in regard to research.

Underlying the nurse–patient relationship is the notion of trust. Trust arises out of the **fiduciary duty** that nurses, and all health care professionals, have toward their patients or clients. A fiduciary duty is one in which the nurse puts his or her own agenda, needs, or feelings aside, in order to place the patient in a position of priority. A fiduciary is a legal term, referring to someone who is entrusted to act in another person's best interests. It is a special responsibility, given to someone because of that person's relationship to another, or by virtue of his or her profession, as in the case of nurses, physicians, and other health care professionals.

The fiduciary responsibility that nurses have with their patients underlies the profession and nursing practice. That ability to act in another's best interest extends to all facets of patient care. Health care research, however, presents unique challenges to protecting that relationship of trust. As nurses become more and more involved in health care and nursing research, they take on new roles in which the fiduciary role looks markedly different. As nurse researchers, the goals of maintaining our fiduciary responsibilities are often intermingled with the goals of seeking new knowledge, obtaining grants, publishing, and presenting our own work. This intermingling of goals can often create conflicts of interest or role confusion.

In any case, nurses must always protect the autonomy and self-determination of the individuals for whom they provide care or involve in research activities. Care must always be taken to ensure that patients understand where the therapeutic relationship ends and the researcher–participant relationship begins. Whether the nurse is providing therapeutic care or is involving a patient in research, there exists a strong ethical obligation to protect the rights of all patients and participants, no matter what the context.

The rights of patients that we protect are the same rights as those of participants in research activities. **How** we protect these rights may differ between these groups, but in some cases, protection of these rights looks very similar. For example, we protect patients' autonomy by ensuring that they are fully informed about therapeutic procedures before they provide an informed consent. We also protect research participants' autonomy by making certain that there are clear, thoughtful, and non-coercive informed consent processes in place for research projects.

It is important to remember that there may be overlap in our clinical or therapeutic activities and our research involvement. This overlap, while unavoidable to some degree, does not change our responsibilities toward others: to protect their trust and autonomy, ensure that we minimize any harm to others, and act in their best interests.

Ethical Issues in Research

Many research texts focus their discussions of ethical issues in research primarily on protection of human rights. This emphasis is understandable because of violations that have occurred. Some of the most cited violations of human rights in research are those that were perpetrated by the Nazis during World War II and that came to public awareness during the Nuremberg Doctor trials. International efforts to provide guidelines for protection of human rights have subsequently been documented in the **Nuremberg Code,** which was developed as a set of principles for the ethical conduct of research against which the experiments in the concentration camps could be judged. This Code emphasizes the importance of informed consent for any participant/subject who is taking part in research. While the principles of autonomy and informed consent are the backbone of the ethical conduct of research, many academic researchers tend to distance themselves from the *Nuremberg Code,* favouring more recent guidelines and documents that are not associated in any way with the atrocities of World War II. The **Declaration of Helsinki** was issued by the World Medical Assembly in 1964 and was revised numerous times with the most recent iteration dated in October 2008 with the World Medical Association's General Assembly in Seoul, Korea. The *Declaration of Helsinki* differs from the *Nuremberg Code* by emphasizing notions of peer review for academic research. The Declaration is highly responsive to modern-day occurrences in the context of research. For example, one iteration of the *Declaration* *of Helsinki* includes statements that object to the phenomenon of researchers who "parachute" into developing countries to conduct research then abandon those same participants after completion of the research. Over the past few decades, this has become a problem, most notably with researchers carrying out drug trials for Human Immunodeficiency Virus (HIV) and AIDS in parts of Africa, only to leave their participants without any therapy after completion of the trial. In any kind of research, participants are giving of their time and often exposing themselves to a certain degree of risk of harm. Therefore, it is considered to be ethically problematic to carry out research on individuals who are vulnerable or less fortunate without commensurate compensation at the very least.

Canadian guidelines for the ethical conduct of research can be found in the *Tri Council Policy Statement* (TCPS) (Canadian Institutes of Health Research, Natural Sciences and Engineering Research Council of Canada, Social Science and Humanities Research Council of Canada, *Tri Council Policy Statement: Ethical Conduct for Research Involving Humans,* 1998 [with 2000, 2002, 2005 amendments]). This guiding document was created in 1998 and has recently been revised to reflect greater attention to issues such as qualitative and social science research, research involving Aboriginal persons and the use of vulnerable populations in research activities.

In spite of these policies and guidelines, ethical lapses continue to occur in research with human participants (Kaplan & Brownlee, 1999; Hilts & Stolberg, 1999; Maloney, 2000a, 2000b). These and other concerns raise questions about whether current regulations adequately protect the rights and welfare of research participants (Moreno, Caplan, & Wolpe, 1998). In Canada, the *Tri Council Policy Statement* (TCPS) is a federal document that provides clear guidelines on the ethical conduct of research and the fair and ethical treatment of participants involved in all types of research (Canadian Institutes of Health Research, Natural Sciences and Engineering Research Council of Canada, Social Science and Humanities Research Council of Canada, *Tri Council Policy Statement: Ethical Conduct for Research Involving Humans,* 1998 [with 2000, 2002, 2005 amendments]). In order to receive federal funding, academic and clinical institutions that conduct research must adhere to these guidelines, and an institutional Research Ethics Board must review all research prior to its being conducted. Health Canada also provides strict oversight on all clinical trials. The mandate of both the Tri-Council Policy Statement and Health Canada's oversight of clinical trials is to protect participants. A new draft of the TCPS was released in 2008 and there are a number of changes that help to ensure protection of participants. For example, new and timely guidelines on research involving Aboriginal persons and participants in qualitative research are included in the new draft. In order to oversee and enforce federal regulations pertaining to research with human subjects, the United States Department of Health and Human Services recently formed an Office for Human Research Protection. Efforts to bolster protections for human research participants focus on education and training of clinical investigators and institutional review board members, auditing records for evidence of compliance with informed consent, improved monitoring of clinical trials, managing conflicts of interest so that research participants are appropriately informed, and imposing monetary penalties for violations of important research practices, such as informed consent (Spicer, 2000).

Think About It

The following are examples of significant and well-known ethical lapses in the conduct of human-participant research:

- Between 1932 and 1972, a group of physicians decided to observe the effect of untreated syphilis in a large group of about 400 mainly African American migrant workers. At the time of the inception of the study, treatments for syphilis were questionable and often toxic, until 1947, when penicillin became the standard and successful treatment. Mainly illiterate, the workers were not informed that they had the disease. They were told that they had problems with their blood and were also told that they were receiving free medical treatment, were provided with rides to and from the medical institutions, and were given funds to cover the costs of eventual funeral and burial rites. They did not receive medical treatment, even in 1947 when the standard proven treatment was widely available. They underwent a great deal of medical testing, had samples of their blood taken, and many understood, mistakenly, that this was a method of "treatment." After the introduction of penicillin to treat syphilis, this study continued for another three decades and the men were never offered treatment. Many continued to be observed and without knowing, spread syphilis to others, until their eventual deaths, usually from complications of the disease.

- Stanley Milgram, a social psychologist, carried out a study at Yale University in 1963 examining human responses to authority. In this study, he recruited participants to take part in an experiment in which they were required to deliver electric shocks to another participant in an adjoining room. The participant receiving shocks was actually an actor hired by the researcher, who did not receive shocks but instead cried out in pain at each "delivered shock." The recruited participants could not see the actor, but could hear the cries of pain and anguish. As the study progressed, participants were instructed to increase the level of joules of delivered electricity, to a point that was clearly potentially fatal. While obedient to the authority figure, as participants were asked to deliver more and more electricity to another person, they became clearly distressed and markedly affected by the level of deception involved in this experiment.

- In the book *The Tearoom Trade* (1970), sociologist Laud Humphreys documented his doctoral ethnographic research, in which he followed men into public bathrooms to observe male–male sexual acts, colloquially referred to as "tearooming." He would then follow the men to their cars, record their licence plates and, with the help of the local department of transportation, access their addresses. Armed with their contact information and knowledge of usually illicit and secretive sexual activity, he would confront the men in their homes and ask that they consent to be interviewed about their sexual behaviour, using false pretences and strong coercive influence.

Each of these examples illustrate significant risks, coercion, and explicit deception, without safeguards for the participants or a reasonable balance of risk and benefits.

What are your thoughts on these research studies?

Do you find it shocking that they occurred so recently?

Do you think that the policies and guidelines in place today are enough to avoid similar ethical lapses?

Principles of beneficence, respect for human dignity, and justice underlie the ethical conduct of research (Canadian Institutes of Health Research, Natural Sciences and Engineering Research Council of Canada, Social Science and Humanities Research Council of Canada, *Tri Council Policy Statement: Ethical Conduct for Research Involving Humans,* 1998 [with 2000, 2002, 2005 amendments]; Newland, 2000). Throughout the international research community, there are also common ethical principles more specific to research and rights of participants that have been articulated and well documented.

Arising out the values of beneficence and respect for human dignity are the following rights and principles: respect for human dignity, respect for free and informed consent, respect for vulnerable persons, and respect for privacy and confidentiality. The principle of beneficence also underlies the aims of balancing harms and risks in research and maximizing benefit while minimizing harm. Respect for fairness and inclusiveness arise out of the principle of justice. A brief discussion of each principle follows.

Beneficence. This principle derives from the maxim that says "above all, do no harm." In research situations this means that researchers need to design and conduct studies so as to protect the participants from potential risks of harm, including physical, emotional, economic, psychological, financial, or social harm. The notions of harm and risk of harm are subjective. In other words, researchers must attend to the perspectives of the participants and what they might consider to be harmful. Harms may be permanent or transient, and may be differently considered by different persons and groups. Moreover, harm and risk of harm occur on a spectrum, from less severe to very serious. For example, asking new immigrants without legal status questions about the services they can access is of significantly more risk than asking permanent residents the same kinds of things. Risks and harms may be related to the research activity or to the attributes or special situations of the participants. More vulnerable participants may be subject to greater potential harms, by virtue of their health status, age, social, or economic status.

Physical harms are not necessarily related to only potential injury or serious adverse effects. They may include fatigue or physiological symptoms related to stress. Emotional or psychological harms may refer to triggering unpleasant or distressing memories, being anxious or embarrassed, or feeling deceived or unduly coerced to take part in research activities. Social harms may include being exposed to others, being misrepresented, having one's reputation harmed, or having one's privacy or confidentiality breached. Financial harms may include lost earnings for time taken for participation in research activities or, more seriously, loss of employment if the confidentiality of sensitive or negative information is not maintained.

In all research activities, the burden of responsibility lies with the researcher to assess potential for harm and risk of harm and to enact all possible strategies to mitigate these harms. Most importantly, the foreseeable harm or risk of harm must be balanced with the potential or anticipated benefits. Participants must have full information about the potential risks of harm as well as anticipated benefits, which should not be overstated, promised, or guaranteed. While it is noted that research endeavours involve a certain degree of uncertainty, there are steps that can be taken by researchers, as well as processes in place, that address ethical obligations around balancing foreseeable risks and anticipated benefits (Canadian Institutes of Health Research, Natural Sciences and Engineering Research Council of Canada, Social Science and Humanities Research Council of Canada, *Tri Council Policy Statement: Ethical Conduct for Research Involving Humans,* 1998 [with 2000, 2002, 2005 amendments]).

Traditionally, research has been designated as either less or greater than minimal risk. The standard of minimal risk implies that participants are not being subjected to a greater probability of harm than they might encounter in a typical day. This, of course, relates directly to the participants and their everyday life. Someone living in an area of civil war, extreme poverty, or strife is subject to a greater daily risk or harm than a person living in a peaceful, democratic, and socioeconomically stable environment.

If a person, by virtue of taking part in a research activity, is potentially being subjected to a risk that is greater than what they might encounter in their daily life, then this would be considered greater than minimal risk. Greater scrutiny of research processes and safeguards as well as enhanced protection for participants would be defensible in this case (Canadian Institutes of Health Research, Natural Sciences and Engineering Research Council of Canada, Social Science and Humanities Research Council of Canada, *Tri Council Policy Statement: Ethical Conduct for Research Involving Humans,* 1998 [with 2000, 2002, 2005 amendments]).

Since our role as nurses compels us to protect those in our care from unnecessary harm or risk of harm, if the risks of research potentially or clearly outweigh the benefits, the study should be redesigned or discontinued.

Respect for Human Dignity. Implicit in this principle is the right to self-determination, which acknowledges the autonomy of the potential participant in research. This means that persons have the right to choose whether they wish to participate in the research; that is, participation is voluntary and free from coercion of any type. **Coercion** includes threat of harm or penalty for not participating in the research, or offering excessive rewards for participation. The right of self-determination means that the person has the right to withdraw from participation in the study at any time without imposed consequences, such as denial of health care or benefits. Voluntary participation requires **full disclosure**, that is, that the potential participant be fully informed of the nature of the study, the anticipated risks and benefits, time commitment, what is expected of the participant and the researcher, and the right to refuse to participate. This is addressed through the process of informed consent, which is discussed below and revisited in Chapter 11.

The *Declaration of Helsinki* (World, Medical Association, 2008) states

> It is the duty of physicians who participate in research to protect the life, health, dignity, integrity, right to self-determination, privacy, and confidentiality of personal information of research subjects. (Article B: 11)

Justice.   The principle of justice includes the rights to privacy and to fair treatment. The nature of research is to gather information about that which is being studied. When persons are the focus of study, the **right to privacy** is a critical issue. Attentiveness to privacy means the participant determines when, where, and what kind of information is shared, with an assurance that information, attitudes, behaviours, records, opinions, and the like that are observed or collected will be treated with respect and kept in strict confidence. Privacy is maintained through anonymity, confidentiality, and informed consent. If even the researcher cannot link information with a particular participant, then **anonymity** exists. **Confidentiality** refers to the researcher's assurance to participants that information provided will not be made public or available to anyone other than those involved in the research process without the participant's consent. Confidentiality is maintained by using codes rather than personal identification on data collection forms and restricting access to raw data to those on the research team who need to use the data.

The **right to fair treatment** is related to the right to self-determination. Equitable treatment of participants in the selection process, during the study, and after the completion of the study is at the basis of this right. Factors to consider in fair treatment include selecting participants based on the research needs, not on the convenience or compromised position of a group of people; equitably distributing the risks and benefits of the research among participants regardless of age, gender, socioeconomic status, race, or ethnic background; honouring any agreements made or benefits promised; treating participants with respect, providing access to research personnel or other professionals as needed; treating persons who decline to participate or withdraw from the study without prejudice; and debriefing as needed to clarify issues or when information had been withheld prior to the study.

CASE PRESENTATION

Protecting Patients Who Are Research Participants

Parvati is a charge nurse in a women's health clinic. David is a close colleague, who is completing his Masters in Nursing. For his thesis, David hopes to examine the experiences of women who present to the clinic reporting domestic or spousal abuse. He hopes to eventually contribute to improving both the direct services and the referrals that the clinic provides for the women, and knows that in order to do this, their experiences and views must be sought. When Parvati asks him about recruiting his participants, he tells her that he will contact any previous clinic patients who have reported potential domestic abuse, after going through the clinic files, as he will have complete access to them, once Parvati approves. He will ask them if they are interested in being interviewed one on one, privately, at a time convenient to them. He'll tell them that it is for his thesis, which is very important both for his own professional advancement and for the clinic population. He is sure that they will wish to cooperate, as many are patients known to him and he feels that they have a good therapeutic relationship, underpinned by mutual respect and trust.

Parvati asks him if the Research Ethics Board at his university reviewed his proposal and David replies that he is in the process of putting his proposal together to submit to them, but is fairly sure that there won't be any ethical problems with the proposal. He is so sure of the project being approved that he thinks he may begin looking through the charts now, before getting explicit approval.

Think About It

What principles guide the ethical conduct of clinical research?

- What ethical principles are involved in this situation?
- What dilemmas do you foresee arising with David's research proposal?
- If you were a member of the university Research Ethics Board reviewing this proposal, what would you recommend and why?
- David wants to begin looking at charts right away. Should Parvati allow him to access the charts for this purpose? What principles would underlie her decision-making process in this situation?

Informed Consent. As noted above, voluntary participation in a research study requires full disclosure. Informing potential participants of the research purpose, expected commitment, risks and benefits, any invasion of privacy, and ways that anonymity and confidentiality will be addressed are included in the process of **informed consent.** The researcher must ensure that the person who is agreeing to participate in the study comprehends the information included in the consent and has a chance to receive clarifications and additional information when needed. Written consent forms should be written in common language without using high-level medical or legal terms, at approximately a grade seven reading and comprehension level. The literacy level of the person signing the informed consent should be determined and recorded, and the person agreeing to participate in the research must be mentally and emotionally competent to make the decision. In addition to having cognitive capability to understand and provide consent, participants must also have the volitional capacity to make informed consent decisions. In other words, consent must be both "free and informed" (TCPS, Section 2, Article 2.1).

While Munhall and Boyd (1999) suggest that the process of informed consent provides a way of including the person as a collaborator in the research rather than as a mere "subject," we must always be acutely aware of coercion or undue influence that may alter a person's abilities to voluntarily provide informed consent. Preexisting relationships, hierarchical relationships, or the use of managers, employers, or those in any kind of "power-over" relationship to recruit participants may result in persons feeling coerced or unduly influenced to participate. In other words, any kind of pressure that is exerted, either explicitly or implicitly, by virtue of a pre-existing relationship, is what may be referred to as coercion. Any kind of coercive factor in recruiting and obtaining consent from potential participants in research projects must be addressed and strategies put in place to mitigate the effects of these factors. One review of nursing research protocols found more ethical concerns arising from the relationship between the researcher and study participant than from physical harm (Olsen & Mahrenholz, 2000). When the nurse who cares for the patient is on the research team and the one obtaining the informed consent, determining whether the patient is giving consent to the "nurse" or to the "researcher" can be somewhat tricky. The nurse-researcher must determine whether the patient truly feels the freedom to refuse to participate.

Article 2.4 of *The Tri Council Policy Statement: Ethical Conduct for Research Involving Humans* (1998, with 2000, 2002 and 2005 amendments) lists the following elements that need to be provided as part of a process of obtaining informed consent:

> **(a)** Information that the individual is being invited to participate in a research project;
>
> **(b)** A comprehensible statement of the research purpose, the identity of the researcher, the expected duration and nature of participation, and a description of research procedures;

(c) A comprehensible description of reasonably foreseeable harms and benefits that may arise from research participation, as well as the likely consequences of non-action, particularly in research related to treatment, or where invasive methodologies are involved, or where there is a potential for physical or psychological harm;

(d) An assurance that prospective subjects are free not to participate, have the right to withdraw at any time without prejudice to pre-existing entitlements, and will be given continuing and meaningful opportunities for deciding whether or not to continue to participate, and;

(e) The possibility of commercialization of research findings, and the presence of any apparent of actually or potential conflict of interest on the part of researchers, their institutions or sponsors.

Source: Canadian Institutes of Health Research, Natural Sciences and Engineering Research Council of Canada, Social Science and Humanities Research Council of Canada, *Tri Council Policy Statement: Ethical Conduct for Research Involving Humans,* 1998 [with 2000, 2002, 2005 amendments].

Nurses who are assisting with research or who work on units where research is being conducted must be familiar with these elements of informed consent. If consent processes and forms do not contain these elements, nurses should bring this to the attention of the investigators or the institutional Research Ethics Board.

CASE PRESENTATION

Juanita is a registered nurse, working in a large urban hospital in a thoracic surgery step-down unit. Today, she notices that two of her patients have been enrolled in a new study, in which they may receive one of the traditional pain medications for post-operative pain or be randomized into a group that receives a new type of analgesic. When Juanita looks up the new drug on the Internet, she notes that it has been used in a limited number of other contexts, but never in post-operative pain management. Juanita knows that pain after thoracic surgery can be excruciating and she is concerned.

She calls the study nurse listed on the patients' consent forms for more information. It turns out that the study nurse is Wayne, a friend from nursing school. When Juanita voices her concern to Wayne more about the study drug, he assures her by reminding her that it isn't an experimental drug any longer but one that is being used in a new way. He also says to Juanita that she likely knows as much as he does about the drug, as he hasn't researched it too much but does know that it is safe in the limited contexts in which it has been previously used.

He recruits patients for the study on top of his work in the cardiac unit, on his days off. He tells Juanita, "The drug company pays me one hundred dollars for each patient who is enrolled, followed up, and completes the study. It only takes a few minutes to sign them up, put a randomization number on their chart, notify the pharmacy, and get the data after surgery. It's pretty easy. You should do it too!"

❓ Think About It

- What issues of concern do you identify in this case situation?
- What ethical principles are being violated or potentially violated?
- Why is Juanita concerned? Is her concern justified? What ethical principle or principles underlie her concern?
- What kinds of potential consequences or conflicts of interest might affect the outcomes of this situation?

Special Considerations: Vulnerable Populations

Nurses must be especially attentive to protection of human rights in research with vulnerable populations. These populations may include physically, developmentally, or mentally challenged persons; young children or elderly persons; those without full legal status or refugees; persons who are living at extremely low socioeconomic levels or who are homeless; those who are dying, sedated, or unconscious; persons who are institutionalized, incarcerated, or highly dependent on agencies; pregnant women, and fetuses. Because people in these populations are potentially more vulnerable to deception and coercion, and may have decreased ability to give informed consent, advocates or guardians who clearly and explicitly have the person's best interest in mind must be involved in decisions regarding their participation in research. An important consideration for research with vulnerable populations is that the less able the person is to give informed consent, the more important it is for the researcher to protect the person's rights (Wilson, 1999). Nurses who work with these populations need to be especially cognizant of their roles as advocates, particularly when research is proposed or being conducted in their settings.

While research on vulnerable persons requires more stringent oversight and monitoring, it also is imperative to allow vulnerable persons to participate in research. Not allowing vulnerable persons access to new and innovative therapies, or to have their experiences documented or voices heard, may be thought of as a form of discrimination and may lead to further marginalization (Mastroianni and Kahn, 2004). For example, conducting research on the kinds of services accessed by persons in Canadian cities without full legal status is essential in order to gain insight into the kinds of services that they might require and the critical needs that they have. As an additional example, consider that without allowing pregnant women to participate in research, we would not have made the advances in obstetric care that have been documented nor would we have knowledge about the effects of particular drugs and treatments upon pregnant women and fetuses. As a final example, it is clear that the health, physical, and emotional needs of persons who are homeless may differ from the needs of those living in relative comfort. Therefore, by allowing those who are homeless to participate in research, their experiences are articulated and specific services that may address their needs might be put into place, with the evidence that such research would present.

More than Protection of Human Rights

Although protection of human subjects is a very important consideration in nursing research, other issues deserve equal attention. Wilson (1999) discusses characteristics of ethical research that go beyond the protection of human rights. These include:

Scientific objectivity—reporting all data, both supportive and unsupportive of hypotheses, and not engaging in misconduct, fraud, or acts of bad faith;

Cooperation—submitting proposals to and following recommendations of those authorized to review the research for protection of human rights;

Nobility—working actively to ensure protection of participants from harm, deceit, coercion, and invasions of privacy, even when this may inconvenience the study;

Integrity and truthfulness—honestly describing the research process, including the purpose, procedures, methods, risks, discomforts, benefits, and findings;

Impeccability—ensuring anonymity and confidentiality of data and using discretion with information learned about people;

Illumination—publishing and presenting research findings in order to enhance nursing's body of scientific knowledge;

Equitability—noting contributions of others in publications and presentations;

Forthrightness—disclosing funding sources and sponsorship in publication and presentation of research findings;

Courage—publicly clarifying any distortions of research findings made by others.

When nurses are working in agencies or institutions where research is being conducted, whether or not they are directly involved in the research, they must be aware of standards for ethical research in order to guard against violations of these standards.

Nurses who participate in conducting research may at times experience role conflict. A nurse is held to standards of professional practice that delineate the nurse's concern as safeguarding the health and well-being of the patient. A researcher is focused on processes and outcomes of a study in which patients may be used as sources of data. A responsible researcher is guided by humanistic values of moral concern in decisions regarding research participants (Fry, 1981). Thus, when there is a question of potential harm to a patient involved in a research study, the nurse's fiduciary duty, advocacy role, and therapeutic imperative take precedence over integrity of the research protocol (Fowler, 1988a; Munhall and Boyd, 1999; Namei, King, Byrne, & Proffitt, 1993). Incomplete knowledge of ethical and legal guidelines related to research is no excuse for a nurse's failing to be a patient advocate in research situations. Although research is necessary for development of scientific and therapeutic knowledge, a balance between principles guiding scientific inquiry and those guiding nursing practice must be maintained.

When nurses are employed, particularly in institutions that are research focused, they need to clarify what is expected of them in regard to research. Nurses should know prior to accepting a position whether they will be required to gather data or administer treatments as part of research protocols, and whether such treatments may have potential risk of harm to patients. Nurses in such settings need to know whether their positions will be jeopardized if they refuse to participate as part of a research team. When participation in research is expected as part of a nurse's job, the nurse must know the protocol, whether it has been approved by the institutional Research Ethics Board, and whom to consult with regarding any concerns about the research process and effect on patients.

Ask Yourself

What Takes Precedence—Research or Nursing Care?

Fowler (1988b, p. 354) poses some questions that are worth pondering:

- Is the good of the patient ever subservient to the acquisition of nursing knowledge?
- Does the therapeutic imperative of clinical care and the good of the patient always preempt the mandate to enlarge the nursing profession's body of knowledge?
- At what point must a nurse stop a specific nursing research project?
- When must a nurse intervene to halt a specific medical research project?
- Are there conditions under which a nurse should not include a specific subject in a study, even though consent has been secured?

ETHICAL TREATMENT OF DATA

Scholarship issues regarding data include how the data is handled during the collection and analysis process and how the data is reported. **Ethical treatment of data** implies integrity of research protocols and honesty in reporting findings. The honesty and integrity of the researcher are of utmost importance in the ethical treatment of data. Taking care to ensure that only those who are involved in the research process have access to the data and to maintain confidentiality were mentioned previously. A critical ethical obligation of qualitative nursing researchers is to present and describe the experiences of others as authentically and faithfully as possible, even when it is contrary to our own aims (Munhall & Boyd, 1999). The imperative to report the findings as accurately as possible is an ethical obligation in quantitative studies as well.

CASE PRESENTATION

Protecting Patients Who Are Research Participants

A classmate and good friend is in the process of doing a research project required for graduation. You know she is frustrated because the on-line survey has not been completed by enough participants. She has sent out many reminders to potential participants but her response rate remains low. She needs to do well on this project in order to pass the final course of her degree and graduate. In order to have a large enough sample, she tells you that she is going to log onto her own survey and fill it in several times herself. She asks if you will do the same, noting that the surveys are anonymous and that several other friends are "helping is out" in the same way. She says that, after all, the objective of the project is simply to demonstrate that one can collect and analyze data. It isn't really, she notes, about the actual data at all, but about the processes. You are aware that the best studies are chosen for presentations at the university Research Day, and have, in the past, been published.

Think About It

Honesty in Nursing Research

- What is your reaction to her plan and request?
- Discuss the ethical issues involved in this scenario.
- Describe what stance you would take, and why it would be ethically justified.
- What would you do in this case and what ethical principles would guide your actions or decisions?

Nurses involved in research are accountable to professional standards for reporting findings. Principles that guide academic honesty apply as well to nurse researchers in reporting outcomes of studies. It is dishonest to exaggerate results or adjust facts of a study in order to maximize or minimize particular outcomes or hypotheses. When information from someone else is included in a report without appropriate referencing, this is plagiarism. In recent years, scientific misconduct has become a concern within the scientific community. Articles have been published in professional journals reporting studies that were never conducted, findings that were fabricated, or findings that were intentionally distorted by researchers (Burns & Groves, 1997; Chop & Silva, 1991; Friedman, 1990; Hawley & Jeffers, 1992; Parascandola, 1999). Although these reports have related more to biomedical studies than to nursing research, such reports present problems to disciplines whose clinical practice may be changed based on research findings. They also serve as a reminder to nurses to be vigilant regarding ethical reporting of research findings.

Ask Yourself

Consequences of Reporting Fraudulent Research

Pause and think about the havoc rendered by publication of fraudulent research.

- How might this affect how others view the integrity of the profession?
- How might this affect a reader's response to other research published in the same journal?
- How would this affect your ability as a nurse to determine whether you should adjust your practice based on reported research?
- Imagine that you have just read the report of a research project for which you gathered data and discovered that the process described was quite a bit different from what you had done, making the results take on a different meaning. How would you react and what would you do?

SUMMARY

Nurses are expected to exhibit principled behaviour in all situations. This chapter has focused on principles related to scholarship issues facing nurses. Nursing students face decisions related to academic honesty before they ever encounter a patient. Because personal values affect professional behaviour, choices made in the academic arena concerning actions such as plagiarism, cheating, or forgery may foreshadow values used to guide future professional decisions. Nurses must be familiar with principles guiding ethical practices in research and reporting of research findings. These principles guide nursing decisions about research protocols, participation, and advocacy for patients related to research issues. Ethical practices regarding scholarship are essential to the integrity of both the professional and the profession.

CHAPTER HIGHLIGHTS

- Veracity and integrity are core principles related to both academic honesty and to ethical treatment of research data.
- Nursing research and researchers must adhere to nursing standards regarding the ethical conduct of research that affirm a participant's right to freedom from intrinsic risk of injury, right to privacy, right to anonymity, and the right to choose to participate or not.

- Protection of human rights, a prime focus of research ethics, is based on principles of beneficence, respect for human dignity, and justice. These principles imply protection from physical, psychological, social, or economic risk of harms, voluntary participation in research; and assurance of privacy, confidentiality and equitable treatment of all research participants.

- Informed consent for research studies, which helps to ensure that a participant's rights are protected, must include the elements promulgated in the *Tri Council Policy Statement*.

- When there is a question of potential harm to a patient involved in a research study, the nurse's advocacy role and therapeutic imperative takes precedence over the integrity of the research protocol. Nurses need to be especially attentive to protection of rights of vulnerable groups in clinical and research settings.

DISCUSSION QUESTIONS AND ACTIVITIES

1. Review your school's policy regarding academic integrity, and discuss ethical principles that are violated in cases of academic dishonesty.

2. Describe factors that persons reviewing cases of academic dishonesty or misconduct should consider.

3. How did protection of human rights come to be required for research involving human subjects?

4. What guidance do nursing standards offer nurses who are participating in or conducting research? What principles underlie the ethical conduct of research? Discuss nursing roles related to these principles and standards.

5. Interview a nurse researcher regarding how human rights are protected in the study. Have all the required elements been included in the informed consent?

6. Give examples of situations in which the nursing roles of patient advocate and researcher might be in conflict. Which role takes precedence and why?

7. Discuss potential effects of unethical treatment of data on patient care.

8. Compare and contrast what the American Nurse's Association (http://www.nursingworld.org), the Canadian Nurses Association (http://www.cna-nurses.ca/cna), and the International Council of Nurses (http://www.icn.ch) say about human rights in research and in nursing practice.

9. Review the second draft of the *Tri Council Policy Statement*. Note the changes and revisions and discuss their timeliness in the context of what you have learned in this chapter. (www.pre.ethics.gc.ca/english/pdf/newsandevents/TCPS_Dec_4_en.pdf)

REFERENCES

Burns, N., & Groves, S. K. (1997). *The practice of nursing research* (3rd ed.). Philadelphia: Saunders.

Canadian Institutes of Health Research, Natural Sciences and Engineering Research Council of Canada, Social Science and Humanities Research Council of Canada, *Tri Council Policy Statement: Ethical Conduct for Research Involving Humans,* 1998 (with 2000, 2002, 2005 amendments).

Chop, R., & Silva, M. C. (1991). Scientific fraud: Definitions, policies, and implications for nursing research. *Journal of Professional Nursing, 7,* 166–171.

Cizek, G. J. (1999). Cheating on tests: How to do it, detect it and prevent it. New Jersey: Lawrence Erlbaum Associates.

Cox, D. H. (2003). Academic integrity: Cheating 101—a literature review. *The News about Teaching and Learning at Memorial, 6*(2). Newsletter of the Instructional Development Office.

Fowler, M. D. M. (1988a). Ethical issues in nursing research: Issues in qualitative research. *Western Journal of Nursing Research, 10,* 109–111.

Fowler, M. D. M. (1988b). Ethical issues in nursing research: A call for an international code of ethics for nursing. *Western Journal of Nursing Research, 10,* 352–355.

Friedman, P. J. (1990). Correcting the literature following fraudulent publication. *Journal of the American Medical Association, 263,* 1416–1419.

Fry, S. T. (1981). Accountability in research: The relationship of scientific and humanistic values. *Advances in Nursing Science, 4,* 1–13.

Hawley, D. J., & Jeffers, J. M. (1992). Scientific misconduct as a dilemma for nursing. *Image, 24,* 51–55.

Hilts, P. J., & Stolberg, S. G. (1999). Ethics lapses at Duke halt dozens of human experiments. *The New York Times,* May 13, A26.

Humphreys, L. (1970). Tearoom Trade: Impersonal Sex in Public Places. Aldine Transaction: Piscataway, USA.

Husted, G. L., & Husted, J. H. (1995). *Ethical decision making in nursing* (2nd ed.). St. Louis, MO: Mosby.

Kaplan, S., & Brownlee, S. (1999). Duke's hazards: Did medical experiments put patients needlessly at risk? *U. S. World and News Report, 126*(20), 66–68, 70.

Maloney, D. M. (2000a). Federal agency has all the legal authority it needs to suspend human subjects research. *Human Research Report, 15*(1), 1–2.

Maloney, D. M. (2000b). Court says state agency avoided usual way of reporting problems with human subjects: *T. D. v. New York State Office of Mental Health* (Part III). *Human Research Report, 15*(2), 7–8.

Mastroianni, A., & Kahn, J. (2004). Swinging the pendulum: Shifting views of justice in human subjects research. In *Health Care Ethics in Canada,* Second edition. Baylis, F., Downie, J., Hoffmaster, B., & Sherwin, S. (eds). Toronto, Canada: Thomson Nelson.

Moreno, J., Caplan, A. L., & Wolpe, P. R. (1998). Updating protections for human subjects involved in research. *Journal of the American Medical Association, 280*(22), 1951–1958.

Munhall, P. L., & Boyd, C. O. (1999). *Nursing research: A qualitative perspective* (2nd ed.). New York: National League of Nursing Press.

Namei, S. K., King, M. O., Byrne, M., & Proffitt, C. (1993). The ethics of role conflict. *Journal of Neuroscience Nursing, 25,* 326–330.

Olsen, D. P., & Mahrenholz, D. (2000). IRB-identified ethical issues in nursing research. *Journal of Professional Nursing, 16*(3), 140–148.

Parascandola, M. (1999). Investigator fraud in clinical research. *Research-Nurse, 5*(2), 1–9, 20–21.

Ryerson University Office of Academic Integrity. (2005). Academic Integrity: A Student Guide. Ryerson: Toronto. Retrieved January 20, 2009, from www.ryerson.ca/ai/students.html.

Simon Fraser University. (2000). Code of academic honesty. Retrieved July 10, 2008, from http://www.sfu.ca/policies/teaching/t10-02.htm.

Spicer, C. M. (2000). Federal oversight and regulations of human subjects research: An update. *Kennedy Institute of Ethics Journal, 10*(3), 261–264.

Wilson, H. S. (1999). *Introducing research in nursing* (2nd ed.). Redwood City, CA: Addison-Wesley.

World Medical Association. (Oct. 2008). *The Declaration of Helsinki.* Seoul, Korea: World Medical Association.

CHAPTER 13

Health Care Changes and Challenges

By Barbara Kupchak

OBJECTIVES

After completing this chapter, the reader should be able to:

1. Identify patterns of health care delivery from ancient times to the present.
2. Discuss historical events that have helped to shape Canadian health care.
3. Examine trends in health care delivery and financing that have emerged in recent history.
4. Describe challenges facing health care delivery systems around the globe.

5. Discuss factors prompting a renewed interest in traditional healing systems worldwide.

6. Briefly describe factors affecting health care delivery for rural and urban aggregates.

INTRODUCTION

The health care delivery system and the way it is financed define the parameters within which nurses and other health care personnel function. Issues of health care delivery and the effectiveness of the health care delivery system are of concern throughout the world. In Canada and most of the Western world, delivery of health care is much like a runaway train of high technology—there is a proliferation of markets for new medications and expensive treatments. Further, the system is challenged to provide for an ever-increasing global population with decreasing resources. At the basis of this global concern is the ever-increasing cost of health care and the issue of its sustainability. Developing countries are recognizing that current and future health care systems have at their foundation expensive medicines and technologies that are imported from more developed regions of the globe. Questions arise about prioritizing health expenditures. Can countries address the health needs of their people without relying on expensive medications and treatments? Can local, existing systems of health care be utilized to provide basic health services to rural and urban poor communities? In developing countries, can traditional methods and systems of health care be utilized to promote health care and prevent disease, thus reducing the burden on the system? Has modern Western health care practice been lax in preserving and utilizing the traditional methods in favour of technology, and, if so, at what cost?

Health care systems must address global changes and challenges if they are to survive in the twenty-first century and beyond. In order to gain an understanding of these changes and challenges, we need to explore the history of various contemporary health care systems and their financing, including traditional methods of health care. In addition, we must look at rural and urban at-risk communities and factors that impede the delivery of health care in an overburdened system.

Ask Yourself

What Cultural Influences Affect Your Health Care Practices?

All persons have roots in beliefs and cultural heritage from their family of origin and place of birth.

- What do you know about the health care practices of your cultural origins?
- Have you or anyone you know ever utilized any healing modalities that are not part of what would be deemed modern health care?

A BRIEF HISTORY OF HEALTH CARE DELIVERY: THE EURO-AMERICAN EXPERIENCE

From the earliest civilizations there is evidence of some type of health care. The methods of health care were often a mixture of religious, civil, and mythological belief that combined to keep away disease, prevent wars, and ensure survival of populations in order to keep the various empires strong. In every culture there have been individuals designated to provide care to the sick. Some were formally trained as nurses and physicians, while others seemed to have been deemed as having a natural gift for the art of healing. Asian and Middle Eastern peoples, such as the Mesopotamians, Babylonians, Hebrews, Persians, Hindus, and Chinese, have recorded some type of system for the delivery of health care. In all of these cultures, religious or civil laws enforced systems of disease prevention in matters of hygiene and diet, some of which were connected to the various religious practices of the ancient civilizations.

Early Eras of Health Care Delivery

Achterberg notes that "the Sumerians, and not the ancient Greeks and Romans, are the parents of Western healing systems" (1990, p. 14). Archeological findings in the area of ancient Sumer, which is located in the vicinity of modern Iraq, include numerous prescriptions and two tablets that are considered to be the oldest medical text in existence (Achterberg, 1990). Sumerian knowledge of healing and theories of disease were dispersed to other areas through trade with the Phoenicians, Greeks, and Egyptians.

The ancient Greek civilization represents a major force in the systematic organization of education, both in secular and scientific fields. The most well-known name in ancient Greek medicine and health care is Hippocrates, known as the Father of Medicine. His approach of separating medicine and health care from religion, magic, and myth was considered purely scientific for his time. He diagnosed from observed symptoms, with emphasis on treating the whole patient, and he promoted continuous bedside care. His method of systematic record keeping of the patient's appearance, vital signs, and general bodily functioning became a standard for health care. Hippocrates approached medicine and health care from the highest ethical standard, believing medicine to be the noblest of arts. In addition, he believed that the physician's conduct should be of the highest quality and above reproach. Hippocrates gave the health care system organized writings of medical books that include detailed descriptive case histories, technical practices, and reports of research on various disease treatments, including treatments that worked and those that did not, in order to avoid repeating errors in care (Kelly, 1985).

As nations and populations expanded, knowledge was disseminated from culture to culture, constantly redefining the approach to health care, research, and practice. Alexander the Great, who conquered Greece in about 339 B.C.E., spread what he learned in Greece throughout the entire known world. He established medical schools in Egypt that included clinics, laboratories, and libraries. Physicians were supported by the government, and could devote their time to practice and research. Gradually, through various wars and assimilation of culture, Greek medicine supplemented or replaced practices throughout the known Western world.

The empire of Rome replaced methods of health care that were based on folklore and magic with a knowledge base developed in Greece. Within this developing culture, medicine and health care soon became a part of the necessary education of upper-class men, and women's health issues and childbearing practices regained importance. Midwives became key figures in the care of women (Kelly, 1985). Important contributions to health care delivery in the Roman Empire include public health sanitation and public health law. The Romans instituted city planning that provided for development of sewage systems, aqueducts, and baths. In addition, they can be credited for the development of hospitals with male and female attendants to care for the sick.

A new era in the care of the sick occurred after Christianity became the official religion of Rome. The Christian attitude of care for persons, based on a strong belief in the sanctity of human life, was derived from Hebrew tradition as well as the teachings of Christ. Bishops assigned individuals to care for widows, orphans, the sick, and the poor. Hospitals to care for the sick and institutions to care for the poor offered combinations of outpatient and welfare services. Monastic orders of monks and nuns, who were generally better educated than the ordinary person, controlled the health care institutions. Their writings documented the care given to the sick and techniques used, which provide early records of diseases, practices, and research for cure and care (Bullough & Bullough, 1978).

Changes from the Middle Ages to the Industrial Revolution

From the eighth to the thirteenth century, during the Islamic Golden Age (also known as the Islamic renaissance), countries in the Islamic empire established bimaristans, from the Persian word for hospitals, differentiated from healing temples and lay hospices, where the ill of all social classes, genders, and cultures were welcomed and treated. Highly organized, the hospitals in the Muslim world insisted on qualified staff (instead of lay or religious healers) including physicians and nurses. These were, essentially, the first public hospitals, according to the modern understanding of the word. Additionally, Muslim physicians also established the first medical degree–granting universities and psychiatric hospitals. Although the Islamic Golden Age is formally noted to have ended in the thirteenth century, some posit that the accomplishments associated with this era continued until the fifteenth and sixteenth centuries.

During the thirteenth and fourteenth centuries, the organization and founding of medical schools and universities and the advent of book binding all worked to promote a better educated health care provider. Nurses, who were not as fully established as physicians, functioned as attendants who made beds and gave baths to the sick.

Amidst the religious revolution that had taken place against the church of Rome (known as the Reformation) in the early sixteenth to seventeenth century, the disbanding of convents and monasteries led to severe impediments in the care of the sick. During this time, some progress was made in midwifery, medicine, and nursing. However, it was not until the mid-nineteenth century and the Industrial Revolution, when the demand for intellectual freedom brought about educational institutions for men, that the health care system as we know it began to emerge.

During the nineteenth century, Florence Nightingale's leadership influenced not only nursing education and nursing care, but also public health and global health care (Nightingale, 1859/1992; Bullough & Bullough, 1978; Selanders, 1998a, 1998b; McDonald, 1998; Dossey, 2000). Nightingale is perhaps best known for crafting the standards of Western secular nursing education and practice. Her leadership was also felt in the area of public policy, social reform, and the utilization of research in clinical practice. She spearheaded improvements in British military medicine, and greatly influenced public health reform in Great Britain and India. She was also a pioneer in using evaluative statistics to monitor the various factors influencing health and the effectiveness of the health care system. Keep in mind, however, that despite the great changes to nursing that Florence Nightingale made, it was the Victorian age. Nurses were still trained to be passively involved in heavy-duty work for low wages. The unpleasant working conditions combined with the lack of respect in many environments meant that many women from higher social classes were not interested in becoming nurses. The profession was seen as one that was for women of lower- or working-class homes.

Ask Yourself

How Have Things Changed?

- Consider the discussion of the early era of the health care delivery system and identify problems in early civilization that might still be seen in today's world.
- Consider how Florence Nightingale's profound influence on health care systems worldwide continues to affect health care today. How can nurses continue this legacy in the twenty-first century?

Changes Influencing Development of Modern Health Care in Canada

Health services in Canada developed from health care models in European countries. These systems share the products of medical innovations that took place from the late nineteenth century to the time of the First World War, a time when major nations were changing from agricultural to industrial economies. Such innovations as the use of anesthesia in surgery and the recognition of bacteria as a causative factor in many widespread diseases provided the impetus that led to the development of the modern hospital as it exists today. The dissemination and incorporation of this knowledge among the large number of practising physicians took at least a generation to accomplish. Consequently, the importance of the place of the modern hospital in society was not felt until the late nineteenth century and into the early twentieth century. At the time of this revolution of knowledge, physicians, who were the primary health care practitioners, engaged primarily in a private practice, fee-for-service system.

Physicians and Hospitals.   While many European nations had both tax-supported charity hospitals and private hospitals for those patients who had the ability to pay for their own health care, Canada opted for a more egalitarian system, in which hospital and physician services have been made available to all persons, subsidized by the government (Anderson, 1963). This model has evolved over the twentieth century, and there have been differences between the provision of care between provinces and territories (some provinces and territories have had and continue to have citizens pay deductibles and co-payments), but the system, at a federal level, has been built upon the principle that health care, and the care provided in hospitals, is a basic right or need that should not be provided based on the ability to pay. The primary purpose for hospitals built in Europe was ministry to the low-income or charity patient, while in Canada, hospitals were built for the provision of health care to all citizens.

The development of hospitals affected European physicians by creating a class of specialists who operated in the general hospital and also had the option of treating private-pay patients. These specialists often created their own cottage hospitals, where they could treat their private-pay patients. All other physicians in that system were excluded from practising in a hospital. In North America, on the other hand, practitioners sought out appointments to the hospital system in order to be able to admit patients, while at the same time maintaining private offices in which to see their patients. This began a new approach to the use of the hospital system, in which resources were used more extravagantly and the system was more democratic in its care of patients than the European system. The North American health care system became immersed in greater use of technology, industrial and management skills, and scientific methods, creating by some estimates the best health care system in the world, and arguably the most expensive (Anderson, 1963).

As an outgrowth of the development of hospitals, a greater awareness of public health problems arose. Prevention programs for the public, such as sanitation, environmental issues, control of communicable diseases, and maternity and infant care, developed. Curative programs, which were generally hospital-based, were supported by government funding. Hospital clinics that provided outpatient services became the primary site of health care for many patients. During that period, physicians provided these outpatient services and, in return, were able to participate in the hospital system, where the latest in knowledge and technologies was being introduced. This information could then be applied to the care of large numbers of patients. Hospitals provided physicians an opportunity to develop their skills through training and to provide service to the public, thus fulfilling the physician's commitment to the public interest (Anderson, 1963).

Ask Yourself

How Do Nineteenth-Century Concepts Affect Twenty-First-Century Health Care?

- What concepts or practices regarding health care from the late nineteenth century and early twentieth century still affect a patient's access to health care today?

- How is the health care delivery system that we know different from the system at the turn of the nineteenth century?

- What is your vision for health care for the remainder of the twenty-first century?

- Public health was emphasized in health care until the 1940s when post-war health care became more institutionally based. How do you see this trend today? Should the focus of health care continue to be institutional and episodic? Is this a sustainable way to manage the kinds of modern health care problems we face in Canada?

- Throughout the twentieth century, the "face" of Canada has markedly changed with many more persons from around the world immigrating to Canada. What do you believe some current health care challenges might be, related to changing demographics of our country?

- What kinds of challenges and concerns do you think a nurse had in 1909 compared to a nurse in 2009?

Twentieth and Twenty-First Century Changes and Challenges

The latter part of the nineteenth century saw many changes in the health care system, especially in areas that we would today call public health. Government programs were set up to improve health for all Canadians and especially the poor and native persons. Programs to improve water quality, sanitation, and spread of disease were initiated by municipal governments. Medical care was still grievously lacking for many, however, and problems like tuberculosis and other infectious diseases still had the greatest impact on the poor. The turn of the century saw the development of an industrialized society, the growth of the economy, and the increased capability of a growing health care system, which began to produce a healthier and more aware population. However, twentieth-century changes created new challenges for the health care system.

In the early part of the twentieth century, a growing nation experienced population increases and a greater influx of immigrants, with over one million immigrants from southern and eastern Europe in 1905 alone. The need for health care and related services warranted attention. Medical schools and nursing schools expanded to provide personnel to meet the demand. Science, technology, public health services, and medicine progressed at an increased rate. Physicians and scientists began to use such diagnostic tools as X-rays. They made strides toward reduction of infectious organisms through the use of rubber gloves. They began to research the causes and cures of diseases such as yellow fever and typhoid and to use radiation to treat breast cancer. Amid such major advances as the discovery of penicillin at the University of Toronto in 1928, the proliferation of science and technology, the advancement of the professions of nursing and medicine, and the changing conceptualization about disease, a phenomenon unique to Canada emerged: the Canadian health care system. This phenomenon has shaped Canadian society in the twentieth century and into the twenty-first century as well. The first public calls for a national health insurance system came in the early twentieth century, when the government did become involved in setting up institutions to care for those with mental illnesses and tuberculosis. While William Lyon MacKenzie King did create a Department of Health within the government while he was in power, a nationally funded and insured health care system did not become a reality until many years later. Today, despite challenges with the system and worries about its sustainability, many Canadians view the health care system as the hallmark of Canada and a fundamental part of widely held Canadian values.

The later part of the nineteenth century and the first two decades of the twentieth century saw the transformation of hospitals from asylums for the poor to modern institutions dedicated to science and improved patient care. While the first institutionalized patients were those with mental illnesses and tuberculosis, now patients with a variety of ailments were treated in government-run hospitals. Physicians expanded surgical interventions such as tonsillectomies, removal of tumours, and many gynecological operations. Nurses began to take a more active role in managing the hospital environment to control infection, and began to have more responsibility for technical management of patient care through duties such as taking the patient's pulse, temperature, and blood pressure (Stevens, 1989). Patterns that developed in the health care delivery system in the early part of the century can still be seen today. Physicians gained a new and strong identity and prestige, and their professional organizations became a powerful force. Physicians gained increased authority in the routine workings of hospital systems, shifting the balance of power from boards of trustees to the medical decision makers (Stevens, 1989).

As a result of battlefield experiences in the First World War, nurses, physicians, and other health care workers designed and set up streamlined, technically proficient, and very efficient specialized hospitals for the acutely ill or injured patient. On the home front, in response to ever-increasing numbers of immigrants, models of health care with emphasis on prevention and community interaction were developed. Prior to the war, the elite area of nursing was public health, with nurses at the forefront of campaigns for infant care and welfare, tuberculosis, and infectious disease. The war, however, emphasized the glamour of hospitals, and by 1920, many general hospitals in this country had schools of nursing attached to them. Hospitals had already realized that classes of student nurses were a good source of free, somewhat skilled labour, and many students spent much of their learning and free time in the hospitals, providing care to patients while learning skills and usually living within the hospital until graduation. Eventually, with the realization that graduate nurses were the mainstay of the front-line labour force in hospitals, many nursing schools were supported to extend their nursing education program to three years. As early as 1909, it was noted that almost all of Canada's nursing schools had extended their programs to this length of time with a strong emphasis on in-hospital training. Like physicians, nurses became caught up in the culture of the acute health care environment and were reluctant to expand their professional interests into public health and the social aspect of health care (Stevens, 1989). The following is a summary of some of the significant events that have influenced health care in Canada since the mid to late nineteenth century.

Figure 13–1 **Selected Significant Events in Health Care History in Canada**

1867–*British North American Act*: Defined Canada as a country. This was renamed the *Constitution Act* in 1982. In this act, provinces have authority over health care but the federal government has a responsibility to fund health care. Public health nursing is on the rise.

Early 20th century–William Lyon MacKenzie King responds to Canadians calling for more government involvement in the regulation, monitoring, and funding of health care and urging government to introduce a national health insurance program.

1928–The discovery of insulin by Frederick Banting and Charles Best, with their colleagues J. J. R. Macleod and J. B. Collip at the University of Toronto. They would later go on to be awarded a Nobel Prize for this discovery that would change health care as well as modernize front-line care for soldiers in the Second World War.

1935–The title "Registered Nurse" was protected by making registration mandatory for its use. At the same time, standards for both the education of nurses and the practice of nursing were established.

1940s–Shift from public health toward institutionalization of health care. Initiation of public immunization programs.

1946–The Saskatchewan Government, led by provincial Premier Tommy Douglas (premier from 1944–1961 and often referred to as the "Father of Medicare" in Canada), introduces the first provincial hospital insurance program in Canada called the *Saskatchewan Hospitalization Act*.

1957–Paul Martin Sr., Minister of National Health and Welfare and known to some as the "Father of Canadian Medicare" from 1946 to 1957 played a key role in the passing of the *Hospital Insurance and Diagnostic Services Act*. The five "pillars" of this act eventually became the five principles of the *Canada Health Act* (comprehensiveness, universality, public administration, accessibility, and portability).

1962–Saskatchewan's doctors' Strike. Physicians in the province went on strike for twenty-three days to oppose government involvement in health care, the same day that the NDP government introduced the first public health care program, the *Saskatchewan Medical Care Insurance Act*.

1964–A Royal Commission on Health Services headed by Justice Emmett Hall (a Supreme Court justice) recommends universal and comprehensive national health insurance program based in part on Saskatchewan's program, in existence from 1946.

1966–Parliament creates a national medicare program (the *Medical Care Act*) under a Liberal minority government with Ottawa paying 50 percent of provincial health costs. Keep in mind that as of circa 2005, the federal government funding now makes up less than 20 percent of the total costs of health care in the provinces and territories.

1974– Marc Lalonde (Minister of Health) publishes *A New Perspective on the Health of Canadians* (also called the *Lalonde Report*). This report clearly cited that factors other than one's biological or genetic "luck" such as social status, environment, education, access to health care, literacy, nutrition, and lifestyle choices such as smoking or alcohol intake, were responsible for health states. This report emphasized that the determinants of health did not simply exist within the health care system, but also in other sectors, such as education and welfare systems.

1977–Trudeau Liberals pass the *Federal–Provincial Fiscal Arrangements* and the *Established Programs Financing Act* (also known as EPF), which represented a change from 50:50 cost sharing between the provinces/territories and federal government to new block funding. While this change provided the provinces with more freedom on how funds were spent, they were still required to comply with the federal guidelines for provision of health care.

1982–The *Constitution Act* is passed. The first part of this act is the *Canadian Charter of Rights and Freedoms*. Preceded by the *Canadian Bill of Rights* (1960), the *Charter* is seen as an explicit articulation of national values and a document that has helped to shape national identity. It outlines the civil and political rights of all Canadians and is recognized as a fundamental document of national unity, declaring freedom as a national core value.

1984–The *Canada Health Act* is passed unanimously by parliament. This document outlines, specifically, the conditions that the thirteen provinces and territories must adhere to, in order to receive federal funding for health care. It is imperative that the provinces provide universal coverage (i.e., to all "insured" citizens) for all "medically necessary" hospital, physician, and allied health services. Ability to pay must not be a barrier to accessing health care, in any way. The five tenets of the *Canada Health Act* include universality, accessibility, public administration, portability, and comprehensiveness.

1996–Paul Martin Jr. creates an amalgamation of two programs, the Established Programs Funding (EPF), established in 1977 (supporting health care and education) and the Canada Assistance Plan, established in 1966 (supporting social assistance) and introduced the Canada Health and Social Transfer payment system (CHST), a system of block payments from the federal governments to the provinces and territories. This caused massive

(Continued)

cuts in the total transfer payments from the federal governments to health and social programs in the provinces and territories.

1997—National Forum on Health releases its report. This forum was established in 1994 to advise the prime minister on ways to reform the ailing health care system and improve the health of Canadians. The report calls for medicare to be more strongly "evidence-based" with improvements in integrated decision making and health information systems.

1998—Marked decrease in Canada Health and Social Transfer payments to provinces and territories.

1999—Marked increase in private-sector expenditures on health care, as noted by Gratzer (2002), who cites an increase in private funding from ~23 percent in 1975 to 30 percent in 1999. These monies go toward the kinds of health care services not covered by provincial health plans, such as laser eye surgery, psychological services, in vitro fertilization, and dentistry. Most people pay for these kinds of services partially out of pocket and partially through private insurance companies, usually provided by their employer.

1999—Health care spending is ~9 percent of Canadian GDP with a total cost of $C 95 billion annually. The majority of the funds are spent on hospital and physician care. Worries about sustainability (which initially began in the 1970s) abound (Martin and Singer, 2003).

1999—Social Union Framework Agreement carried out between Prime Minister Cretien and the premiers of the provinces and territories (except Quebec). This agreement, while not health care–specific, emphasizes the importance of social programs, equality of opportunity for all, and a reduction in barriers due to ability or mobility issues.

1978—In the Declaration of Alma-Ata (World Health Organization, 1978), the World Health Organization calls for "Health for all by the year 2000" with a call to all countries to improve primary care and health promotion along with ensuring that essential health services for all persons are provided, e.g., safe water, adequate sanitation, maternal and child health care, immunization, control of infectious disease, adequate nutrition, and safe environments.

2000—First ministers announce the Primary Health Care Transition Fund (an investment of $C 800 million to improve primary health care, increase health promotion and injury prevention programs, increase the number of services offered on a 24/7 basis, establish more interdisciplinary teams, and facilitate intersectoral collaboration with a goal of helping those in the health care sector work with those in other sectors to improve health of citizens and address issues of basic health promotion, e.g., education, social services, labour, sanitation, etc.

2000—Alberta Premier Ralph Klein introduces legislation to allow private hospitals and a resultant two-tiered system in Alberta with the goals of improving efficiency, reducing wait times, and delivering health care in innovative ways.

2002—The Royal Commission on the Future of Health Care in Canada conducts cross-country public hearings led by Commissioner Roy J. Romanow QC. The final report, entitled *Building on Values: The Future of Health Care in Canada* was tabled in Ottawa on November 28, 2002.

2002—Senator Michael Kirby publishes a document on health care reform initiatives entitled "The Health of Canadians: The Federal Role" tabled in October 2002.

2003—First Ministers' Health Accord announced. The commitments of this accord include a significant increase in health care funding over the next three to five years. Programs such as primary health care, home care, and catastrophic drug coverage are targeted as key areas for reform and increased funding. Accountability and transparency are emphasized along with a proposed change to the way in which the federal government transfers funds to the provinces and territories, called the Canada Health Transfer, effective in April 2004. The accord also calls for better methods of reporting back to Canadians on how their tax dollars are spent on health care by the production of an annual report.

2007—The Canadian Medical Association releases a report in support of private health care as a means to improve a non-sustainable health care system.

2008–9—Total Canada Health Transfer payments from the federal government to the provincial and territorial governments total about $C 37 billion.

Source: Compiled by author from information provided by Ministry of Health and Long Term Care, Ontario; Department of Finance Canada; Health Canada; Canadian Nursing Association; Canadian Institute for Health Information; Canadian Broadcasting Corporation Archives; and World Health Organization.

Figure 13–2 **A Review of the Federal and Provincial Responsibilities for Health Care**

How the Work of Health Care Is Divided between the Federal and Provincial or Territorial Governments

The federal government is responsible for the following:

1. Deciding on and administering the principles for health care through the *Canada Health Act*.

2. Ensuring that provinces follow the set principles for the delivery of health care and adjusting federal to provincial payments based on this.

3. Assisting with the financing of provincial health care delivery of services.

4. Delivering direct health care services to veterans, native Canadians, persons living on reserves, military personnel, inmates of federal penitentiaries, and RCMP officers.

5. Some roles such as health protection, disease prevention, and health promotion are shared responsibilities but the federal government plays an important role.

(Continued)

The provincial and territorial governments are responsible for the following:

1. Delivering and managing insured health services such as hospital and physician care
2. Planning, financing, and evaluating hospital and physician care
3. Managing some public health and prescription care.

(Health Canada, 2004a, 2004b.)

HEALTH CARE PERSPECTIVES: A GLOBAL CONCERN

The challenge to provide health care for populations across the globe requires increasing effort and creativity. Many variables play a part in this challenge, including economics, cultural factors, epidemics, environment, war, and national crises. The problems are further compounded by the relationship, or lack of relationship, between modern medicine and traditional healing systems, and preventive methods of health promotion contrasted with curative methods of treating illness. These factors all affect the functioning of health systems in various countries around the world (Bodeker, 1996).

All industrialized nations, with the exception of the United States and South Africa, have comprehensive national health care programs. The countries that operate with nationalized systems include Australia, Austria, Belgium, Bulgaria, Canada, the Czech Republic, Denmark, Finland, France, Germany, Great Britain, Greece, Hungary, Ireland, Italy, Japan, the Netherlands, New Zealand, Norway, Poland, Portugal, Romania, Russia, the Slovak Republic, Spain, Sweden, and Switzerland. However, even with health care programs in place, all are not equal and do not function as smoothly as one would hope (Shikles, 1991).

One way to measure the health of nations is to look at the rates of infant mortality. While the numbers since 2004 have not changed markedly, they do reflect differences in resources, both financial and human, and access to the basic determinants of health. Infant mortality is expressed as the number of infants per 1000 live births who die under one year of age. As of 2007, Canada's rate of infant mortality was 5.08. This can be compared to the United States (6.30), the United Kingdom (4.93), and the European Union (6.38). Singapore has the lowest infant mortality rate of 2.3 while currently the highest rates are found in Afghanistan (154.67), Sierra Leone (156.48), and Angola (182.31) (Central Intelligency Agency, 2008).

The following examples outlining challenges and triumphs in the provision of health care across the globe demonstrate the inequities in health care between many developed and developing countries. If we examine the Russian health care system, we can look back to the early 1990s, when the Russian government mandated obligatory health insurance to replace the state-funded health care system. Reforms of the system included a shift from a national system, with fairly equitable access to care, to a decentralized and fragmented variety of state systems. Despite these reforms, however, there is still great dissatisfaction with the new system and Russia continues to suffer from a health care system that is in grave danger of being overtaxed (Twigg, 1999).

In 1992, Erlanger reported a critical shortage of essential drugs; basic sterile equipment such as syringes, antibiotics, x-ray equipment; and basic medical supplies in Russian hospitals. Hospitals were unhygenic, personnel were overworked, and there was a neglect of sanitation procedures. Rural areas in the former Soviet Union fared much worse. Some rural clinics had nonfunctioning or nonexistent sewage systems. Some lacked piped-in water, or if water was piped in there was no system for heating it safely. Many hospital personnel, such as physicians, nurses, and technicians, had gone on strike because of poor working conditions and poor rewards for service. In this crippled health care system, there is no cohesive public health policy, and nurses are often paid less than a housemaid, and physicians less than a bus driver (Erlanger, 1992; Nursing and health in Russia, 1998). In Russia, many nursing administrative positions are in fact held by physicians, who are paid more than a salaried nurse, still making only enough to manage a modestly appointed lifestyle. Many physicians, in order to make a better income, take extra jobs teaching nursing or providing direct nursing care. Most nurses report to a physician or to a nurse manager, who in turn reports to a physician in charge. The hierarchy of many Russian hospitals means that physicians may hold nursing positions from the bedside all the way up to director of nursing (Uhlich, Michaud, & Giblin, 2007).

Questions arise regarding whether market-based medical insurance is the best solution to Russia's health-financing problems, given the persisting problems with overall political and economic reform (Burger, Field & Twigg, 1998; Twigg, 1999). Recent reforms in Russia have meant an increased investment in health care with a total expenditure of about $C7 million (145 billion rubles) on the health care system in 2006–2007. However much of those funds were apparently spent on high-tech medical centres and modern equipment along with salary increases for medical personnel. While this investment did help a markedly ailing system, the most recent investments were seen as political maneuvers and short-term solutions. Attention on how to restructure the health care system is more critical at this point. Like many other countries, most Russian health care is provided in hospitals, and not enough attention is given to public health and non-acute care (Womack, 2008).

South Africa, while technically an industrialized nation with many natural resources, is plagued with health care problems similar to those occurring in many developing countries. The government of South Africa has as its long-term goal affordable and accessible health care for all its citizens. This goal is far from being realized, however, because the rise in urbanization and the proliferation of developing-country illness is causing a deterioration in the process of organizing health care for all. In their present system, physicians and nurses are overworked, there is unequal access to public health services, hospitals are overcrowded, and much of the equipment is nonfunctioning or outdated (Bloom & McIntyre, 1998; Randolph, 1991).

The health care system of Cuba has been lauded by both the World Health Organization (WHO) and the United Nations as a major achievement for the country's citizens (Shikles, 1991). This system provides services from primary care to the most sophisticated procedures, available free to urban and rural citizens alike. Upheld as a model for other developing nations, the Cuban system greatly reduced rates of infant mortality and communicable diseases such as diphtheria, malaria, polio, and whooping cough. Primary-care clinics abound in rural areas and are open around the clock. Nurses and physicians make house calls to older or very ill residents. However, over the past fifteen years a shortage of medical supplies has threatened this model health care system (Barry, 2000). Factors affecting the supply shortage include the U.S. embargo and absence of aid from the former Soviet Union. Barry cites examples of lye ingestion in toddlers related to very limited availability of soap, and blindness related to decreased access to necessary nutrients, as some of the profound effects of the shortages on nutrition and overall health of vulnerable populations.

As was mentioned earlier, most industrialized nations have some type of universal health coverage. These systems vary in regard to the amount of government and private pay insurance, and some countries have a combination of several methods. Germany, France, and Japan have systems of health care coverage that mandate benefits coverage, the cost of which is shared by employees, employers, and government tax revenues. Medical care is offered through private physicians and through private and public hospitals. Patients may choose their providers. Most people in these countries have health insurance coverage through their place of employment. Health insurance is offered to the citizens of these countries through multiple third-party insurance agencies.

In Germany, France, and Japan, reimbursement rates are standardized for physicians and hospitals through a negotiation system between hospitals, physicians, third-party payers, and the government. Similar problems to those existing in the United States exist, such as high costs and increased spending for technology. However, every citizen has some type of health care coverage. In an attempt to hold down rising health care spending, all have instituted direct controls on the price of health care. The controls apply to all of the health care systems in the respective countries, and policies are strictly enforced to comply with the set limit on health care spending (Shikles, 1991).

Great Britain, like Canada, has developed a national health care system that provides health care for its citizens. The government-run plans provide cradle-to-grave services that are financed through taxes. These plans enable patients to receive services free, and to choose their own hospitals and physicians. The plans pay salaries to physicians and operate their own hospitals.

As we know, in Canada, citizens can go to physicians or hospitals of their choice when they need care. Physicians bill the province for patient care. Patients do not pay for services, nor are they required to fill out endless forms. Negotiations for fees, cost-containment measures, and salaries take place between the provinces and the health care system.

Citizens of Great Britain again, like citizens of Canada, consider health care to be one of their basic rights, and they value and respect their health care systems. Major political parties in these countries support the systems, and physicians and hospitals seem generally satisfied as well, since they receive a guaranteed payment. Businesses applaud the programs because payment is spread across society, and they do not have to carry a large part of the payment burden for employees (Beatty, 1991).

There are both champions and critics of the national health insurance systems like those in Canada and Britain. Some say the systems are sound, while others say they are flawed. Some critics of Canada's health care system cite that the system sets up a system of rationing because of insufficient funds for specialized health care. It has been said that waiting for care in these systems sometimes means death. Access to certain procedures and technologies is limited. Waiting lists reached crisis points in the 1980s and 1990s in areas like cardiac surgery and orthopedic surgery. Critics say that there is an unequal access to health care from province to province, depending on the affluence of the province. Even within provinces, inequalities abound between persons living in resource-rich urban centres versus those who live in remote rural areas. Some Canadian citizens who can afford to pay out-of-pocket go to the United States for specialized care and surgeries. In all instances, the increase in health care spending due to the high cost of technologies and research is having an impact on these systems in much the same ways as it is across the globe (Walker, 1992; Farrell, 1998; Katz, Verrilli, & Barer, 1998).

Ask Yourself

Access to Health Care—Rights and Responsibilities

Much of the discussion regarding the health care delivery systems in many countries in the world is a commentary on access to what is termed *modern medical care*.

- How does access to health care affect an individual's participation in the health care system?

- What is our individual responsibility in the big picture of these vast health care systems?

- Do you consider health care a basic right? If it is a right, what are our individual responsibilities in ensuring this right for all citizens?

- Many people consider health care as a privilege instead of a right. Is there a difference? If so, what do you think is the difference between these two terms?

- Think of yourself and those you care about who live in Canada. What does health care and access to health care mean to you and your family? What would you do if you lived in a different place in which health care was inaccessible or unaffordable to you? How would you feel?

- Nurses often act as advocates for individual patients and groups of patients. Do you see one role of nurses as being advocates for health care as a right for all?

- What kind of health care problems do you see, in your practice or your community, that arise from sectors other than health care?

ALTERNATIVE TRADITIONS OF HEALTH CARE

Indigenous populations in cultures throughout the world have traditional forms of health care that view humanity as connected to the wider dimensions of the earth and nature. In developing countries, these forms of traditional healing systems provide comprehensive approaches to prevention of illness and promotion of health that go beyond the scope of modern medical care. The World Health Organization (WHO) refers to these systems as holistic—that is, viewing a person in totality within a vast ecological spectrum, and emphasizing the notion that illness or disease occurs as a result of an imbalance between the person and his or her ecological systems (WHO, 1978). While many western nations are embracing the notion of holistic care, there are cultures and systems that have been providing and emphasizing holism in health care for a much longer period of time.

An important component of traditional systems of health care is their basis in models that take into account mental, spiritual, physical, and ecological factors in assessing health and well-being. A basic concept of all traditional health care systems is that of balance between mind and body; function and need; and individual, community, and environment. Illness or disease is thought to be a breakdown in the balance in one or more of these areas. Treatments are designed to restore health and balance between the individual and his or her internal and external environments. While these models of traditional health care systems have been considered primitive and unsophisticated by modern practitioners, an increasing number of developing countries are showing a new interest in program development toward revitalizing these traditional systems. There are several factors at work in promoting this resurgence of interest.

The majority of rural populations of developing countries cannot afford Western types of medical health care. Rural people have to travel many days to reach the larger health care centres, resulting in loss of wages in addition to money spent for travel and medicines. In Asia, the traditional systems are being incorporated into other, more formal health care systems to provide for care and ease the burden of cost. India has over 200,000 traditional practitioners. In Thailand, the Ministry of Health promotes the use of traditional medicinal plants in primary health care, state-run hospitals, and health service centres. In Korea, twenty percent of the national health care budget is directed to traditional health care services. Health insurance coverage is available for Chinese medical treatments and traditional health care methods (Bodeker, 1996).

In Africa, governments are facing huge bills for the AIDS crisis. These governments are exploring their traditional indigenous medicinal treatments for inexpensive and effective ways to relieve the suffering of patients with AIDS. Health care providers in Uganda have been active in promoting research into traditional medicine for treating people with AIDS.

China has had a policy of integrating traditional health care into the national health care policy for over forty years. The Chinese are trying to combine the modern and the traditional as formal components of health care provision. In China, traditional health care providers perform the majority of care to the poor and rural communities. The country physicians are educated in a three-year program that includes a combination of traditional medicine and modern medicine. Modern Western medicine is being strongly pursued at great financial cost to the government, but at the same time hospitals and health care systems offer a choice to patients. Persons who take advantage of these choices are often the older and the less affluent. As the country is opening up to capitalist beliefs and free enterprise, some Chinese citizens who now have the financial means to make different choices are choosing Western methods of treatments, and often ignore the tried and true Chinese methods for status reasons. The younger generation of Chinese seem to believe that what is Western is always better. In observing some of the health care delivery in China, there is evidence that the government, while allowing the practice of ancient Chinese medicine, is putting a strong emphasis on a belief that technology is the answer to health care in this heavily populated country. This is especially disconcerting in view of the fact that Chinese medicine and the tradition of health care with alternative choices have been functioning well for two thousand years, and Western health care providers are beginning to research and utilize these traditional systems of care in order to offer them to their patients.

Ask Yourself

What Do You Know About Traditional Healing?

Traditional methods of healing and health care have kept indigenous populations healthy and functioning for thousands of years. Many countries are trying to reinstate these practices to promote health and reduce the cost of health care and health care delivery.

- How do you think traditional and modern healing systems should relate to each other?
- What traditional methods of health care are available in your community or nearby area?
- With what traditional or folk health practices are you familiar? Have you or persons you know utilized these practices?
- How would you feel if a patient preferred a traditional or folk method of healing over a conventional medical treatment? How would you approach this issue?
- Many of us turn to nonconventional methods for treating ailments such as common colds or flus. Think of your own practices for treating common nonacute illnesses. Would any of these practices be seen as "odd" or "eccentric" to someone else?
- What are some strategies to best incorporate traditional practices into health care?
- What kinds of practices or research can we do to foster collaboration and integration?

CHALLENGES FOR RURAL AND URBAN AGGREGATES

Problems in the delivery of health care to populations around the world occur not only because of expensive technology or lack of money to pay for insurance in some countries, but also because of geographic barriers. Accessibility is one of the five key features of the *Canada Health Act* (1984). In this section, it is noted that "reasonable access" to health care must exist for citizens without financial barriers (which might include extra billing or user fees in this context). However, the act does not directly address geographical accessibility. As urban populations continue to grow, much of the acute care services are focused on these populous areas and often affiliated with universities located in larger cities. Small local hospitals often cannot afford the expensive technology and qualified staff. Often patients from rural areas who require surgeries, transplants, or procedures such as MRIs or CT scans are taken into larger teaching hospitals in urban centres for this kind of care. This is expensive and time consuming, contributing to increased morbidity and long waits for care. Rural populations in Canada and abroad often have to do without services because of lack of providers and facilities within a reasonable distance from their homes. Health care for persons in these populations requires a day off work for travel and waiting in crowded waiting rooms. Many rural areas lack health care personnel, and emergency care is often nonexistent. Many rural areas do not have 911 services available or, if they do, may face long waits through difficult terrain or seasonal challenges such as snow or heavy rains that may make roads inaccessible. In the far north, in areas that are accessible only by small planes, waits for basic medical supplies have an effect on physician and nursing care. Certainly a patient living in the north of Canada will face a longer and more difficult wait for open heart surgery than a patient waiting in a downtown Montreal or Toronto hospital, simply by virtue of their geographic location. Patients often delay treatment or do not become involved with prevention or health education plans because they require so much effort to accomplish.

The urban poor face similar access problems, not because care is geographically distant, but because access may require trips to busy centres, often with long waits for care. While there may be more centres and providers in urban centres, queues for care and long waits at appointments may result in a different kind of burden for the urban poor. Like their rural counterparts, the urban poor may be required to take time from work in order to see a provider. For someone working at a job with a minimum hourly wage, it is much more difficult to leave work for a number of hours or a day in order to wait to see a health care provider, compared to a person in a better paid or more autonomous position. Prescribed care such as psychology, dental care, physiotherapy, or occupational therapy, not covered by the Canada Health Act may be unaffordable to those working in minimum wage jobs with no health benefits.

Large immigrant populations live in overcrowded situations in some urban settings and, in some cases, persons living without legal status may be unable to access care or make use of a strong community network. In addition to financial constraints, there may be language and cultural barriers as well as lack of knowledge about how to access a highly complex health care system.

SUMMARY

Historical awareness enables us to have a more informed view of circumstances in the present. Contemporary issues and concerns regarding health care delivery and financing are related to the historical interplay of advances in scientific and medical knowledge, social and political climate, and waxing and waning of economic and other resources. Current parameters in which health care providers function are changing. Acute-care hospitals are changing the focus of, and in some cases limiting, services; and many people are looking to the traditional healing systems of various cultures to provide needed health care services. Although some countries ensure access to basic health care services for their citizens, many individuals throughout the world have limited or no access to basic health care. Questions regarding access to and availability of resources are not new, but they must be addressed anew in light of the various currents within contemporary society. The future of the system is uncertain, and we must consider whether issues of the past are destined to repeat themselves. Perhaps we can take what is positive from the past, and blend this with both traditional and modern healing approaches in order to rescue a flawed health care system in this country and around the world.

CHAPTER HIGHLIGHTS

- Systems of health care, which have existed to address societal needs for healing from early civilization to the present, have been influenced by cultural, political, economic, religious, and scientific factors throughout history.

- Scientific and medical innovations, coinciding with the shift in Western nations from agricultural to industrial economics in the latter nineteenth and early twentieth centuries, provided a basis for modern-day health care. Societal changes such as wars, women working more outside the home, and the influx of immigrants have raised new issues and concerns for health care delivery at various times in Canada history.

- Expansion of hospital and other health care services has reached a point of crisis in which out-of-control health care costs have prompted many to seek solutions through proposals for health care reforms.

- Some nations provide basic health care services for their citizens, while people in many areas suffer from limited access to or availability of such services. People in both developing and industrialized countries are exploring ways to incorporate traditional and modern healing practices into contemporary health care systems, in an effort to utilize the benefits of both systems in meeting the health care needs of society.

- Problems of access to and payment for health care services are of special concern among rural populations and the urban poor.

DISCUSSION QUESTIONS AND ACTIVITIES

1. Interview or read a biography of a person who worked as a nurse during or within the decade following the Second World War, and discuss nursing roles and duties, types of health concerns for which patients were hospitalized, and what were considered new therapies at the time. Compare the information you obtain to your experience of health care today.

2. Review nursing and medical journals and texts from the earlier part of the twentieth century regarding issues of concern in practice and to the profession. Compare and contrast these issues to issues of current concern.

3. Imagine that it is the year 2040 and you are being interviewed by a nursing student about factors that affected health care delivery and financing in your early days in nursing. What would you say?

4. Discuss global issues related to health care delivery. Which of these issues would have the greatest impact on your nursing practice and why? Use the Internet to investigate health care issues in a nonindustrialized country. Share with classmates how these issues might affect your nursing practice.

5. Describe the impact of health delivery and financing on patient care and outcomes. Identify potential ethical dilemmas related to current systems of delivery or financing.

6. How should traditional and modern healing practices and practitioners relate to each other?

REFERENCES

Achterberg. J. (1990). *Woman as healer.* Boston: Shambhala.

Anderson, O. W. (1963). Medical care: Its social and organizational aspects. Health services systems in the United States and other countries—critical comparisons. *The New England Journal of Medicine, 269,* 839–843.

Barry, M. (2000). Effect of the U.S. embargo and economic decline on health in Cuba. *Annals of Internal Medicine, 132*(2), 151–154.

Beatty, P. (1991). Canada's health care system is sound. In G. McCuen, ed., *Health care and human values* (pp. 162–176). Hudson, WI: GEM Publications.

Bloom, G., & McIntyre, D. (1998). Towards equity in health in an unequal society. *Social Science and Medicine, 47*(10), 1529–1538.

Bodeker, G. C. (1996). Global health traditions. In M. S. Micozzi, ed., *Fundamentals of complementary and alternative medicine* (pp. 279–290). New York: Churchill Livingstone.

Bullough, B., & Bullough, V. (1978). *The care of the sick: The emergence of modern nursing.* New York: Prodist.

Burger, E. J., Field, M. G., & Twigg, J. L. (1998). From assurance to insurance in Russian health care: The problematic transition. *American Journal of Public Health, 88*(5), 755–758.

Central Intelligence Agency. (2008). Rank order—infant mortality rate. *The World Factbook*. Retrieved January 25, 2009, from https://www.cia.gov/library/publications/the-world-factbook/rankorder/2091rank.html.

Dossey, B. M. (2000). *Florence Nightingale: Mystic, visionary, healer*. Springhouse, PA: Springhouse Corporation.

Erlanger, S. (1992, May). Cuts gut Russian health care. *The New York Times*. Retrieved January 25, 2009, from http://query.nytimes.com/gst/fullpage.html?sec=health&res-9EOCE7D81338F93AA35756COA964958260.

Farrell, M. (1998). Trends in the global healthcare environment: The developed countries. *Contemporary Nurse, 7*(4), 180–189.

Health Canada. (2004a). *Health care system: Federal role in health*. Retrieved January 25, 2009, from http://www.hc-sc.gc.ca/hcs-sss/delivery-prestation/fedrole/index-eng.php.

Health Canada. (2004b). *Health care system: Provincial/territorial role in health*. Retrieved January 25, 2009, from http://www.hc-sc.gc.ca/hcs-sss/delivery-prestation/ptrole/index-eng.php.

Katz, S. J., Verilli, D., & Barer, M. L. (1998). Canadians' use of U.S. medical services. *Health Affairs, 17*(1), 225–235.

Kelly, L. Y. (1985). *Dimensions of professional nursing* (5th ed.). New York: Macmillan.

McDonald, L. (1998). Florence Nightingale: Passionate statistician. *Journal of Holistic Nursing, 16*(2), 267–277.

Nightingale, F. (1859/1992). *Notes on nursing: What it is and what it is not* (Commemorative ed.). Philadelphia: Lippincott.

Nursing and health in Russia. (1998). *International Nursing Review, 45*(3), 89–93.

Randolph, E. (1991, November). Soviet hospitals besieged by filth, shortage of drugs. *Washington Post*.

Selanders, L. C. (1998a). Florence Nightingale: The evolution and social impact of feminist values in nursing. *Journals of Holistic Nursing, 16*(2), 227–243.

Selanders, L. C. (1998b). The power of environmental adaptation: Florence Nightingale's original theory for nursing practice. *Journal of Holistic Nursing, 16*(2), 247–263.

Shikles, J. L. (1991, November). Health care spending: The experience of France, Germany and Japan. *U.S. General Accounting Office Report*.

Stevens, R. (1989). *In sickness and in wealth*. New York: Basic Books.

Twigg, J. L. (1999). Obligatory medical insurance in Russia: The participant's perspective. *Social Science and Medicine, 49*(3), 371–382.

Uhlich, C., Michaud, S. L., & Giblin, C. (2007). Canadians partner with Russians to advance nursing reform. *The Canadian Nurse, 103*(6), 10–13.

Walker, M. (1992). How they don't do it in Canada. *Reason,* 35–42.

WHO (1978). *Traditional medicine*. Geneva: WHO Publications.

Womack, H. (2008). Russia's next president needs to tackle health reforms. *The Lancet, 371*(9614), 711–714.

World Health Organization. (1978). *The declaration of Alma-Ata*. Retrieved January 25, 2009, from http://www.wpro.who.int/rcm/en/archives/rc32/wpr_rc32_ro5.htm.

SUGGESTED READINGS

Bullough, B., & Bullough, V. (1994). *Nursing issues*. New York: Springer.

Castro, J. (1994). *The American way of health*. Boston: Little, Brown.

Dauner, C. D. (1994). *The health care solution*. Sacramento, CA: Vision.

Kalisch, P., & Kalisch, B. (1989). *The advance of American nursing* (2nd ed.) Boston: Little, Brown.

Knowles, J. H., ed. (1977). *Doing better and feeling worse*. New York: Norton.

Kovner A. (1995). *Health care delivery in the United States* (5th ed.). New York: Springer.

Long, R. E., ed. (1991). *The crisis in health care*. New York: Wilson.

Rosenberg, C. E. (1987). *The care of strangers*. New York: Basic Books.

Wekesser, C., ed. (1994). *Health care in America: Opposing viewpoints*. San Diego, CA: Green-haven Press.

PART IV

Global Issues That Impinge on Nursing Practice

P art IV recognizes each person as part of an interrelated global population affected by many interacting forces. Focusing on nursing, this part begins by addressing challenges and changes in health care delivery. This section then explores local, national, and global issues. These chapters encourage nurses to examine their views on what constitutes a responsible professional and citizen. Additionally, this section encourages active participation in political advocacy for issues of social justice and an awareness of economic, social, gender, transcultural, and spirituality issues.

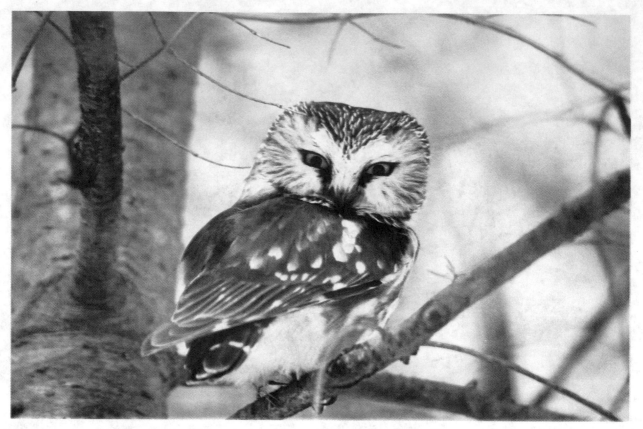

CHAPTER 14

Health Policy Issues

OBJECTIVES

After completing this chapter, the reader should be able to:

1. Understand what makes an issue "political."
2. Distinguish between politics and policy.
3. Identify basic legislative processes that affect health policy in Canada.
4. Give examples of specific political issues related to health care.
5. Discuss your personal stand on various political issues in relation to ethics.
6. Describe the health policy process.
7. Discuss the role of ethics in policy making.
8. Explain the role of nurses in the policy-making process.
9. Describe various methods of influencing public policy.

INTRODUCTION

We can view health policy and politics in a number of different ways. Some perceive health policy as a political process, strongly influenced by ideology and party politics. Others see the health policy-making process as a thoughtful one, by which decisions are based on data and the rational analysis of needs, outcomes, and costs (Donley, 1996). In reality the health policy process is a combination of both informed rational judgments and ideological partisan politics.

Nurses have become more involved in the political process, particularly in the realm of health policy. Nurses view health, at least in part, as dependent upon various environmental factors that can be altered by health policy decisions. Recognizing our role as advocates for patients' health, and acknowledging the importance of being involved in regulatory processes, we are assuming more responsibility in the political arena. This chapter features examples of selected political issues in the discussion of the process of creating health policy, and describes specific methods that nurses can utilize to influence policy.

POLITICS

Politics, political action, political issues, policies—what do these terms mean and how are they different? Furthermore, why are they so important to consider in nursing and health care? Whether you are a nurse at the bedside in an intensive care unit or a rural visiting home care nurse, your work, your scope of practice, and the structures within which you practise are all affected by politics and government policies.

Politics refers to anything that involves groups of persons making decisions or influencing how decisions are made or resources are allocated. The term implies both action and thought. It is, essentially, a neutral term although many people use the term with a negative connotation, e.g., "She is too caught up in the politics of all this." Certainly, politics and the activity of being political can be seen in a negative light, but this depends on your experience, biases, and how invested you are in the issue or end. Typically, people tend to act in a "political" way when the issue is one that will have an effect upon their own personal or professional lives. Otherwise, they tend not to pay attention to many political issues.

Policies are plans of action that guide actions—of governments, institutions, corporations, communities, etc. Policies often reflect the values and beliefs of the majority or of those directly responsible for creating the policy. Many times, when governments put policies in place, they reflect the overarching values of the government in power and may be altered when a different governing body comes into power. In Canada, our political parties hold very different views on many issues, for example, social policy issues like welfare and education, the environment, and gun control. Different political parties may take different stands on an issue either because they understand the available evidence differently, have different priorities, or have different moral or ideological points of view.

Many types of policies exist. We can have *social policies, public policies, or institutional/organizational policies*. The process of creating different policies may be similar; however, their jurisdiction and enactment might be markedly different. Some policies may be formed by governmental bodies as legislation while others may be mandated by institutions or communities. A good example of a social policy would be setting an age of consent or having an age limit on the purchase of alcohol or tobacco. Our non-smoking policies across Canada would be good examples of public policies. One major topic for social, public, and institutional policies is health. Health policies are any policies related to health care, health promotion, or health research. Health policies of special interest to nurses include those related to the provision of physician and hospital treatment in Canada along with province-specific decisions on coverage of related services, such as eye care, chiropractic care, nursing services, home care and long-term care. Institutional or organizational policies are those that refer to workplace, professional, or association issues. For example, hospitals may have a policy on the nurse–patient ratio on a particular unit (institutional policy) that has an impact upon how many shifts a nurse might work in a designated period of time, while the professional nursing union has specific policies on how many shifts in a row any nurse can work (organizational policies).

How Laws Are Made in Canada

In Canada, there are two main ways in which laws are created, through either the judicial system (known as "**common law**") or through the legislative or administrative system of the government (known as "**statutory law**"). **Common law** (sometimes called case law) developed originally in England, and is a system of laws derived from the decisions of courts and judges. This is in contrast to the laws set out by the government through acts, statutes, codes, or laws that enable, command, or enact, which is known as **statutory law**. Traditionally, statutory law may be seen as more important because there is less room or freedom for interpretation by judicial bodies. While there is room for interpretation in common law, the notion of precedent acts as a regulating force by establishing principles by which courts and judges make decisions in subsequent cases.

As noted in chapter seven, the **common law** is a tradition followed in all Canadian provinces, except Quebec. How the common law system is set up, at a federal and provincial level, is outlined by the terms of the *Constitution Act* (1867) which divides judicial responsibility between the levels of government. Within the provincial judicial systems, courts and judges make decisions at various levels. Each level must answer to or abide by the decision of a more superior court. For example, a decision in a lower court in British Columbia may be overturned by a higher court such as the British Columbia Court of Appeals. One important thing to note, however, is that a decision made at the highest level of a provincial court is not binding in other provinces, so a decision made at the highest court in Nova Scotia would not apply to Ontarians, although it may be considered as relevant or persuasive if the same issue were to be heard in an Ontario Court of Appeals. The highest course of appeal is the Supreme Court of Canada and the federal government decides who will serve as members of this court.

Statutory law refers to the body of law laid down by the legislature, either by the Parliament of Canada or by one of the provincial or territorial legislatures. At the federal level, bills (which eventually become laws) are passed by a complex process that involves a number of federal governing bodies within **Parliament**, which is made up of three parts: the **Governor General of Canada**, the appointed **Senate**, and the elected **House of Commons**. The governor general represents the queen and is responsible for calling Parliament together, reading the Speech from the Throne (outlining the priorities of the elected government), and approving all bills passed through the Senate and the House of Commons. The Senate (also referred to sometimes as the Upper Chamber) consists of members appointed by the governor general at the advice of the prime minister. Senators represent areas of the country and may serve up until age 75. They are not replaced if and when a new government is elected. The House of Commons is made up of elected officials from various ridings (electoral areas) across Canada. Normally, a member of the House of Commons serves for the period of time that the current government is in power, which is normally no more than five years.

So how does a law get introduced and eventually passed? Usually it is introduced as a proposal or a "**bill**" in the House of Commons (or the Senate, then the House of Commons). Once introduced in the House of Commons, the proposed bill goes through a series of three "readings," which means that the proposed bill is debated, discussed, revised, and amended. At each reading, the bill is voted on by the members. At the final or third reading in the House of Commons, if the bill is voted to be passed, it moves forward to the Senate and then the governor general, who gives the bill **Royal Assent**. Until a bill is given Royal Assent, it cannot become a law. Royal Assent is a formal completion of the legislative processes and is carried out in Commonwealth countries by the representative of the sovereign. It represents the authority granted to the representative—in this country, our governor general—to act on behalf of the queen to assent to legislation. It is rare, if not unheard of, that a bill passed by a House of Commons would be met with dissention by the governor general as she or he acts upon the advice of the prime minister. Therefore, many people view the Royal Assent of legislation as a mere formality.

Nurses should also have some basic knowledge about various types of law. **Civil law** deals with the rights of individuals and may refer to issues of **contracts** and **torts** (wrongs or harms done to others). **Criminal law** refers to the system that defines particular crimes and regulates the apprehension, charging, and procedures of trying suspected offenders. Criminal law also includes the system by which decisions are made regarding the punishments of persons convicted in the courts of committing a criminal act. **The *Criminal Code of Canada*** (a federal act) is the formal articulation of all offenses and procedures. Turn to Chapter 7 for a more detailed description of the various types of law that are relevant to nursing practice.

Think About It

In Canada, there are two main forms of legislation—**acts** and **regulations**. **Acts** are usually passed in federal Parliament or a provincial legislature. **Regulations** are usually made within the confines of a specific act and are often referred to as "delegated" or "subordinate" legislation for this reason. Note, though, that both acts and regulations are legally binding.

(*Continued*)

The Canadian government enacted the *Tobacco Act* in 1997. This act controls the sale, promotion, and labelling of tobacco products. It was put in place to protect the public, and specifically youth, from the proven dangerous effects of smoking on health. Some of the tenets of this act include restrictions on tobacco companies regarding how they advertise or market their products, requiring that they do not promote tobacco through lifestyle ads, ads targeted at youth, or ads depicting the use of tobacco as glamorous or exciting. Furthermore, tobacco companies may not sponsor youth-related activities or lend their name (and funds) to a cultural or sports facility.

In 2008, two new provisions of the *Tobacco Act* came into effect. One prohibits the public view of tobacco products in almost all places that sell them. A second provision prohibits workplace smoking rooms.

In addition to the *Tobacco Act*, each province and territory has legislation governing smoking. For example, in 2002, Newfoundland passed its *Smoke-Free Environment Act*, amended in 2005 to ban smoking in all public places, including bars. Quebec's *Tobacco Act* (2006), requires a smoking ban in all indoor public places with a ban on designated smoking rooms, effective 2008. Ontario has the *Smoke-free Ontario Act* which also bans smoking in all public and work places as of 2006. The act now also prohibits smoking in vehicles, in reserved seating in open-air stadiums, and in underground parking lots. Finally, Saskatchewan's *Tobacco Control Act* has a complete public ban on smoking, including casinos, private clubs, and bingo halls. This contrasts with neighbouring Alberta, which still allows smoking in casinos, bingo halls, and bars.

- What is your stand on smoking in public areas?
- Reflect on your stand and what kinds of experiences or beliefs have influenced you and your views on smoking.
- Do you think that these types of legislation limit the autonomy of persons?
- How do these kinds of laws protect those most vulnerable?
- What do you think should be more important for governments, protecting the autonomy of individuals or protecting the vulnerable? Why? Use the smoking laws to illustrate your views.

Nursing as a Political Force

Knowing all that goes into passing bills and enacting legislation, you might be asking yourself how these processes are relevant to individual nurses. Certainly, nurses can and should be involved in the passing of both public and private bills by helping to elect members of Parliament through their individual votes, lobbying for bills to be proposed or passed, and acting as expert witnesses during the process of parliamentary debate and discussion of bills, as they are moved through the House of Commons on their way to becoming laws.

Nurses can lobby for bills to be proposed or introduced through Parliament. For example, nurses in Canada were an active part of proposing mandatory bicycle helmet laws for children. In everyday practice, nurses see individual effects of many kinds of public and social issues (e.g., second-hand smoke, riding all-terrain vehicles [ATVs] without helmets, lack of access to healthy options, lack of clean water, etc.) and they often have good ideas about strategies to reduce both morbidity and mortality that can be translated into legislation protecting public interests. Nurses also have strong opinions about professional issues that have legal implications and are usually governed by provincial acts, issues such as scope of practice and entry to practice. As knowledgeable consumers of health care, professionals whose practice is regulated by the government and morally and ethically sensitive advocates for patients, nurses *should* be highly politically involved. Furthermore, as the largest group of health care professionals in Canada, made up of women and men from diverse backgrounds and experiences and espousing varying values, beliefs and opinions, nurses are highly representative of the Canadian public at large.

There are many kinds of political issues that should be and are of interest to nurses. We have identified four categories of political issues in Figure 14-1, including political–ethical issues, political–social issues, professional issues with professional implications, and those involving public health. Nurses' opinions on these issues may be based on both personal and professional experiences, ethical orientation, religious or spiritual beliefs, cultural norms, and other factors that have an impact on how persons develop their own sets of values, norms, and beliefs. Naturally, there is much debate and discussion arising from healthy diversity of opinions about many of the issues identified in Figure 14-1.

Figure 14–1 **Selected Examples of Political Issues**

Many of the political issues listed below are not exclusively "social" issues or "ethical" issues. In fact, many fall into more than one category. For example, issues around genetic testing certainly have ethical implications but they are also considered to be social issues as they have implications for the health of groups of persons. As another example, the mandated use of child seats or motorcycle helmets is a social issue (because it represents a limit on personal freedom) with public health implications.

The following are examples of some political issues in Canadian health care.

Political–ethical issues
- Abortion
- Genetic testing and research
- Reproductive technologies
- Contraception
- Organ procurement and transplantation
- Informed consent
- Age of consent
- Euthanasia and assisted suicide
- Access to care

(Continued)

Political–social issues

- Privacy of health records
- Tobacco legislation
- Accessibility for persons with disabilities
- Health of Aboriginal persons
- Urban and rural health priority setting
- Health care reform initiatives
- Listing and delisting of provincially covered health services

Political issues with professional implications

- Entry to practice
- Scope of practice
- Use of advanced practice nurses and prescriptive authority
- Use of nonregulated health care professionals
- Research funding
- Safety and workplace legislation

Political issues involving public health

- Bicycle helmet laws
- Seatbelt and child safety-seat laws
- Clean air legislation
- Water quality
- Disaster readiness and pandemic flu planning
- Pollution control
- Treatment and reporting of STIs
- Mandatory reporting of child abuse and neglect
- Mandatory gunshot wound reporting
- Mandating and/or availability of flu shots
- Food safety and labelling
- Substance abuse and "clean needle" or harm reduction programs

HEALTH POLICY

Because health plays a critical role in the physical, psychological, and economic condition of individuals, it affects society in general. The central purpose of health policy, therefore, is the improvement of the overall health of the population. Health policy is far reaching; it influences the behaviour and decisions of people in relation to their environment and living conditions; it affects lifestyle and personal behaviour; and it affects availability, accessibility, and quality of health care services. Health-related issues receive considerable attention in the policy-making forum.

Different people define health in different ways. Different definitions of health include notions of normality, and of illness, and the factors affecting these notions. The most popular definition of health affects the kinds and degree of investment society is willing to make in health care and social programs and the programs that are eventually funded. For example, if our society defines health narrowly in terms of illness, policy makers might choose to fund programs that focus on treatment of illness, but neglect programs that support health-promoting behaviours. In contrast, a society that defines health positively, in terms of wellness, would place more emphasis on funding programs to prevent illness or maximize health potential.

Health policies are formal and authoritative decisions focusing on health. Health policies are made in both the legislative and judicial branches of government, and are intended to direct or influence the actions, behaviours, or decisions of others. Policy comprises of a very large set of decisions. Examples of health policies include legislation rules and regulations designed to guide decision-making for the government, and various governmental programs related to health. **Statutes** or **laws** are pieces of legislation that have been enacted by legislative bodies and approved by the government. **Rules** or **regulations** are policies that are established to guide the implementation of laws and programs. **Judicial decisions** are authoritative court decisions that direct or influence the actions, behaviours, or decisions of others.

Although there is significant potential for overlap, health policies fit into two basic categories: allocative and regulatory. **Allocative policies** determine how priorities are set; that is, where resources are allocated. Resources may be financial resources, human resources, or time. This is the area in which we see distributive justice in practice. In most countries, including Canada, special attention is given in these policies to facilitate access to goods and services for the disadvantaged, marginalized, or vulnerable. Allocative policies are based upon fundamental beliefs about which distinct group or class of individuals or organizations should receive the benefits. Policy makers realize that some will receive benefits, some will not, and others will bear the expense. Ideally, these decisions are based upon public objectives (Longest, 1995). In Canada, with a publicly funded health care system (often called "medicare"), we are not forced to make decisions about how health care, specifically physician and hospital care, is allocated. However, decisions about where to build hospitals, what programs to offer at specific hospitals, how many physicians to put into place at centres, are all decisions about allocation that affect health care. A person living in a particularly underserved rural area does not have the same access to physician care, specialty care, or acute care services that a person living in downtown Toronto or Montreal would have. This is a direct result of resource allocation decisions.

Similarly, while physician and hospital care is covered under the *Canada Health Act,* medications are not (except for inpatients in hospitals). Each province decides on a prescription drug benefit plan and these vary between provinces as do requirements for co-payments by individuals. Many provinces have plans with some coverage for prescription drugs for the elderly or those on social assistance. Many persons who have chronic illnesses or devastating acute health care events, must often pay for their own medications. The way in which provinces decide upon how to cover prescription drugs is also an example of an allocation decision.

Regulatory policies are those designed to direct the actions, behaviour, and decisions of individuals or groups. Examples of regulatory policies include acts that regulate the practice of health care professionals, such as physicians, nurses, midwives, dietitians, pharmacists, physiotherapists, chiropractors, etc. Here are a few examples: In Ontario, there is the *Regulated Health Professions Act* (1991); Manitoba has the *Regulated Health Professions Statutes Amendment Act* (1998) and Alberta has the *Health Professions Act* (1999). Workplace regulations aimed at safe workplaces and procedures are also examples of regulatory policies. One example is the *Occupational Health and Safety (OHS) Regulation Act*. There are many acts in Canadian health care that might be considered regulatory policies. Figure 14–2 provides a brief description of a few of these regulatory acts.

As with all policies, the purpose of regulatory policy is to ensure that public objectives are met. Many nurses do not realize the impact regulatory policies have on nursing practice. Following are selected examples of recently debated regulatory policies: policies that would allow women unrestricted access to their choice of ob-gyn providers, including advanced practice nurses; policies to require health records privacy; and policies to protect workers from accidental needlestick.

Figure 14–2 **Examples of Regulatory Acts in Canada**

Assisted Human Reproduction Act
- This act is concerned with the health and safety of women involved in and children born as a result of assisted reproduction, which may include or restrict technologies and activities such as in creation of embryos in vitro, surrogate mothering, or sale of fertilized embryos or gametes (ovum or sperm).

Controlled Drugs and Substances Act
- This act is concerned with the production, sale, export, and import of narcotics (e.g., heroin, morphine, methadone) and controlled substances (e.g., ketamines, fentanyls).

Food and Drugs Act
- This act concerns the manufacturing, sale, labelling and safety of food, natural health products, drugs, and medical devices in Canada.

Quarantine Act
- This act allows the Minister of Health in the event of an outbreak of an infectious or highly contagious disease to quarantine persons, set up quarantine stations, and designate quarantine officers as required.

Canadian Environment Protection Act
- This act addresses issues pertaining to environmental and human health protection alongside sustainability of environmental development.

The Health Policy Process

Health policies are those that affect health in any way, either directly, as with immunization programs, or indirectly, as with statutes that describe scope of practice of health care providers. The process of health policy includes three distinct phases. These phases are both consecutive and circular. The first phase is that of **policy formulation.** This phase includes such actions as agenda setting and the subsequent development of legislation. The second phase is that of **policy implementation.** This phase follows enactment of legislation, and includes taking actions and making additional decisions necessary to implement legislation, such as rule making and policy operation. The final stage is **policy modification.** The purpose of this stage is to improve or perfect legislation previously enacted. This might entail only minor adjustments made in the implementation phase, or it may involve major changes or the elimination of particular statutes (Longest, 1995).

Policy Formulation. The first phase of policy making is policy formulation. This phase is divided into two distinct sequentially related sets of activities: agenda setting and legislation development (Longest, 1995). At any point in time, there is a complex mix of three variables: health-related problems, possible solutions and alternatives, and diverse political interests. As agenda setting progresses, the emerging issues can proceed to the development of legislation.

Problems. The existence of real or perceived problems is the impetus for the policy formulation phase of policy making. Problems may become evident in a number of ways. Some problems occur as the result of the interaction of certain variables related to previous policy. In the late 1980s and early 1990s, long waiting lists for cardiac and orthopedic surgical procedures across Canada resulted in a number of new policy initiatives related to resource allocation, triage of patients, and the management of queues. Other problems may gain attention as they reach unacceptable levels. Growth in the number of HIV-positive persons and the rate of spread of the virus is an example of such a problem. Other problems emerge as a result of some specific event that forces public attention. In 2003, there was a global outbreak of Severe Acute Respiratory Syndrome (SARS). While there were reported and suspected cases across Canada, a total of 44 persons died in the Greater Toronto Area and significant policies were put into place (quarantine, hospital visiting), on an emergent basis during the epidemic and afterwards as precautionary measures in the case of possible future outbreaks. Nevertheless, the mere existence of problems is not always sufficient to ensure the formulation of legislation. There must also be feasible solutions to the problems and the political will to enact legislation.

Solutions. Someone must come up with an idea to solve a problem before legislation is initiated. The process of offering solutions to problems involves generating ideas for solving the problems, refining the ideas, and selecting from among the options (Longest, 1995). A significant example of the generation of ideas to solve real and potential problems in health care would be the Commission on the Future of Health Care in Canada (Romanow, 2002).

Political Circumstances. Even if we identify a serious problem and offer feasible solutions, we may not be able to influence legislation. Legislation can progress through the process only with the sponsorship and support of influential policy makers who believe in the issue and invest time and energy. Potential sponsors are sensitive to political will. Factors that influence political will include public attitudes, concerns, and opinions surrounding an issue; the preferences and relative ability to influence political decisions; the positions of key political leaders on the issue; and other competing items on the policy agenda. Longest (1995) believes that creating a political thrust forceful enough to cause policy makers to formulate and implement new policy is often the most difficult problem. Nurses are a significant percentage of the voting population. We are in a good position to influence political decisions collectively and enhance the political will essential to formulate health policy.

Policy Implementation.

Policy implementation immediately follows the enactment of legislation. Because legislation seldom contains explicit language on how it is to be implemented, details are left to the process of rule making. A formal part of the implementation phase, the dissemination of rules is accomplished by specific implementing organizations. For example, the provincial governments, while involved in passing legislation related to the regulation of nurses, leaves the implementation, promulgation, and enforcement of specific legislation related to the licensing and regulation of nurses to the provincial and territorial colleges and Associations of Nursing. Thompson (1991) calls the interaction between some implementing organizations and affected interest groups "strategic interaction." Interest groups routinely seek to influence rule making, because they are so often the targets of rules established to implement health policies. Lobbying is one of the major means by which interest groups attempt to influence policy makers. Lobbying is especially intense when various interest groups disagree upon the formulation of a particular policy.

Policy Modification.

As the third phase of the policy-making process, policy modification occurs when outcomes, perceptions, and consequences of existing policies indicate that either the original problems still exist, or new problems have arisen from unforeseen circumstances or from the policy itself. The policy modification phase is intended to be a kind of feedback loop, into the agenda-setting and legislation-development stages of the formulation phase—potentially creating new legislation—and into the rule-making and policy operation stages of the implementation phase, stimulating changes in rules or operations. Many programs are routinely amended, some of them repeatedly, over a period of many years. These modifications may reflect, among other things, the development of new technologies, changing economic conditions, and public demand (Longest, 1995).

Ethics in Policy Making

Because policy affects people's lives and relationships and is often part of the distributive justice process, policy making is an inherently ethical endeavour. The outcomes and consequences of most health policy affect large groups of people. There are two equally important functions of ethics in public policy making. In the policy formulation phase, ethics can guide the original development of new policies. Ethics is also useful in the policy modification phase as a means to legitimately criticize policies that are already implemented (Thompson, 1985). There is, however, some practical difficulty in adhering strictly to specific ethical principles during the policy-making process. Discussing the complexity of policy making and ethics, Beauchamp and Childress (2001) write:

> Policy formation and criticism involve more complex forms of judgment than ethical principles and rules can handle on their own. Public policy is often formulated in contexts that are marked by profound social disagreements, uncertainties, and different interpretations of history. No body of abstract moral principles and rules can determine policy in such circumstances, because it cannot contain enough specific information or provide direct and discerning guidance. The specification and implementation of moral principles and rules must take account of problems of feasibility, efficiency, cultural pluralism, political procedures, uncertainty about risk, noncompliance by patients, and the like. Principles and rules provide the moral background for policy evaluation, but a policy must also be shaped by empirical data and by information available in fields such as medicine, nursing, economics, law and psychology. When using moral principles or rules to formulate or criticize public policies, we cannot move with assurance from a judgment that an act is morally right (or wrong) to a judgment that a corresponding law or policy is morally right (or wrong). The judgment that an act is morally wrong does not necessarily lead to the judgment that the government should prohibit it or refuse to allocate funds to support it. (pp. 8–9)

Beauchamp and Childress are not suggesting that health policy is so complex as to prohibit the strict and exclusive use of specific rules or principles in guiding policy formulation; rather, the authors suggest that ethical considerations must be accompanied by the rational use of empirical data.

Research and Policy

In order to prevent policies based upon unsubstantiated beliefs or personal values, when we are interested in an issue, we must furnish officials with important and reliable information. If they have reliable facts and research findings, policy makers are able to identify problems, make comparisons, confirm trends, and establish policy based on evidence (Donley, 1996). Because time is a precious commodity, officials are often more interested in empirical research findings than unsubstantiated personal opinion. Pender (1992) suggests that nurses who plan to discuss policy with officials carefully review research findings that pertain to the issue and be ready to quote a few particularly compelling or attention-getting statistics. Cost savings often gets attention when other facts elicit little response.

The federal government recognizes the importance of health care research in the development of policy. Here are three examples of how research and policy interact in Canada. The Policy Research Initiative (PRI) is a neutral research organization within the federal government responsive to emerging issues in Canadian society. The broad aims of this initiative are twofold: To connect those involved in policy research, both from within the government and external to it, with those in the policy-setting areas in government and to advance research on emerging and pressing issues. Furthermore the PRI helps to ensure effective knowledge transfer between policy makers and researchers. The Canadian Policy Research Network (CPRN) is an independent, not-for-profit organization funded by a variety of sources, including federal and provincial governments. This organization conducts research and public consultatory processes to find out what kinds of socioeconomic issues are important to the public, e.g., health care, education, sustainable environments and communities, family supports, etc. The network makes its research and data available to the federal, provincial, and local governments to assist in policy-making processes. Finally, organizations at a provincial level such as the Institute for Clinical Evaluative Sciences (ICES) in Ontario function independently to provide scientific research data to assist policy makers in health care delivery. ICES profiles its research work through publications such as atlases and investigative reports as well as peer-reviewed journals in health care. Organizations at a provincial level, such as ICES, can also be mandated by the government to conduct research in specific areas of interest or in areas that require more urgent data in order to make effective policy decisions on an urgent or emergent basis (e.g., SARS).

There are many research policy centres in universities across Canada that provide training and conduct research on health policy issues. Some examples are the Centre for Health Services and Policy Research at the University of British Columbia, the Canadian Research Institute for Social Policy at the University of New Brunswick, the Children's Health Policy Centre at Simon Fraser University and the Health, Law and Policy Group at the Faculty of Law in the University of Toronto.

NURSING, POLICY, AND POLITICS

Not since the days of Lavinia Lloyd Dock have nurses been so actively involved with policy making and politics. It is through the perspective of knowledge, experience, and intimacy with the health care needs of the population that nursing is in the unique position to bring balance to the policy making process (Murphy, 1992). Moreover, professional codes of ethics identify the goals and values of the profession, and explicitly call for nurses to be involved in policy formulation. For example, the ICN *Code of Ethics for Nurses* (2000) calls for nurses to share with society the "responsibility for initiating and supporting action to meet the health and social needs of the public, in particular those of vulnerable populations." The Canadian Nurses Association notes that "If we think of health as something broadly defined and influenced, we begin to arrive at the inescapable conclusion that to be concerned with health is to be concerned with the social context, and that nursing is, indeed, a political act." (CNA, 2000).

The formulation of health policy requires strong nursing leadership and an understanding of the nature of local and national policy making and priority setting. Calling for the political empowerment of nurses, Batra (1992) charges that if we are serious in our efforts to promote health, we must understand the crucial role of public policy. To do this, we must develop the ability to think, teach, research, and act in ways that are relative to policy; we must be aware of the impact that policies have on health and on our clinical practice; we must conduct research on health policy issues; and we must find strategic ways to influence state and national policy agendas. Recognizing health problems as policy issues allows nurses to move into the realm of policy formulation.

Nursing's Political Strengths. There are notable strengths with which nursing enters the political arena. First, the most sizable group of health care providers, the nursing profession boasts an extremely large number of political constituents. Acting together, the nation's nurses have the potential to be a formidable political force. Second, nurses have traditionally been perceived in a favourable light. Nurses are viewed as much less self-interested than any of the other major health-related interest groups (Hadley, 1996). Third, once nurses become involved in health policy, they usually continue to be active (Gebbe, Wakefield, & Kerfoot, 2000).

Nursing's Political Weaknesses. The profession also has a number of political weaknesses. First, relatively new to the political arena, many nurses are not astute or comfortable in policy making or lobbyist roles. Second, there has historically been a lack of ideological and political unity within the profession, a weakness Hadley (1996) believes stems from the lack of uniform educational requirements and titles. Third, though nurses comprise the largest number of professionals, there are fewer dollars in nursing coffers specifically earmarked for intense lobbying than in those of many other special-interest groups. Finally, in nursing education, we have not typically provided education on how to be politically active. While programs now include courses on current trends and issues, very little attention is still given to teaching nursing students how to engage in political activism. We do equip nursing students with skills and knowledge in advocacy; however, it is often related to advocacy for individual patients and not groups or communities. Fortunately, some programs now include more emphasis on political activism, recognizing the evolving roles of nurses in a variety of communities.

Policy Goals for Nursing

How do nurses become aware of the issues that are important and require energy and focus? Each of us has the responsibility to reflect upon problems and potential solutions. In addition, one of the major functions of professional organizations is to provide leadership and assistance to members in political and other matters. In the Canadian Nurses Association's most recent revision of its *Code of Ethics for Registered Nurses* (2008), nursing practice is defined as "direct care (which includes community and public health), education, administration, research and policy development." (p. 1)

Think About It

Nurses Take Positions on Political Issues

The Canadian Nurses Association has been a powerful lobbying force for many years. Issues of interest to members of the organization are freely accessible through the CNA's website at http://www.cna.aiic.ca. The site includes a section entitled "Nursing and the Political Agenda" with links to public opinion polls on current political health care issues. The CNA also has a number of position statements, fact sheets, research summaries, presentations and briefs, and open letters to governments. The CNA has been actively involved in political activism and advocating for policy in a number of areas, including environmentally responsible activity in the health care sector, screening for alcohol and drugs in the workplace, promoting culturally competent care, ensuring patient safety, monitoring entry to practice, and providing care at the end of life. The CNA has also been actively involved in presenting briefs to the government on current issues. These briefs, found on the website, address many diverse interests, e.g., Brief to the House of Commons Standing Committee and Human Resources, Social Development and the status of Persons with Disabilities; and the Brief to the National Advisory Committee on SARS and Public Health: Lessons Learned and Recommendations. Through these briefs and their presentations, the CNA demonstrates political activism, solidarity, and leadership.

These are only a few examples of the kinds of issues the CNA has been involved in over the past decade.

- What are the reasons for the CNA to publish position statements and fact sheets? Who benefits and why?

- Should nurses be concerned with issues such as mandatory gunshot wound reporting or screening for drugs and alcohol in the workplace? Why or why not?

- What are the socio-political issues that you feel are most important in health care today, nationally, in your province or territory and in your city or community?

- Think of one socio-political issue that is important to you today. How would you begin to think about being politically active and advocating for health policy for this issue?

LOBBYING

Sometimes nurses are legitimate members of governmental or institutional policy-making bodies. More often, the nurse's role in policy formulation, implementation, and modification is that of lobbyist. "**Lobbying** is the art of persuasion—attempting to convince a legislator, a government official, the head of an agency, or a state official to comply with a request—whether it is convincing them to support your position on an issue or to follow a particular course of action" (deVries & Vanderbilt, 1992, p. 1). Though many special-interest groups employ lobbyists, every nurse can be a lobbyist and should lobby on issues of concern. Lobbyists have a powerful voice in determining the policy-making process, from agenda setting to policy modification. In fact, some nurses believe it is a nurse's duty to participate in political **activism**. Hagerdorn defines activism as "a passionate approach to everyday activities that is committed to seeking a more just social order through critical analysis, provocation, transformation, and rebalancing of power" (1995, p. 2). Activism promotes "exposing, provoking, and unbalancing the social power that maintains people in a state of disease, while simultaneously nurturing caring" (1995, p. 2). Others believe that constrained, subtle, and persistent political activity is more effective in the long term than overt activism.

To be effective in the political domain, nurses are charged to become politically astute. According to Jennings, "One can have the best policy proposal on the table but if he or she doesn't know how to play the political game, all will be lost. Nurses must be very adept at discerning who has the power in the policy arena and how to link to that source" (1996, p. 4). Knowing the "power players" and understanding the processes in the political arena is one of the most important steps in the lobbying process.

Methods of Lobbying

The most familiar type of lobbying is the face-to-face approach. This process involves either meeting directly with a policy maker to request a desired action, or testifying at a hearing. When possible, both paid and volunteer lobbyists should utilize the face-to-face method of lobbying. A second form of lobbying is **grassroots lobbying.** Grassroots lobbying involves mobilizing a committed constituency to influence the opinions of policy makers. Different types of grassroots lobbying include organized letter writing and implementing campaigns designed to mobilize public opinion.

One of the most important facets of lobbying is knowing whom to lobby. In seeking help to promote a particular legislative agenda, nurses want to begin by enlisting policy makers who have the following characteristics: (1) legitimate power, (2) an interest in the problem, (3) an affinity for nursing or for health care issues in general, (4) time and energy to invest in the process, (5) the respect of colleagues, and (6) committee or other positions that are appropriate to the particular legislation. Finding an official with all of these characteristics will greatly improve the probability of legislative success. New lobbyists waste time and energy lobbying officials who are uninterested, have conflicting loyalty, are powerless, or are not respected by their colleagues. The first step in lobbying is to connect with the appropriate policy makers.

The Lobbying Campaign. Once nurses have identified the appropriate policy-making officials and are familiar with the issues and the legislative and regulatory process, the lobbying campaign can begin. There are two basic types of lobbying: direct and indirect. Indirect lobbying strategies are geared toward influencing public opinion, which in turn will influence policy makers. Methods of indirect lobbying include media broadcasts; newspapers and other written materials; dissemination of the results of opinion polls; paid advertisements; educational campaigns; and organizations' agendas. Direct methods include party platforms, political elections, influence of committees, agency regulations, face-to-face lobbying, letter writing, and contact with policy makers during social events (deVries & Vanderbilt, 1992). For more information on lobbying, check the CNA publication *Getting Started: A Political Action Guide for Canada's Registered Nurses.*

Preparing for Political Action of Any Kind

There are three steps in preparing to engage in political action of any kind, including lobbying, for a specific cause (CNA, 2000). These involve thoughtful assessment of the situation and context in which policy making occurs related to the specific issue with which you are concerned.

- Conduct research and educate yourself in order to speak in a knowledgeable and informed way. You also need to have a good understanding of the processes and levels of government in order to aim your lobbying actions most effectively.

- Enlist interested and informed allies to your lobbying cause. There is strength in numbers, and governments will pay attention to large interest groups and groups that have persons with particular expertise.

- Make sure you have identified the "right" group of decision makers before you begin lobbying. Is this really the group that can help enact the change you want? Is there more than one decision-making group you should be targeting? Should you be involving private industry or corporations as well?

Letter Writing.   Handwritten, personal, mass letter writing is a powerful grassroots lobbying technique. Certain letter writing techniques have been found to be more effective; here are some practical tips for letter writing:

- Whenever possible, individualize and legibly handwrite or type letters on personal stationery. Though more effective than no letters at all, form letters are much less likely to be read by officials than individualized letters.

- Write the letter in your own words, using your own thoughts and logic and drawing pertinent inferences.

- Identify yourself as a nurse and state your reason for writing in the first paragraph, including the title and number of the legislation in which you are interested.

- Be specific and include key information and examples supporting your position.

- Be explicit. Tell the official exactly what you want. If you are writing to ask for cosponsorship or a vote for or against a bill, say so.

- Be brief but informative. Keep your letter to a maximum of one to two pages.

- Include only one topic in each letter.

- Never threaten or use hostility. This immediately destroys your chances of developing a cooperative relationship.

- Offer your assistance as a resource.

- Promptly thank the official for favourable votes.
- Using technology to communicate with large groups of people is highly effective. Legitimate websites, blogs, wikis, and discussion boards can get messages out or enlist allies. Carefully choosing the places you want to send your message and how it is communicated is key to maintaining credibility.
- It helps to have a strong and dependable media outlet through which to communicate your message. Garnering media attention toward your issue can be an essential way of reaching larger groups of persons. Of course, newspapers, television, or radio news programs can have specific political agendas and perspectives so research these and develop trusting and sustainable relationships with media personnel who you feel may be able to present your issue effectively (CNA, 2000).

Personal Visits. A personal visit is usually a more powerful lobbying tool than letter writing. Whenever possible, nurses should seize the opportunity to meet with policy makers face to face. Following are a few suggestions for personal visits with policy-making officials:

- Be prepared. Develop your plan of action and know what you intend to say.
- Be on time for your appointment and be patient if the official is late.
- Be courteous, greet the official with a firm handshake, introduce yourself, and present your business card.
- Identify the subject of the meeting and present your facts in an orderly, succinct, and direct fashion.
- Support your position with personal experiences and anecdotes; use valid research and statistics when appropriate.
- Keep your presentation simple. Avoid technical language and professional jargon. Your goal is to inform and influence, not to impress.
- Close the meeting strongly and effectively, asking for the official's support.
- Leave a short fact sheet summarizing the issue and your position. Include the names and telephone numbers of contact people.
- Send a letter within a few days thanking the official for the meeting, restating your position, and including any information requested during the meeting.

? Think About It

Be Careful of Your Wording

Nurses must be careful in choosing words to use when lobbying. One nurse relates a story of her first experience testifying before a government committee. Feeling her presentation was well prepared and would be effective, the nurse decided at the last minute to substitute the words *nurse voters* for the word

(Continued)

nurses. There were many people giving testimony that day. Following the completion of the testimony phase, the legislators were given an opportunity to make comments or ask questions. There were no questions. Every comment was directed toward the nurse, who was surprised to learn that the legislators perceived the term *nurse voters* to indicate a veiled threat. They did not hear the substance of the presentation, but rather the perceived threat, "If you do not support our position, we will vote you out of office." By unintentionally giving this impression, the nurse ruined a productive relationship with these legislators. The legislation that the nurses were supporting failed.

- Why do you think the nurse changed the wording of her presentation in the first place?

- What words would you have used?

- Describe similar circumstances in which you were speaking and the reaction of the listeners was based upon their inferences from your choice of words rather than their intended meaning.

- How can nurses avoid mistakes of this sort?

Political Campaigns

One very effective direct lobbying technique is for nurses to become involved in either supporting candidates or themselves running for elective office. According to Wakefield (1990), nurses are encouraged to get involved in lobbying for specific legislation, not realizing that the ability to influence decisions occurs long before the issues are revealed to the public. Wakefield suggests that nurses become involved in campaigns and elections. This can be done in any number of ways. First, nurses should become involved in political-party organizations. Political-party activity serves as a vehicle for developing important relationships with elected officials and involvement in a political party is essential to building a political network. Second, nurses can become involved through provincial nurses' associations. These organizations provide an opportunity to meet candidates, form relationships, and offer candidates forums. Forums remind a candidate that nurses are an organized group interested in politics and public policy and acquaint nurses with the candidate's position on important issues. Third, nurses can become actively involved in campaigning for candidates who support their positions on various health care issues. This may take the form of campaigning door to door, stuffing envelopes or publicly endorsing candidates. Actively supporting candidates for public office helps to forge relationships with officials and elect candidates to public office who will sympathize with issues important to nurses. Involvement with political parties and the consequent relationships with public officials can also lead to either nurses' candidacy and election to public office, or nurses' appointments to important policy-making positions.

SUMMARY

There are many political issues that are important to nurses. Most issues for which nurses are actively concerned are related to health policy: issues of a moral nature; issues related to professional regulation; issues related to public health; and issues related to distributive justice. Fulfilling the role of advocate, nurses are challenged to become politically active: to know and become involved with important issues; to learn the political process; to form relationships with public officials; and to become astute in methods of influencing health policy.

CHAPTER HIGHLIGHTS

- The term *political* relates to the policy-making process within the government.
- Political issues are those that are created, affected, or regulated by any of the government branches.
- Political parties are organized groups with distinct ideologies that seek to control government.
- Health policies influence the actions, decisions, and behaviours of people in the domain of health.
- Society's definition of health reflects the extent to which society is willing to go toward maximizing the health of citizens.
- Allocative health policies are designed to provide benefits to a distinct group.
- Regulatory policies are designed to influence others through directive techniques.
- The process of health policy includes the phases of policy formulation, policy implementation, and policy modification.
- There are two important functions of ethics in public policy making—guiding the original development of policy and criticizing previously implemented policy.
- Nurses are able to affect health policy through various political means.

DISCUSSION QUESTIONS AND ACTIVITIES

1. Explore the CNA's website at http://www.cna-aiic.ca. Review some of the presentations and briefs. How do some of these issue relate to current issues in nursing ethics?
2. Discuss the issues listed in Figure 14–1 in class. How do classmates' positions compare to those of the major political parties? Are each student's opinions politically consistent from issue to issue?
3. Discuss the following question in class: What purpose do political parties serve?
4. Compile a list of political issues and classify them as to the branch of government with which the issue is most closely aligned—administrative, judicial, or legislative.

5. Discuss methods for influencing health policy in the administrative and judicial domains.

6. Compile a list of at least five political issues related to health that have been decided within the judicial domain. How have the judicial decisions affected health care delivery?

7. Compile a list of political issues related to moral values. Discuss the role of the professional organization in guiding members' actions related to these moral issues.

8. Discuss popular definitions of health and determine how each definition, if adopted by government, would affect health care delivery.

9. Discuss the role of ethics in policy making.

REFERENCES

Batra, C. (1992). Empowering for professional, political, and health policy involvement. *Nursing Outlook, 40*(4), 170–176.

Bavier, A. (1995). Where research and practice meet: Opportunities at the Agency for Health Care and Policy and Research. *Nursing Policy Forum, 1*(4), 20–38.

Beauchamp, T. L., & Childress, J. F. (2001). *Principles of biomedical ethics* (4th ed.). New York: Oxford University Press.

Canadian Nurses Association. (1997). *Getting started: A political action guide for Canada's Registered Nurses*. Ottawa: Canadian Nurses Association.

Canadian Nurses Association. (2008). *Code of ethics for Registered Nurses*. Ottawa: Canadian Nurses Association.

C.N.A. (2000). Nursing as a political act. *Nursing Now*. May 2000. Ottawa: CNA.

Curtin, L. (1996). *Nursing into the 21st century: Health care reform, restructuring, practice, leadership*. Springhouse, PA: Springhouse.

deVries, C. M., & Vanderbilt, M. W. (1992). *The grassroots lobbying handbook: Empowering nurses through legislative and political action*. Washington, DC: American Nurses Association.

Donley, R. (1996). Shaping health policy. *Nursing Policy Forum, 2*(1), 12–19.

Emerson, R. (1995). What is success? In W. Bennett, ed., *The moral compass: A companion to the book of virtues*. New York: Simon & Schuster.

Gebbe, K. M., Wakefield, M., & Kerfoot. (2000). Nursing and health policy. *Journal of Nursing Scholarship, 32*(3), 307–315.

Hadley, E. (1996). Nursing in the political and economic marketplace: Challenges for the 21st century. *Nursing Outlook, 44*(1), 6–10.

Hagerdorn, S. (1995). The politics of caring: The role of activism in primary care. *Advances in Nursing Science, 17*(4), 1–11.

International Council of Nurses. (2000). *The ICN code of ethics for nurses*. Geneva, Switzerland: International Council of Nurses.

Jennings, C. (1996). Politics and nursing do mix! *Nursing Policy Forum, 2*(3), 4.

Longest, B. B., Jr. (1995). *Health policymaking in the United States*. Ann Arbor, MI: AUPHA Press/Health Administration Press.

Murphy, N. (1992). Nursing leadership in health policy decision making. *Nursing Outlook, 10*(4), 158–161.

Pender, N. (1992). Making a difference in health policy. *Nursing Outlook, 40*(3), 104–105.

Romanow, R. (Commissioner). (2002). *Building on values: The future of health care in Canada*. Ottawa: The Romanow Commission.

Thompson, D. (1985). Philosophy and policy. *Philosophy and Public Affairs, 14*(2), 205–218.

Thompson, F. J. (1991). The enduring challenge of health policy implementation. In T. J. Litman & L. S. Robins, eds., *Health politics and policy* (2nd ed., pp. 148–169). Albany, NY: Delmar.

Wakefield, M. (1990). Political involvement: A nursing necessity. *Nursing Economics, 8*(5), 352–353.

WEBSITES

Institute for Clinical Evaluative Studies (ICES)
http://www.ices.on.ca

Canadian Policy Research Networks (CPRN)
http://www.cprn.ca

Policy Research Initiative (PRI)
http://www.policyresearch.gc.ca

Centre for Health Services and Policy Research at the University of British Columbia
http://www.chspr.ubc.ca

Canadian Research Institute for Social Policy at the University of New Brunswick
http://www.unb.ca/crisp/index.php

The Children's Health Policy Centre at Simon Fraser University
http://www.childhealthpolicy.sfu.ca

Health Law and Policy Group at the University of Toronto Faculty of Law
http://www.law.utoronto.ca/healthlaw

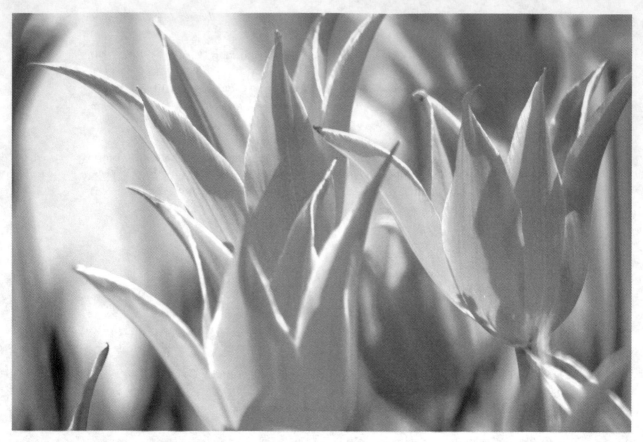

CHAPTER 15
Economic Issues

OBJECTIVES

After completing this chapter, the reader should be able to:

1. Describe the role of economics in health care.
2. Explain the concept of distributive justice.
3. Discuss utilitarian, libertarian, communitarian, and egalitarian theories.
4. Discuss basic questions related to the distribution of health care resources.
5. Describe recent trends in health care economics and the relationship of economic trends to the delivery of health care.
6. Discuss ideas around Canadian health care reform.

INTRODUCTION

Nursing, other health care professions, and the overall health care delivery system exist to deliver health care to society. Over the past several decades, dynamic forces have worked together to create a complex system that has been called one of the best in the world. From advances in knowledge and technology to changes in health care financing, the system has experienced rapid and drastic changes. It is not unusual to hear the term "crisis" used to describe the state of the current health care system. The crisis in health care refers to the ability we have to sustain a system that is incredibly costly, while assuring high quality and access to health services. With an ever-increasing demand for a finite amount of services alongside cuts from the federal governments to support health care, the system is strained at best, ailing at worst. Dramatic costs of new technologies and the push to use them in the management of illness and disease is driving the cost of health care up significantly. The high cost of technology-rich acute care means that resources for areas like public health, population health, and health promotion—all areas in which illness and disease prevention are integral—are few. Thoughtful, systematic, ethical priority setting at all levels of care—the bedside, institutions, and agencies as well as governments—is necessary to try to devise solutions to the current problems in health care.

OVERVIEW OF TODAY'S HEALTH CARE ECONOMICS

Though given its own twists, the history of economic thought is closely associated with the utilitarian movement in the last century (Honderich, 1995). One of the main assumptions in traditional economics is that we should judge the institutions of a society by the preferences of the people that those institutions affect. There are different ways to judge the total preference of society. One method claims that one arrangement is better than another only if it satisfies the preferences of some people and does not frustrate the preferences of any others. This idea is at the centre of what is known as welfare economics. Another method suggests that institutions are properly judged only according to the preferences of the people they affect; therefore, the institution of health care should be judged by the people it serves. Discussion and debate about the current state of health care economics is integral to the process of evaluating the present system and formulating one that is more just.

Today's problems in the health care system have a long history, with many intervening factors. We have produced a system with progressively higher standards that require the most and the best care for a large segment of the population, regardless of cost. This spiralling pattern is combined with irresponsibility caused by a third-party reimbursement system that (in the past, at least) did not require providers or patients to be careful of cost. This has led to a skewed model that focuses heavily on technology and personal autonomy, and ignores basic principles of social responsibility and distributive justice. This system features an odd split between those who make the spending decisions (patients, physicians, and allied health care professionals) and those who must actually pay for the costs of those decisions (provincial governments and private insurance companies). (Morreim, 1995). Moreover, there are staggering contrasts within this system. In some instances, hundreds of thousands of dollars are spent on what is recognized as futile care, yet many wait for urgent care in long queues.

Within the traditional fee-for-service system, ethics is predominately driven by codes of ethical behaviour and patients' rights statements, with a strong focus on the principle of autonomy. This model focuses on the individual patient, protects physician autonomy, promotes treatment that offers potential benefit or prolonged life, and assumes unlimited resources. Clearly, there are ethical problems associated with this model, including both overutilization and rationing on the basis of financial means (Biblo, Christopher, Johnson, & Potter, 1995).

Ask Yourself

Paying for Futile Care

One often hears stories about elderly patients with terminal illness, and even "do not resuscitate" status, who remain in intensive care settings for extended periods of time, often because of family members who insist that everything be done for their loved one.

- Is the expenditure of expensive health care resources appropriate for these types of situations? Explain your position.
- Who should bear the financial burden for futile care?
- What are the ethical principles that conflict in situations of this sort?

In many other countries, health care is also a priority from an economic perspective. Globally, costs are increasing with the use of more advanced technology.

Three basic types of health care systems exist. First there is the national health systems model, in which health care priorities are set and services are organized and delivered by a national system, either in a centralized way, like in Cuba and Russia, or in a decentralized, more local way, as in Sweden and Finland. In the public insurance model, as Canada has, health care services are publicly financed but delivered by others; in this case, provincial and territorial governments and institutions. Finally, in an entrepreneurial model, patients need to be able to pay for health services, which are provided by private providers in a relatively free market. The United States is a prime example of such a model of health care.

The health care systems model in the United States is a source of constant debate. In an essay on reforming American health care, deBlois, Norris, and O'Rourke (1994) discuss the problems with the U.S. health care financing system. While some of the problems are unique to the American system, others are shared by all types of health care systems. Though most people agree that modern health care in the United States is highly sophisticated and technologically advanced, they also recognize that there are many deficiencies in the system. First, health care services and resources are inaccessible to nearly 20 percent of the population. Second, health care costs are accelerating at an unsustainable annual rate, consuming a huge portion of the gross domestic product. Third, the high cost of health care threatens the competitiveness and profitability of business and industry. Fourth, the benefits to the individual and corporate providers within the system are often pursued at the expense (and sometimes harm) of persons who are in need of health care. DeBlois et al. (1995) propose that the real problems with the current American system are related to its priorities and the values and commitments that support them, the most significant of which are

1. an extreme form of individualism that routinely prefers individual interests over concerns about the community of persons;
2. an endorsement of profit making as a primary motive for providing health care services; and
3. an uncritical acceptance of technology as morally neutral and as unambiguous in the service of human goods and goals. (p. 55)

DeBlois et al. (1995) charge that the health and well-being of people subjected to a system under the influence of these values are often threatened by the kinds of services offered, the manner in which they are provided, and the priorities that determine both. Further, if improvements in the system are intended to promote health and well-being of people, efforts need to be ethically grounded and challenge the values that drive this type of system.

Challenging the status quo and the overarching values is an important part of examining a health care system, critically and ethically. While the U.S. system values individualism, the Canadian system espouses a more communitarian-based value system, in which the health of individuals, groups, communities, and citizenships are valued above individual freedom and liberty. In the U.S. system, despite the emphasis on liberty and freedom of individual choice, many people are left without freedom of choice and without funds to afford basic health care. Still others, who can afford a minimum of care, find that they are plunged into debt or financial collapse when faced with a catastrophic illness. These are not choices but severe consequences of such a system.

DISTRIBUTIVE JUSTICE

The ethics of **justice** relates to fair, equitable, and appropriate treatment in light of what is due or owed to persons (Beauchamp & Childress, 2001). As mentioned in Chapter 3, the relevant application of the ethical principle of justice within the health care system focuses on the fair distribution of goods and services. This application is called **distributive justice.** Beauchamp and Childress (2001) define distributive justice as fair, equitable, and appropriate distribution of diverse benefits and burdens such as property, resources, taxation, privileges, and opportunities. Because there is a scarcity of resources and competition for resources and services, it is impossible for all people to have everything they might want or need. It is important to remember that, in Canada, while health care is of paramount importance, other social programs such as welfare, education, and the public retirement income system are also important to maintain health and security of persons. Each time we claim that more funds must be provided for health care, we need to reflect upon the fact that necessarily means funds will be taken away from another type of social program. With the way that health care funds are provided by the federal government to the provinces and territories, each individual province or territory is responsible for deciding how resources should be divided between various social programs. Is education more important than health care? We know, for example, that literacy and education are determinants of health, and neglecting them will have negative effects on the health and well-being of citizens. We also know that if we neglect to provide adequate health care and disease prevention, children may be prevented from being able to go to school. Simply put, it is difficult to say that one kind of social program should be prioritized over another without devastating effects on groups of persons and individuals.

One of the primary purposes of government is to formulate and enforce policies that deal with distribution of scarce resources. To put it simply, distributive justice deals with how the "pie" of health care will be divided among many hungry persons. One can choose to divide the pie equally in similar-sized pieces or to give more to those who are younger, sicker, or more vulnerable. There is no easy solution nor is there a solution that will please everyone. Many people have divergent opinions on what constitutes "fair" distribution of a scarce resource like health care. Some say that funds should be focused on acute care while others claim that disease prevention must get more resources. Many argue that we should spend more money on children's care and cancer, while others say that more resources should be diverted to care of the elderly and frail persons. If we return to our analogy of a pie being divided up between a number of hungry persons, we can easily see how we might have markedly different approaches to dividing up the pie, depending on who is responsible for decision making. Some may feel that those who are most hungry should have the most, while others might feel that the children, by virtue of being at a stage of high growth and development, need the most pie. Others may choose to give everyone an equal piece simply to avoid making judgments about what attribute (hunger, age, health) is most important when rationing out pie, or, for that matter, health care resources. Daniels (1994, p. 27) states

> Rationing decisions, both at the micro and macro levels, share three key features. First, the goods we often must provide "legal services, health care, educational benefits" are not sufficiently divisible (unlike money) to avoid unequal or "lumpy" distributions. Meeting the educational, health care, or legal needs of some people, for example, will mean that the requirements of others will go unsatisfied. Second, when we ration, we deny benefits to some individuals who can plausibly claim they are owed them in principle; losers as well as winners have plausible claims to have their needs met. Third, the general

distributive principles appealed to by claimants as well as by rationers do not by themselves provide adequate reasons for choosing among claimants. They are too schematic; like my "fair equality of opportunity" account of just health care, they fail to yield specific solutions to these rationing problems. Solving these problems thus bridges the gap between principles of distributive justice and problems of institutional design.

Three areas of health care are relevant to questions of distributive justice: Which population groups should be the recipients of health care resources? What percentage of society's resources is it reasonable to spend on health care? Recognizing that health care resources are limited, which aspects of health care should receive the most resources? These are important questions, both practical and ethical in nature.

Many people may think, in Canada, everyone gets an "equal" share so why should we be concerned with how resources are allocated? However, history has demonstrated that, even in a system based on universality and reasonable access—two key principles of the *Canada Health Act* (1984)—there are still those who get more or less benefit from the health care system. People living in remote areas in the north, or rural areas, even in dense provinces such as Ontario or Quebec, have difficult accessing specialists and even family doctors for routine care. Those living in provinces such as Prince Edward Island have no access to a number of important specialties and are forced to travel long distances to access care that someone living in downtown Edmonton or Vancouver could access quite easily. Keep in mind, as well, that the *Canada Health Act* and the universal health care system covers only hospital and physician care. Allied health services, such as psychological services, occupational or physical therapy, vision care, prescriptions, and dental care are not covered by the *Canada Health Act* and are considered out-of-pocket expenses, unless you are fortunate enough to be covered for these kinds of health expenditures through your employer (or your spouse's or parents' employer). Many persons have jobs that do not provide benefits and therefore have difficulties paying for dental care, glasses, psychological treatment, or physiotherapy if they require it. These types of allied services are necessary for many people; however, the requirement to pay for these services means that often those who need them will be denied. Furthermore, some provinces still require a type of out-of-pocket payment, called a premium, on a monthly basis to subsidize health care. Alberta is one province that, up until 2009, still requires citizens to pay monthly premiums. In some areas in Canada, many persons live who do not have legal status, i.e., they have immigrated to Canada and have not been able to achieve legal status. In some urban areas, there are large numbers of persons without legal status and although they are living here in Canada, and many times have complex health needs related to difficult situations from which they have fled, they cannot access health care as our system is set up for Canadian citizens and not visitors or foreigners, without cost.

So, even in what many consider to be a "fair" and "equitable" system, there are still inequities and problems with how health care is distributed; it is necessary that we examine these inequities and problems through an ethical lens.

Entitlement

In deciding questions of distributive justice, we must ask, "Who is entitled to these services?" As with all of ethics, there is no universally accepted answer. Distribution of limited resources is the function of various levels of governing bodies. In attempting to distribute limited resources fairly, leaders will seek systematic means of deciding. Historically, these questions have been answered by such **material rules** as to each person an equal share, to each person according to need, to each person according to merit, to each person according to social contribution, to each according to the person's rights, to each person according to effort, to each person according to ability to pay, or to each person according to the greatest good to the greatest number. Most societies will utilize several of these principles in establishing public policies.

Ask Yourself

Is Health Care a Right or a Privilege?

- Discuss whether you think health care is a right or a privilege. Explain your thinking.

- Should all people have access to the same health care services? Should ability to pay ever influence access to health care services?

- If you believe health care is a right, to how much health care is each person entitled?

- What about the fact that many people are born into situations of destitution, war, and poverty and cannot afford or access quality health care? As citizens of a country with highly developed health care, what do we owe others?

- In Canada, some health care services are not universally covered, such as dental care and reproductive technologies like in vitro fertilization. Do you think that either of these two services should be covered by the health care system? If so, why? Did you feel that one should be covered and not the other? Again, ask yourself why.

- Cosmetic surgery procedures are, for the most part, not covered by our public health care system. However, some procedures that are cosmetic in nature, but done for reasons of repair after a trauma or accident, are covered by public insurance. Do you agree with this? Why or why not?

Right to Health Care.   In examining who should receive care, we ask questions about the basic right to health care. Is health care a right or a privilege? This is a question that is debated fiercely in the media, in the professional and political arenas, and around the dinner table. Is society responsible for providing health care for all citizens, and, if so, to what degree? Should each person be eligible for minimum basic health care, or should everyone be allowed to have everything there is to offer, from organ transplants to tummy tucks to in vitro fertilization, if they wish? Which is preferable—a strict free-market system that would provide health care services only to those who can pay, or a system responsible for the health care needs of all citizens? If health care is a right and health care resources are scarce, what resources should be allocated to which group of people? These and other questions fuel the debate about the right to health care even in Canada.

Discussion of health care as a right is not new. On December 10, 1948, the General Assembly of the United Nations adopted the Universal Declaration of Human Rights, which identifies medical care as a necessary social service ensuring the right to a standard of living adequate for health and well-being (Giesen, 1994).

The issue of health care as a right has some basis in constitutional law. In Canada, our most important Constitutional document is the *Charter of Rights and Freedoms*. While many Canadians consider health care to be a right, there is nothing in the *Charter* that describes such a right (Kirby, 2002, Volume 6, Chapter 5). As Kirby goes on to explain, the *Canada Health Act* notes that the goal of intact and strong Canadian health care policy is "to protect, promote and restore the physical and mental well-being of residents of Canada and to facilitate reasonable access to health services without financial or other barriers" (Kirby, 2002, Volume 6, Chapter Five, p. 100). While this language notes the importance of health care and access to care without the ability to pay being a factor, it does not confer a right to health care. Yet as Canadians, we use that language frequently to describe our feelings about health care and health policy. There is no legal document actually describing a right to health care in Canada. Although policies and government agencies exist to provide health care and ensure access to some health services, this does not mean health care should be a right, backed up by the legal or constitutional systems. However, that Kirby also notes some people who have been denied access to particular services or who have been forced to seek services in other jurisdictions as a result of local cuts or services not locally provided, have turned to the *Charter of Rights and Freedoms* to try to stake their claim to a right to health care.

? Think About It

A Constitutional Right to Health Care?

One commonly cited case in Canada is *Auton (Guardian ad litem of) v. British Columbia (Attorney General)*. In this case, Connor Auton, a preschooler diagnosed with autism spectrum disorder, was denied access to intensive behavioural intervention therapy (IBI) in his home province of British Columbia. Connor's parents, believing that they had a constitutional right to health care for Connor, which, they felt, should include IBI therapy, cited section 15(1) of the *Charter of Rights and Freedoms,* citing that failure to provide this therapy to their son violated this section of the *Charter,* which states that individuals should have equal treatment without being discriminated against for reasons of race, birthplace, skin colour, religion, gender, age or disability. As a person with a diagnosed disability, for which there was documented treatment along with

(Continued)

documentation demonstrating the importance of early preschool intervention, Connor, his parents claimed, was being discriminated against by not being able to access appropriate care that should have been made available to him. While the provincial courts concluded that Connor did have a right to IBI therapy and it should be provided, the Supreme Court of Canada overturned the decisions of the lower courts to conclude that there is no constitutional right to receive therapy for children such as Connor.

- When you read cases like this one, do you think that Canadians have a "right" to health care? If so, what does that mean to you?
- How far would you go to fight for access to health care services?
- Do you think that the lower or higher courts were right in this case? Why?

In the United States, the President's Commission for the study of Ethical Problems in Medicine and Biomedical and Behavioral Research reported that neither the Supreme Court nor any appellate court has found a constitutional right to health care, but many federal and state statutes have been interpreted to provide statutory rights in the form of entitlements to some vulnerable groups. As a consequence, these groups have benefited from many legal decisions. Bandman and Bandman (1978) argue that the common welfare clause of the *Constitution* implies the protection of basic needs, including a right to the protection of health.

Health care as a right is not a universal belief. There are those who believe that health care is a privilege to be enjoyed by some, but beyond the common advantage of all citizens. The entrepreneurial model of libertarianism declares that health care is not a right, but a commodity that must be purchased on the open market like any other service. This model compares the health care professional's right to conduct a practice and charge fees with other businesses's right to do likewise. It can be argued that this model provides health care only for those who can pay, or for those who are given health care services as a gift. It is hypothesized that, as a result of a free market system of health care delivery, supply-and-demand and pricing competition would result in lower health care costs. This in turn would result in health care services becoming more accessible to a larger portion of the population. Except for the fact that professionals can choose to provide services free of charge, this model makes little allowance for children and the very poor (Bandman & Bandman, 1978; Beauchamp & Childress, 2001). The working poor (i.e., those who have full-time jobs but may just barely be able to afford the necessities of living, remain in debt, and cannot see relief) make up a significant percentage of the population. For individuals and families like that, having to pay for health care would be devastating and unrealistic. In Canada today, families like this would, of course, have access to physician, hospital, and allied health care services, but may not be able to afford dental care or eye glasses. So inequities abound in all systems, even ones that "seem" to be more fair.

How Much and to Whom?   If one accepts that health care is a right or that society has an ethical obligation to provide health care services to vulnerable populations, then one is required to examine the question of how much health care is to be provided, and to whom. There are two broad views about the right to access to health care: some believe all should have equal access to health care, while others believe the right extends only to a decent minimum of health care with an understanding that priority setting may mean queues or marked differences in access to care. Consider the following case.

CASE PRESENTATION

Lucy is a twenty-three-year-old woman with a history of depression who has been hospitalized with episodes of severe depression, suicide attempts, and incidents of "cutting" herself. She had to drop out of university and spent a great deal of time in an inpatient unit getting treatment for her depressive episodes. She is now on antidepressants, feeling well, and able to live independently in the community. She would like to return to school to become a physiotherapist but is concerned about a number of significant scars on her arm from cutting herself. She is worried about the stigma of having them seen by her fellow students or friends and feels that she may not be able to cope with this. When she sees a plastic surgeon to have surgery to repair and cover the scars, she says, "I think I can finally move forward in my life, if only we can make these scars less visible."

Tenille is a thirty-five-year-old woman, who, along with her partner, Carlos, has been trying to conceive a child for a number of years. Tenille has had a barrage of tests that demonstrate she is capable of conceiving and Carlos also has had tests to confirm his fertility. Tenille and Carlos both work at a shipping factory, in the offices. While they make a good living, they cannot afford the costs of monthly in vitro fertilization, which, their doctor has told them, is their only chance to have a child.

George is 78 years old and a retired mechanic. He and his wife, Jacqui, have saved for many years in order to be able to retire somewhere warm and sunny. They spend ten months of the year in Florida, in Fort Lauderdale, where they purchased a small condominium. They return home to Canada for one month at Christmas, to see their children and grandchildren and one month in the summer, when it is too hot in Florida for Jacqui, who has asthma. They still maintain a small apartment in Winnipeg but only spend two months a year there. While they are in Florida, George sustains a heart attack. The cardiologist tells him that he has serious triple vessel disease and requires bypass surgery. George insists that the doctor make arrangements to fly him home to Winnipeg, where he can have his surgery and "be at home."

- Should all of these treatments and interventions be provided without charge to the individuals? Why or why not?

- Are these "medically necessary" treatments? If so, what makes a treatment "necessary," in your opinion?

- What would be your reasons for not covering any of the three treatments described above? How would you justify your decision?

Fair Distribution

Few people would argue that there are enough resources to pay for all services. Think about your household budget. If you have only $300 to spend on Christmas gifts for your three sisters and you also need to purchase groceries for the week and antibiotics for yourself, it would be foolish to spend $150 on one gift. By doing that, you would ensure that your sisters would not be treated equitably, that you probably would not be eating very well for the next week, and that you would not feel well anyway, since you could not afford your prescription medication. The same principle applies to health care dollars. The limited public budget must be divided among many interests. In order to maintain a functioning infrastructure, the government must ensure that public schools, highways, police, education, social assistance, and other services in the public domain have a proportionate share of the total budget. Policy makers are charged with the difficult task of making equitable decisions about distribution of resources. These decisions must balance health care spending with other programs, and must carefully avoid both extravagant excess spending and frugality that threaten the health of citizens.

Distribution of Resources

Limited health care dollars must be spent wisely. There are several different criteria that have been proposed to make distributive justice decisions. One method involves making judgments about cost in relation to predicted benefit. For example, we could question the practice of allowing patients in the last stages of terminal illness to monopolize limited and expensive intensive care beds, thus utilizing the most expensive kind of health care for the least benefit. Some propose that the best way to avoid making arbitrary decisions in these kinds of situations is to set mandatory guidelines. For example, some suggest that expensive therapies, such as dialysis or organ transplant, be reserved only for those below a certain age. A second method involves making judgments about the usefulness of given therapies. Immunizations, for example, are cost effective and benefit a large percentage of the population. Some would suggest that the most utile therapies (the ones that are less costly and nearly guaranteed to help a large number of people) are the ones that should have priority.

Theories of Justice

Distributive justice is based upon common morals and ethics. Several theories have been proposed to determine how resources and services should be distributed. Utilitarian, libertarian, communitarian, and egalitarian theories are examples of popular theories of justice. Because of society's fragmented beliefs about social justice, no single theory can be expected to bring coherence to the situation.

Recognizing that no single theory will satisfy society by fulfilling all principles, we suggest that several theories of justice be used to understand competing social goals.

Egalitarian Theories. **Egalitarian** theories are related to the concept of equality, in which people who are similarly situated should be treated similarly, though much depends on what kinds of similarity count as relevant and what constitutes similar treatment (Honderich, 1995). Promoting ideals of equal distribution of social benefits and burdens, egalitarian theories recognize the social obligation to eliminate or reduce barriers that prevent fair equality of opportunity. These theories are cautiously formulated to avoid requiring equal sharing of all possible social benefits. A leading proponent of egalitarianism, John Rawls suggests that in making decisions of justice, one should examine the situation behind a veil of ignorance. In this hypothetical situation, "no one knows his place in society, his class position or social status, nor does anyone know his fortune in the distribution of natural assets and abilities, his intelligence, strength, and the like" (1996, p. 567). This veil of ignorance ensures that no one is able to design principles to favour his or her particular condition. Supporters of Rawls's theory recognize a positive social obligation to eliminate or reduce barriers that prevent fair equality of opportunity, and suggest that health policy formulated according to egalitarian principles would guarantee a safety net or minimum floor below which citizens would not be allowed to fall (Beauchamp & Childress, 2001).

Utilitarian Theories. Based, in general, upon the rule that it is good to maximize the "greatest good for the greatest number," **utilitarian theories** favour social programs that protect public health and distribute basic health care equally to all citizens. This is based on the belief that the outcome of these programs maximizes utility. Although these theories are the basis of many social programs, there are problems in their application. For example, because utilitarianism places aggregate social good before individual rights, a utilitarian model may support maximizing utility while limiting resources directed toward some of society's sickest and most vulnerable populations (Beauchamp & Childress, 2001).

Libertarian Theories. **Libertarian theories** propose that the just society protects the rights of property and liberty of each person, allowing citizens to improve their circumstances by their own effort. Libertarian theories support a private citizen's or group's right to own and manage a health care business. Libertarian theory does not classify health care as a right, but rather as a commodity that operates on the material principle of ability to pay either directly or indirectly through insurance. Strict libertarians view taxation as an unjust redistribution of private property, but do not oppose other methods of distribution if they are freely chosen. Market strategies and managed competition are proposals in the United States that are influenced by libertarianism (Beauchamp & Childress, 2001).

Communitarian Theories. **Communitarian theories** place the community, rather than the individual, the state, the nation, or any other entity, at the centre of the value system. Less fully developed than utilitarianism or libertarianism, communitarianism emphasizes the value of public goods and maintains that values are rooted in communal practices. Communitarians believe that human life will go better if collective and public values guide peoples' lives. They have a commitment to facilities and practices designed to help members of the community develop their common goals and interests and hence their personal lives (Honderich, 1995). Modern communitarian writers disagree on the application of these theories to health care access. Some propose a federation of interlinking community health programs that are democratically administered by citizen-members. In this model, each individual program would determine which benefits to provide, which care is most important, and whether expensive services will be included or excluded. Another communitarian theory holds that community tradition includes commitments of equal access to health care, and suggests that as long as communal funds are spent, services must be equally available (Beauchamp & Childress, 2001).

Ask Yourself

Making Fair Decisions

- Which theory of distribution appeals to you as the most fair and equitable? Why?

- Do you think the theory you chose would be fair to all people in all circumstances? Discuss your thinking.

- Could you combine two or more theories to make a system that is fair and equitable?

RECENT TRENDS AND HEALTH ECONOMIC ISSUES

Questions of ethics and distributive justice began to be discussed well before the mid-1990s. Claims that Canada was experiencing a crisis in health care economics escalated in the last two decades with increasing demands for covered services and long waiting lists for procedures such as hip and knee replacements and cardiac surgery. Skyrocketing expenditures and a general tightening of health care dollars resulted in fiscal scarcity. The federal government has responded by attempting to gain control over expenditures. The tightening of health care budgets, while consistent in a number of sectors (public health, health prevention) is most noticeable in acute care. Sacrificing, in part, the traditional focus on the welfare of patients many hospitals, devised ways to cut costs, improve profits, and increase efficiency by contracting out services such as laundry, catering, and cleaning.

With excessive health care costs, long queues for care and demands by the public for more accountability and transparency in the 1980s, the broad concern that was the system, as it was, was unsustainable. While the system still costs less than other kinds of systems—such as an entrepreneurial model based in the private market, as exists in the United States—rising costs in a country like Canada, in which funds are shared between social programs, meant that there was also a significant threat to other public sectors that make up part of our social safety net, such as education, old age benefits, and welfare. The public felt at that time that there was not enough accountability on behalf of the government, that misspending or overspending might be occurring, and that there was not enough public consultation on how priorities in health care should be set.

In the early 1990s, the federal government reduced transfer payments to the provinces and territories in an attempt to control spending and reduce a large deficit. Over the next few years, these transfer payments for health care, education, and other social services, were further reduced. In turn, the provinces and territories were forced to cut spending in these sectors to accommodate the decreased federal funding. Sharp cutback strategies included hospital amalgamations, reductions in beds on units, pressure to reduce lengths of stay for patients, and longer waiting lists for nonurgent or nonemergent surgeries as well as a movement of care from the hospital to outside the hospital system, which is not covered by the *Canada Health Act* and therefore must be paid for by private insurance coverage or by individual patients. The system truly was in crisis. These cutbacks resulted in decreased satisfaction and worrying concerns on behalf of the public. With the public concerned by an aging population; the costs of increasing technologies; an evolving shortage of qualified health care providers, like family physicians and hospital-based nurses; and long waits and lack of access to care, it was clear that some kind of reform was needed.

Some of the broader problems in the system included things like fragmentation of care, lack of coordination of care, and episodic and illness-based care with a lack of focus on preventative care. All these problems, some of which persist today, result in higher costs and a system that is, therefore, difficult to sustain.

At the level of health policy at this time, there were three important issues in the area of reform. First, there was a feeling that there was an ongoing, growing political assault on the Canadian health care system. Noted erosion in other publicly held value-based programs, such as education, social programs, and care of the environment, meant that the perception, at a policy level, was that social programs reflective of Canadian values and beliefs were no longer a governmental priority. Second, with changing values, stronger trade relationships with the United States, and demands for choice, came the rise of a greater emphasis on providing health care through a "free market" approach; to provide people with choices if they want them, and possibly consider the creation of a two-tiered system. Alongside these kinds of pressures, the force of globalization added demands for greater harmonization between different, interacting markets. Much of the force of globalization is of course driven by the strongest players, so the call for harmonization was, and remains often, to adhere primarily to U.S. norms (Spalding, 2000). From a policy perspective the concern with how health care is provided is an important one, but the issues are greater than simply the "site" of care. The issues were, and continue to be, much larger. Concerns with efficiency are reflected in the broader discussion on the possibilities of a two-tiered system. Concerns over site of care (i.e., hospital versus the community), are in turn reflected in discussions about considerations of other types of health care systems and markets. Policy makers ask themselves serious and difficult questions about the implications of introducing other kinds of delivery methods in order to save the system money. Should we make health care an industry? Should we inject it with additional funds from the private sector? Should the patient now be a client or consumer of health care?

As a result of the pressures to reform the health care system, two important reform documents were produced in Canada. Both released in 2002, the *Romanow Report* and the *Kirby Report* called for significant changes in the way that health care is delivered in the county. Both are available on-line, in French and English.

Challenges to the Health Care System, According to the Romanow Commission Report

- An overall lack of accountability in the health care system
- Lack of transparency over spending, priority setting, decision making
- Lack of seamlessness between services, sectors, disciplines
- Increased pressure to privatize services
- Focus on illness-based, acute and episodic treatment
- Accessibility is not consistent as those in rural and remote areas have decreased access to services
- Resources are not being used optimally or appropriately
- *Canada Health Act,* while perhaps somewhat outdated and restrictive, has values that need to be reaffirmed but the act must also be modernized, reflecting current contexts (e.g., more appropriate definition for "medically necessary" health care in light of ongoing debates and divergent opinions on what this term means)
- Poor information dissemination and poor management of health information leading to lack of continuity of care
- More emphasis on primary health care/health promotion and shift away from hospital care and disease treatment
- Not enough focus on the long-term strategies for increasing sustainability of system and better health of all Canadians
- Waiting lists need to be better and more consistently managed
- Needs to be increased acknowledgment of diversity of needs across cultures, ages, areas, abilities, etc.
- National platform needed for home care
- Coverage of home care services through the *Canada Health Act*
- Need for improved and better covered community mental health care and palliative care services
- Need more integration between "pharmacare" (i.e., the provision of drugs) and medicare
- No national "drug agency" to oversee and monitor pharmaceutical activity/quality/delivery
- Poor Aboriginal health.
  (Romanow, 2002)

While it is clear that there are problems in our system, as with any high-cost, high-demand system, there are different kinds of problems in all sorts of health care systems. Evaluation and reform of health care systems is an ongoing activity, all over the world. If we look at the United States, for example, with each presidential election, candidates bring forth their ideas for new and innovative ways to provide health care. Often there is acknowledgment that a "Canadian-style" system may be a direction to aim toward; however, it would require significant overhauling of the managed-care system.

Interestingly, when we look at other systems of providing health care, we note that different kinds of inequities and challenges prevail. The American managed-care system is defined by Chang, Price, and Pfoutz as a "health care system willing to be held accountable both clinically and financially for the health outcomes of an enrolled population for a capitated (fixed) payment" (2001, p. 299). It is further described as an integrated form of health care delivery and financing that represents attempts to control costs by modifying the behaviour of providers and patients. Managed care moves away from a system focused on patient and provider autonomy and instead aims to focus on cost-based analysis of effectiveness of care and quality of priority setting and decision making. While there are many claims that managed care helps cut costs, in fact, it costs significantly more than the Canadian system, by virtue of skyrocketing administration costs. Compared to Canada, in which ~9 percent of our GDP is spent on health care, the American system costs ~14 percent of the GDP. Furthermore, administrative costs, as noted, are markedly lower—10 percent in Canada, compared to 24 percent in the United States (Spalding, 2000). Many Canadians view the American system as being one driven by the patients' ability to pay as opposed to the Canadian system, guaranteeing reasonable access to care, regardless of income or ability to pay.

Managed care has profound ethical implications. Based on the assumption that the basic ethical criterion for the planned organization of the system and allocation of resources in any health care setting at the policy level is the well-being of the group of individuals for whom the decisions are being made, balanced by the requirement of respect for individual needs, some scholars involved in bioethics at the Center for Practical Bioethics in Kansas City, Missouri, have commented on the relationship between this ethical criterion and a managed-care system.

The Center for Practical Bioethics has developed a list of considerations to be used by managed-care organizations for guidelines on how to ethically ration care:

1. Caring is an ethical imperative for health care providers because it is an essential benefit.

2. The first duty or obligation of any health care professional is to provide treatment that is clearly of benefit.

3. It is never ethically defensible to ration palliative care.

4. Futile treatment is of no benefit and should not be provided. However, care must be taken when defining a treatment as futile that the point of view of the patient is considered.

5. Treatment of marginal benefit needs to be carefully evaluated so that decisions are not inappropriately influenced by concerns such as subjective quality of life judgments of anyone other than the patient, cost constraints, or defensive medicine.

6. Individuals should make for others only those rationing decisions they are willing to impose upon themselves.

7. Populations that are especially needy or vulnerable should be given special consideration in order to be able to compete for the benefits society has to offer.

8. In rationing decisions, people ought not to be discriminated against without cause.

9. Lifestyle choice in and of itself is not a reason for denying care. However, it is ethically justifiable to provide positive incentives to support the development of healthy lifestyles. (Biblo et al., 1995, pp. 19–20)

CASE PRESENTATION

Challenges in Our Health Care System

Many rural hospitals have centralized services for dialysis, where patients from a large geographical area come to be dialyzed. As the patient population and the acuity changes, the nurses on these units have to set priorities as there are a limited number of dialysis machines and, therefore, a finite number of dialysis spots each week.

In this case, the weekly schedule for this particular dialysis unit at a rural hospital is very full and the nurse manager has to make some difficult decisions about how dialysis can be provided to a larger number of patients than there are available spots. So he decides that the unit will make some patients wait until they are demonstrating signs of fluid overload (i.e., difficulty breathing) to be dialyzed.

Mr. M is a dialysis patient who has been on the unit for a number of years. He is a retired principal of a local high school and many of the nurses know him well. Mr. M has a history of not managing his disease well and, despite getting lots of good advice from the nurses, has been quite negligent at managing aspects of his own health. He has been bumped off of the dialysis schedule this week to make room for a very ill young woman, Miss S, who has just arrived in Canada from Ghana, where she was unable to access adequate medical care for her congenital kidney disease, which has worsened suddenly. She is not a Canadian citizen, and is now staying in the county with refugee status, with her sister, to access dialysis. She has a young son at home being cared for by her aunt, and she is a single mother. She is quiet and scared when she comes to the unit with her sister.

Some of the nurses on the unit go for their coffee break and they discuss that they are upset that Mr. M, a likeable and familiar patient, will have to wait to be dialyzed. He has required more frequent dialysis lately and they know that he will be uncomfortable and in some degree of distress at home while he waits. One nurse says, "He's been paying taxes all his life! Why should he wait?" Another nurse adds, "But he's contributed to his disease. Hers isn't her fault!" Everyone seems to have a different opinion about who should have been a priority for dialysis.

Think About It

- Do you think that the right decision was made to make Mr. M wait for dialysis to make room for the acutely ill Miss S? Why or why not?

- If paying taxes is a justification for receiving better health care, then what about children? Should we deny them care because they haven't yet paid taxes?

- One nurse states that Mr. M has contributed a great deal to the local community whereas Miss. S has not. Do you think that this should be a consideration in deciding who gets dialyzed first?

- What criteria would you use if you were the nurse manager and had to make this difficult decision?

SUMMARY

Because health care is a scarce resource, citizens rely upon social institutions to make fair and equitable distributive justice decisions. There is little consensus on basic ethical questions such as How should people receive health care resources? Is there a right to basic health care? How much should be spent on particular health care services? What percentage of the society's overall resources should be invested in health care? Egalitarianism, utilitarianism, libertarianism, and communitarianism are theories that attempt to describe fair means of distributing resources. Recent focus on problems related to the sustainability of Canada's health care delivery system has prompted debate on practical issues of distributive justice and accountability. In any health care system, when setting priorities or making decisions around reform, close attention must be paid to overarching values and ethical standards in health care.

CHAPTER HIGHLIGHTS

- The history of economic thought is closely associated with the utilitarian movement in the last century.

- The traditional health care system in Canada is a public insurance model.

- Justice relates to fair, equitable, and appropriate treatment in light of what is due or owed to persons, and recognizes that giving to some will deny receipt to others who might otherwise have received these things.

- Distributive justice is the fair, equitable, and appropriate distribution of benefits and burdens. Theories of distributive justice seek to render diverse principles coherent.

- Egalitarian theories are related to the concept of equality in which people who are similarly situated should be treated similarly.

- Utilitarian theories are based upon the rule that it is good to maximize the greatest good for the greatest number.

- Libertarian theories propose that the just society protects the rights of property and liberty of each person, allowing citizens to improve their circumstances by their own effort.

- Communitarian theories place the community, rather than the individual, the state, the nation, or any other entity, at the centre of the value system.

- Scarcity of health care resources has led to a rethinking of the structure of health care economics.

- Managed care gives rise to ethical problems associated with balancing utilitarian views of cost-effective care with a respect for persons and the traditional view of a duty to care.

- Health care evaluation and reform is an ongoing activity in Canada, in order to ensure high quality and ethical care.

DISCUSSION QUESTIONS AND ACTIVITIES

1. Discuss current problems in health care economics with classmates. Is there a consensus regarding root causes, right to health care, or the role of the government as a payer for health care services?

2. Go to the library and find a basic economics text. How does the health care system differ from other free-market systems? Should it? Why or why not?

3. Discuss the influence of utilitarian theory on the economics of the current health care system.

4. How do patient and provider autonomy affect health care delivery and financing?

5. Define distributive justice. In class, discuss the material rules of distributive justice. Which material rule is most popular among classmates?

6. What method of distributing goods and services do you think is fair and equitable? Do your classmates agree with your theories?

REFERENCES

Bandman, E. L., & Bandman, B. (1978). *Bioethics and human rights: A reader for health professionals*. Boston: Little, Brown.

Beauchamp, T., & Childress, J. (2001). *Principles of biomedical ethics* (4th ed.). New York: Oxford University Press.

Biblo, J. C., Christopher, L. J., Johnson, L., & Potter, R. L. (1995). *Ethical issues in managed care: Guidelines for clinicians and recommendations to accrediting organizations*. Kansas City, MO: Bioethics Development Group.

Chang, C. F., Price, S. A., & Pfoutz, S. K. (2001). *Economics and nursing: Critical professional issues*. Philadelphia: Davis.

Daniels, N. (1994). Four unsolved rationing problems: A challenge. *Hastings Center Report, 24*(4), 27–9.

deBlois, J., Norris, P., & O'Rourke, K. (1994, Autumn). *A primer for health care ethics: Essays for a pluralistic society,* pp. 5–6. Washington, DC: Georgetown University Press.

Giesen, D. (1994). A right to health care?: A comparative perspective. *Health Matrix, 4*(2), 277–295.

Honderich, T., ed. (1995). *The Oxford companion to philosophy.* New York: Oxford University Press.

Kirby, M. J. L. (2002). The health of Canadians: The federal role. *Final Report.*

Morreim, E. H. (1995). *Balancing act: The new medical ethics of medicine's new economics.* Washington, DC: Georgetown University Press.

Rawls, J. (1996). A theory of justice. In J. Feinberg, ed., *Reason and responsibility: Some readings in basic problems of philosophy* (pp. 567–572). Belmont, CA: Wadsworth. (Reprinted from J. Rawls, *A theory of justice,* 1971, Cambridge, MA: Harvard University Press)

Romanow, R. (Commissioner). (2002). *Building on values: The future of health care in Canada.* Ottawa: Romanow Health Care Commission.

Spalding, K. (2000). Introduction to politics and health policy. Lecture in course entitled "Nursing and the health care system: Policy ethics and politics." Faculty of Nursing, University of Toronto.

CHAPTER 16

Social Issues

By Mary Jo Butler

OBJECTIVES

After completing this chapter, the reader should be able to:

1. Explain how social conditions such as poverty, homelessness, intimate-partner violence, an increasing elder population, and racism affect health.
2. Apply the concept of justice to vulnerable populations, elaborating on the implications for society and the health care system.
3. Discuss the application of beneficence and nonmaleficence to vulnerable groups in light of today's health care system.
4. Identify the pros and cons of promoting autonomy for health care decision making among vulnerable populations.

5. Analyze evidence of victim blaming within the health care system.

6. Illusrate application of the concepts of advocacy and nonviolence to care of vulnerable populations.

7. Examine current research for application to culturally diverse groups.

INTRODUCTION

Health is unquestionably a product of the person and environment interchange. Thus, social conditions that alter the person and environment interchange process are critical concerns for nurses and nursing students. Nurses confront social issues that shape the health and health care management of individuals on a daily basis. These social issues may create conflicts in values and ethical dilemmas that must be addressed in order to determine appropriate health care interventions for involved individuals. The purpose of this chapter is to help clarify the principles inherent in decision making when social issues create ethical dilemmas for the nurse.

SOCIAL ISSUES

Many pervasive social issues are of special concern to health care providers today. Poverty, homelessness, intimate-partner violence, an increasing elder population, and racism are examples of some of these very important concerns. Each of these issues is reviewed briefly in this chapter, along with the dominant guiding principles for related ethical decision making.

Poverty

Poverty and homelessness continue to be prevalent in North America, and in Canada specifically.

Poverty, growing worldwide, is known to have a negative impact on both the health of individuals and the receipt of health care services (Catley, 1992). Poorer people are often sicker than people with adequate financial resources. While poverty is detrimental to the health of all individuals living with inadequate resources, it produces a next generation of citizens with more health problems than usual. Poverty can affect health in many ways, not just physically. Psychological effects of poverty include helplessness and lack of control over one's daily life, both of which are strongly correlated with poor health outcomes (Wallerstein, 1992). Children living in poverty have a higher incidence of conditions associated with trauma, drugs, burns, mental illness, and HIV infection (Wessell, 1992). Children living in poverty are more likely to experience poor nutrition, inadequate exercise, and diseases from environmental factors such as vermin or lead. They are also more likely to sustain physical injuries, be harmed in a fire, on be victims of homicide, compared to children not living in poverty (CICH, 2001). They are more likely to grow up with chronic illnesses that require extensive health care resources. In Canada, the rate of children living in poverty is increasing

(14 percent of children live in after-taxes poverty) (Canadian Institute of Child Health, 2000). While the rate is lower than in the United States (22 percent), it is still higher in countries such as France (seven percent), Sweden (three percent) and the United Kingdom (ten percent). It is estimated that in 1996, one in four children lived in poverty in Canada. Children of lone-mother families, Aboriginal children, and children from visible minorities are all at a significantly higher risk for living in poverty, according to the most recent *Health of Canada's Children*. According to CICH, "Children who live in poverty encounter more hurdles to healthy development and are, consequently, at an elevated risk for a wide range of negative health outcomes" (Canadian Institute of Child Health, 2001b, p. 2).

In a discussion on poverty in Canada, Raphael notes that while there are many discourses about poverty, or ways to think about the notion of poverty, many of these discussions are at the level of the individual living in poverty (2001). While he acknowledges that in fact, poverty does have a marked effect on the health and well-being of individuals, he instead suggests that we think about the kinds of community, social, economic, and environmental structures that can "support or limit the health status of those living in poverty." (p. 224).

According to Raphael (2001), there are three main reasons Canadians should be concerned with economic inequality and poverty: (1) It contravenes international notions of basic human rights; (2) it may also strain the health care system and social safety net of the country through the increased health care needs and problems of those living in poverty; and (3) the connection between the degree of economic inequality and both higher mortality rates (at all ages) and lower life expectancy is clear, thus posing a threat to all Canadians living in situations of economic disadvantage.

CASE PRESENTATION

Socioeconomic Influences on Health

Martha D is a sixty-nine-year-old woman who lives in a substandard third-floor walk-up, cold-water apartment in a housing project with a high crime rate. She draws a small monthly welfare cheque that does not cover living expenses. Her income is supplemented by housing assistance, and by working as a nanny for three small children for twenty hours a week. Ms. D earns minimum wage for her job as a nanny, and accepts cash for her work to avoid any interference with her welfare cheque. She uses public transportation to go to and from her job, spending $5.00 each working day on bus fare.

Martha helps her alcoholic single daughter, age forty-seven, with two teenage children, especially when her daughter is experiencing a drinking binge. The children frequently stay with Martha and rely on her for food, shelter, and love. Martha's husband is an alcoholic and has not been home for two years; however, he does occasionally call from a homeless shelter or treatment facility. Neither her daughter nor her husband contribute to household expenses, but Martha remains devoted to her family, especially her two grandchildren.

Martha D is 5'8" tall and weighs 285 pounds. She has hypertension, with her blood pressure ranging from 200/90 to 250/110. She is on medication for her blood pressure, and the physician has linked her with a home health nurse to encourage a diet and simple exercise regime for her obesity and hypertension. Ms. D is beginning to show signs of Type II diabetes and has been encouraged to lose weight and adhere to a diabetic diet. In addition, Ms. D has some small ulcerations on her left ankle.

The home health nurse visits Ms. D and instructs her in the care of her ulcers, advising her to keep her left foot elevated as much as possible. The nurse spends considerable time explaining a 1200-calorie diabetic diet with moderate sodium restriction to Ms. D, and talks with Ms. D about the need to begin walking as soon as the ulcers on her foot heal. Ms. D lets the nurse know she used to attend a weight control group and understands low-fat and diabetic diets. However, she says coming home to her usual dinner of high-fat, prepared foods is her only daily pleasure. "I've lived sixty-nine years on this diet, don't wish to change, and have nothing to lose if I remain on it the rest of my life." She also points out that it is not safe to walk in her neighbourhood, so she stays inside. In addition, she indicates that she is too tired to exercise after working all day.

? Think About It

Who Decides What Is Best for a Patient?

- Consider Ms. D's decision to ignore recommendations regarding diet, exercise, and, perhaps, care of her ankle ulcerations in relation to autonomy, beneficence, and nonmaleficence.

- What two principles are "at odds" here?

- Since the principle of beneficence requires actively doing good for Ms. D, who decides what is good?

- How would the home care nurse decide how to best help Martha?

Homelessness

Homelessness is a difficult social phenomenon to capture, characterize, or assume we can understand. There are many assumptions about persons who are homeless—that they all have issues with drug addictions or that they are persons who chose to reject other lifestyles. Many of these assumptions are simply not true and instead represent a lack of insight into the increasing phenomenon of homelessness in Canada. While acknowledging the difficulty in capturing an accurate number of homeless persons, Murphy (2000) estimated that, in 2000, there were between 15 000 and 20 000 homeless persons in urban centres across Canada. This number is increasing and today, the numbers of homeless persons in Canada may be closer to ten times Murphy's original estimate. Additionally, Murphy notes that while these numbers represent those who do not have a permanent address, there are many more people living in what most of us would classify as barely acceptable housing with substandard amenities, poor construction, health hazards, and hygiene risks. The numbers of those living in inadequate housing is even more difficult to capture accurately than perhaps the numbers of homeless persons.

There are many complex causes of homelessness and to characterize all those living on the street or in shelters as having similar issues and personal histories would be markedly inaccurate. Men, women, children, and families are affected by homelessness, and causes are the result of multiple factors. Some hypotheses for the increasing rates of homelessness in urban centres across Canada include the lack of affordable housing for those living on lower incomes, the gentrification of downtown areas with the resultant displacement of persons living in poverty, and the trend toward community living and the de-institutionalization of those with mental illnesses.

Like those living in poverty, homeless people suffer from acute and chronic health problems. Burg (1994) categorizes their health problems as those resulting from limited access to care, those coincident with homelessness, and those associated with the psychosocial burden of homelessness. Health problems resulting from limited access to care include exacerbated or advanced conditions that would have responded to early and thorough intervention. Health problems coincident with homelessness include illnesses resulting from living with inadequate nutrition, warmth, hygiene, safety, and other basic needs. Health problems associated with the psychosocial burden of homelessness are primarily mental illnesses, suicide, assault, and substance abuse, which can dull the anxiety of homelessness.

Mondragon (1993) describes the pervasive assumptions that undergird some models of health promotion. These assumptions view health as the absence of disease and associate common diseases with controllable risk factors. Thus, the key to improved health is deemed to be the provision of knowledge and skills to individuals. It is assumed that people will use self-determination, individualism, and responsibility to secure adequate housing, employment, and proper nutrition. While this model may benefit people with good education, a continuum of options, and resources to elicit change, it is less relevant to those with limited choices by virtue of their socio-economic status.

CASE PRESENTATION

Few Choices

Diane is a forty-two-year-old woman with a history of mental illness, asthma, and former drug dependency who has been living, sporadically, for the past three years, on the streets. She occasionally has been admitted for acute exacerbations of her illnesses and for problems with her medications. For the most part, however, she is able to survive and look after herself with the resources available to her, including street health nurses, shelters, and soup kitchens. She is able to work occasionally cleaning a local church and is paid in cash, which she carefully carries with her and spends judiciously.

Christopher is her primary outreach nurse from the local clinic. He meets with Diane, usually in a local coffee shop, once weekly. This week, when they meet, it is apparent that Diane is upset. She tells Christopher that the women's shelter has closed temporarily and the women who depend on this shelter are now sleeping in the men's shelter down the street. She tells Christopher that "the neighbourhood is changing" and she doesn't feel safe any longer. Christopher knows that there have been issues with violence in the men's shelter and the supervision is less than ideal. However, it is now November and the weather has become cold and rainy.

Diane tells Christopher that she feels she cannot sleep in the men's shelter. She was a victim of intimate-partner violence a number of years ago and cannot expose herself to that risk again. She informs Christopher that she will sleep in the park across town because she feels safer and knows of hidden spots in which she can make a place to sleep. She tells Christopher that she has a male friend who has told her he will be with her at night to help and protect her. Christopher knows that Diane's friend is a drug dealer with a history of violence and feels that will put Diane at risk for returning to taking street drugs. Additionally, sleeping in the park across town means that she cannot meet Christopher regularly anymore as it will be difficult for her to get to the park and back again for their weekly meetings.

Christopher asks Diane to reconsider. Given the challenges of managing her medications, her risk for entering into drug use again, the obvious health and personal safety risks of sleeping in the park, and the loss of the regular contact with her primary nurse, Diane's plan hardly seems like a good idea, and Christopher tells her so. He tells her that he is concerned about her and that he feels she would be exposing herself to a number of serious risks with her plan. He also tells her that he is worried that her male friend is coercing her into moving across town. Christopher tells Diane that he would be willing to speak and work with the shelter managers to make sure that improved safety measures are taken, especially with the influx of women clients.

Diane listens to Christopher but insists that this is the plan she must follow, despite the risks.

Think About It

- How would a deontologist analyze this case and reflect on what action, if any, Christopher should take?
- How should we decide what is in Diane's best interests?
- Given that Christopher feels Diane is not making rational or sensible choices, what might he do, if anything? What would he be justified in doing? What would be ethically problematic and why?
- Would restricting Diane's autonomy, at this time, be either reasonable or in her best interests?

Intimate-Partner Violence

A third common social condition affecting health and health care delivery is intimate-partner violence, the most common but least reported crime in North America. Estimated numbers of abused women range from two to twelve million per year. Intimate-partner violence flows from a historical position of sexism. Eisler (1987) describes how select tenets of Judaism, Christianity, and Islam support patriarchy, the inferiority of women, and women as the property of men. In the United States it was legal for a husband to beat his wife to maintain his authority until 1899 (Diehm & Ross, 1988). Remnants of these beliefs are still threaded through society, affecting the way families socialize their children and the way communities tolerate gender inequity. Butler and Weatherley (1992) and Roberts (2000) indicate that women have long been defined by the mothering role and dependence on men in North American society. While these role definitions are changing, events in society continue to perpetuate gender inequity. As long as gender inequity exists, intimate-partner violence will remain a social problem.

Women are not the only victims of intimate-partner violence. Men can also be victims of violence in their homes; however, women remain at greater risk, almost three times more at risk than men for being victimized, sexually assaulted, or killed by an intimate partner. Fewer than one-third of all victims of intimate-partner violence ever report their problem or seek help. This may be due to any number of reasons, including embarrassment, fear for their own safety or the safety of children involved, or a suspicion that the judicial system will not be able to protect them from violence.

The vast majority of abused women eventually leave their abusive partners. However, leaving is a process that takes time, energy, and resources. Many abused women will leave and return to their abusive partners several times before permanently terminating the relationship. Esposito (1993) attributes this to the inability to find housing or suitable jobs; the fear, loneliness, or poverty that results from being out on their own; concern for children who are experiencing relocation and other difficulties; relentless pressure from family and friends to try harder to make the relationship work; or poor support from the criminal justice system. It is sometimes easier to return to a familiar though unpleasant situation than to start over and deal with numerous unknowns.

Since sex is the risk factor, intimate-partner violence affects women of all socio-economic, racial, and ethnic groups (Esposito, 1993; Ewing, 1987; MMWR, 2000). Many women living in violent relationships will experience poorer health. Women living in abusive situations experience acute traumatic injuries and chronic physical and emotional problems (Butler & Weatherley, 1992; Kernic, Wolf, & Holt, 2000). They are especially vulnerable to battery during pregnancy and at a higher risk than nonbattered women for poor pregnancy outcomes (Bohn, 1990). The health care system may add insult to abused womens' injuries. The women often feel humiliated by and blamed for the abuse by a health care system that minimizes the abuse, makes insufficient referrals, and fails to acknowledge abuse as the culprit (Campbell, Pliska, Taylor, & Sheridan, 1994). As a result, women leave health care settings without having the intimate-partner violence addressed, remaining isolated and uninformed about their options (Fishwick, 1995).

CASE PRESENTATION

Suspicions of Abuse

Maria P is a twenty-five-year-old woman who made an initial visit to the clinic for prenatal care when she was eighteen weeks pregnant. She has returned for a second prenatal visit at twenty-two weeks gestation. Maria has a four-year-old son and a two-year-old daughter. Her record indicates she had several bruises, lacerations, and a black eye during her last pregnancy that she attributed to clumsiness. Her two-year-old weighed four pounds, eight ounces at birth and was seventeen inches long.

As part of routine prenatal care for the most recent pregnancy, Maria was tested for HIV antibodies. The test was positive, and the physician and nurse conveyed this information to Maria during her second prenatal visit. Maria, of course, was upset. She admitted that her spouse has been physically abusing her for some time and that both have used intravenous drugs in the past. She has had no sexual partners other than her spouse.

The nurse encourages Maria to tell her spouse that she is HIV positive so that he can be tested for antibodies. She also encourages use of condoms during sexual intercourse to help avoid transmission to her spouse should he not be infected. Maria insists that her husband refuses to use condoms as they interfere with his pleasure. In addition, she says he would "kill" her if he knew she was HIV positive.

The nurse encourages Maria to go to a shelter for abused women and links her to both a counsellor and a social worker who help her devise a safety plan. However, Maria ultimately decides to go home because she cannot abandon her children, and she does not want them in a shelter. She knows she cannot make it on her own, as she has neither income nor job skills. She requests that the clinic not interfere and that they allow her to decide if, when, and how she will notify her spouse about her HIV status.

Think About It

When Patient Choices Place Them at Risk for Harm

- Consider the principle of autonomy when determining the appropriate decision in this situation. Remember that confidentiality is an inherent part of autonomy.

- What do you think is in Maria's best interest, at this point? How best can the clinic nurse support her?

- If it is revealed that Maria's children have witnessed her being abused by her spouse, is this a situation which a registered nurse is mandated to report?

- Can the nurse force Maria to seek help or go to a shelter? If not, how can she best support Maria and help to ensure her safety?

Increasing Elder Population

In addition to poverty, homelessness, and intimate-partner violence, the elderly are a growing population worldwide (Catley, 1992). In Canada, our elderly population is rapidly growing, as baby boomers age. People are living longer due to healthier diets, vaccines, and improvements in the environment (Windom, 1988). Certainly, advances in health care knowledge have contributed to greater longevity. However, many elderly, especially from minority populations, live without pensions and on incomes below the poverty level (Hall, 1993). The elderly have much higher rates of poverty; notably, those who are elderly and living alone, unattached to families, have a significantly higher rate of poverty than any other age group. Data gathered from 1994 to 1996 demonstrate a poverty rate of 47.9 percent for elderly persons living alone with no connection to family compared to the already significant rate of poverty of seven percent for those elderly persons living with someone else (Canadian Council on Social Development, 1996). Vast numbers of the elderly are socially isolated, in need of work to survive, and susceptible to economic hardship. Chronic illnesses; pain, especially from arthritic processes; frailties; and disabilities may occur with increasing frequency as people age (Tebb, 1995). Health problems contribute significantly to the social isolation and financial burden that may accompany aging.

The assumption in current prevailing health care models is that the frail elderly will be cared for at home by friends and family to alleviate strain on the health care system. In reality, family members may be unable to provide needed support due to geographical distance from the frail elderly family member or personal responsibilities. Skaff and Pearlin (1992) describe how caregivers of the elderly experience emotional and financial strain. The caregivers often have to help with finances of the elderly, since their fixed incomes cannot cover the basic cost of living as well as health care expenses. Reliance on friends and family for health care of the frail elderly is especially problematic for the elderly without the necessary social or financial resources. The shift to caring in the home and the emphasis away from institutionalized care has two distinct effects. While many elderly persons would prefer to live in their own home, they may require either intensive or specialized care, if they are frail or ill. Lay family members may not be able to provide the level or intensity of care required. More emphasis and resources need to be directed toward strengthening and supporting home care initiatives (Romanow, 2002).

CASE PRESENTATION

Aging, Poverty, and Illness

Mr. Chang is a sixty-five-year-old widower with chronic kidney disease. He is supposed to receive dialysis three times a week but frequently misses his appointments due to no transportation or not feeling well. His only hope for a cure is a kidney transplant, which Mr. Chang really wants. Mr. Chang is very frail with many health problems. He lives alone in a small garage apartment. The landlord is threatening to evict Mr. Chang because he is behind in his rent payments. Mr. Chang lives on a small pension. As Mr. Chang lives in Ontario, most of his prescription costs are covered by the Ontario Drug Benefit Program. However, some costs and health products are not and Mr. Chang has to pay for these expenses out of his pensions.

A home health nurse used to transport Mr. Chang to dialysis occasionally, as Mr. Chang lives outside the city limits and is unable to access public transportation services. The nurse also helps Mr. Chang with his ADLS and showers. Additionally she provides strong support to him and assists him with his medications. Finally she has helped advocate for Mr. Chang with his landlord. The clinic does not believe Mr. Chang is a candidate for a transplant, due to his fraility. Due to cuts in home care, the nurse is no longer able to visit Mr. Chang unless he has a specific need such as a dressing change or intravenous medication. Therefore, she can no longer visit Mr. Chang nor transport him to dialysis. No volunteer organizations for transport to hospital exist in Mr. Chang's area.

? Think About It

What Health Care Should Society Provide for Its Citizens?

- Consider the principle of justice in deciding if health care is a right or a privilege. If health care must be rationed, who decides what services an individual will receive?
- Should we, as a Canadian society, be willing to provide health care for all?
- Is there a level of care that society should provide to all citizens? Explain.
- What is fair for Mr. Chang?

Racism

Racism is another social concern that affects health. The term "race" generally refers to an attribute that allows classifications of human beings on the basis of certain biological characteristics (Melville, 1988). Although no racial group of people ascribes to the same cultural beliefs and practices, it is often race that stereotypes a group of people or engenders ethnocentric beliefs and moral conflicts in values. Brown (1991) believes racism is an ethical problem based on inadequate respect, violation of personal boundaries, and an imbalance of power.

Racism exists today despite strong legal frameworks, policies, and laws opposing racism and racially based discrimination in Canada and in countries around the world (Minister of Public Works and Government Services, Canada, 2005). The International Convention on the Elimination of All Forms of Racial Discrimination, ratified by Canada in 1970, calls upon governments to eliminate racial discrimination and ensure equality for all in terms of human rights and freedoms. The *Canadian Charter of Rights and Freedoms* outlines the fundamental rights of all those living in Canada and it is entrenched within the constitution. Specifically, Section 15(1) states "every individual is equal before and under the law and has the right to equal protection and equal benefit of the law without discrimination" (1982). Furthermore, Section 35 confirms the historical and treaty rights of Aboriginal persons. Other relevant legislation includes the *Canadian Human Rights Act;* the *Canadian Bill of Rights;* the *Employment Equity Act;* the *Official Languages Act;* the *Canadian Multiculturalism Act;* the *Immigration and Refugee Protection Act;* and the *Citizenship Act.* A link to each of these is provided at the end of this chapter.

Racism in Canada persists. In a 2003 Ipsos-Reid survey sponsored by the Centre for Research and Canada and *The Globe and Mail,* over 70 percent of respondents felt that racism persists in Canada. In other research, almost forty percent of visible minorities reported that they felt they had been discriminated against because of ethnicity or culture. This includes 50 percent of blacks and over 30 percent of South Asian and Chinese persons (Statistics Canada, 2002). Almost half of all Aboriginal persons not living on reserves reported being a victim of racial discrimination in a 2003 report (Minister of Public Works and Government Services, Canada, 2005). Furthermore, in a separate survey one year earlier, more than half of all the Canadians surveyed felt that racism separates Aboriginal persons from the rest of Canadian society (Minister of Public Works and Government Services, Canada, 2005). The reality is that the stereotypical "face" of Canada has changed and nearly half of all Canadians are from an ethnic origin other than British, French, or native-born Canadian. We are a multicultural society and enjoy the advantages of this. However, not all persons are able to enjoy the advantages of a rich multicultural society, experiencing racial and ethnic discrimination in various contexts and situations in their daily lives.

Poverty and racial discrimination can be linked by virtue of barriers to opportunities and advantages. The 2001 Census report notes that over 20 percent of all immigrant families in Canadian cities are low-income families. The rate for non-immigrant families in the same geographic areas is almost ten percent lower (Census of Canada, 2001).

There is significant interface of poverty, homelessness, intimate-partner violence, an increasing elderly population, and racism. Poverty underpins homelessness. Women experiencing intimate-partner violence move frequently and often deal with homelessness and poverty as they try to improve their situations (Kanna, Singh, Nemil, & Best, 1992). Goodman (1991) provides data that poverty and homelessness are linked to a high abuse rate, and Campbell (1993) in one US-based study, indicates that violence and poverty are linked, at least among African Americans. The elderly are often made homeless as they face mounting health care and medication costs and living costs on a fixed income. Persons experiencing poverty, homelessness, aging, intimate-partner violence, and racism are vulnerable to poor health and inadequate health care delivery. Often these vulnerable groups are the least powerful and vocal persons in society, yet they are the groups most affected by ethical decisions regarding health and health care (Wessell, 1992).

These social situations represent examples of classism, sexism, and racism. Each indicates prejudice or discrimination against a particular class, gender, or racial group. The implication is that one group of people is held to standards espoused by another group. Statistical data on these social situations, and the health of persons experiencing the social situations, explain why a feeling of helplessness may emerge when social situations are so intrinsically intertwined with health. Yet treating a person's symptoms without attending to the root causes of the problem may be viewed as inadequate health care.

ETHICAL PRINCIPLES APPLIED TO SOCIAL ISSUES

The common principles most essential in unravelling ethical dilemmas encompassing social issues include justice, nonmaleficence, beneficence, and autonomy. A brief discussion of each principle follows.

Justice

Justice is the duty to treat all people fairly without regard to age, socioeconomic status, race, or gender. This implies a fair distribution of the benefits and burdens among members of a society, with equal treatment to all or to those most in need. A frail elderly man, beloved by his family, might receive an expensive but desired transplant procedure based on justice, even though there is only a moderate chance that the extensive surgery will prolong life or improve the quality of life.

Ask Yourself

Who Should Receive Limited Health Care Resources?

- In this day of declining health care resources, should those with the greatest need or those who have contributed to society receive expensive restorative procedures? Or should these procedures be available to all? Support your position.
- When thinking about this question, also consider how you think all health care resources should be allocated, if not by need?

Nonmaleficence

Nonmaleficence is the duty to prevent or avoid doing harm, whether intentional or unintentional. This could mean ensuring a seriously ill research participant has full information on the risks of entering a clinical trial. It might also entail ensuring a safe, hygienic environment before hospital release of a newborn infant and mother suffering from poverty or homelessness.

Beneficence

Beneficence is the duty to actively do good for patients. It requires a careful consideration of the best interest of others and the ability to see issues and challenges from the perspective of another. Thus, the homeless woman with leg ulcers and diabetes who walks all day and stands in lines in poor shoes and in all types of weather to secure free meals and safe sleeping quarters will receive treatment for the leg ulcers that will ensure adequate diet and rest, elevation of the legs, and proper hygiene. Treatment would have to go beyond the usual prescriptions for drugs and address the social conditions contributing to the physical problems.

Autonomy

Autonomy is the patient's right to self-determination without outside control. Related to this principle are the principles of veracity, privacy, confidentiality, and respect for all persons. Little (2000) reminds us that we must develop our sense of autonomy. She suggests that autonomy involves a set of skills that people possess to greater or lesser degrees. These skills often require someone to help us cultivate them, a context that sustains them, and help in exercising them when we are in a vulnerable position. One of the skills is the capacity to think through different options and imagine possibilities. Our social context, however, can get in the way of seeing our options. Autonomy would direct us to work with an abused woman to develop a stronger sense of herself and to help her to see various options and available support. Autonomy would also honour her choice to return home, even if her safety is a concern, continuing to offer support as she struggles with difficult decisions. We must always consider how factors, such as the chronic stress of living with abuse, affect a person's ability to act autonomously (Limandri & Tilden, 1993).

? **Think About It**

The Impact of Social Conditions on Vulnerable Groups

Consider how social conditions affect other vulnerable groups such as children, people with mental health challenges or physical disabilities, and people who are institutionalized or incarcerated.

- Discuss the factors that make these populations vulnerable.
- Describe the issues related to these populations that give you concern as a nurse.
- Discuss the ethical concerns related to the needs and care of people in these groups.
- How would you apply principles of justice, nonmaleficence, beneficence, and autonomy to health care concerns with people in each of these groups?

PERSONAL IMPEDIMENTS TO INTERVENING WITH VULNERABLE GROUPS

Working with persons who are poor, homeless, experiencing intimate-partner violence, or vulnerable requires exploration of personal values to ensure that one's own attitudes, values, and beliefs do not interfere with health care. Price, Desmond, and Eoff (1989) caution that victim blaming is a real phenomenon that can colour attitudes and interactions.

Victim Blaming

Victim blaming tends to hold the people burdened by social conditions accountable for their own situations and responsible for needed solutions. Victim blaming is often evident in language. If there is evidence of personal or systemwide victim blaming, a new world view may be needed. However, it is important to note that when we hear a nurse voicing notions of victim blaming, this is likely a direct result of his or her own experiences and challenges, so sensitive exploration of attitudes is required. A desirable world view would see all persons as autonomous beings who deserve to be treated with dignity and fairness. Unfortunately, the health care system may not be designed to extend the needed degree of autonomy to all persons. Nurses and other health care providers are generally educated to make decisions, considering the best interests of others. Sines (1994) describes how prominent power relationships interfere with therapeutic practice and desirable client outcomes. To respect others by allowing them to make choices and decisions, when they are capable of doing so, requires an attitude of caring with a focus on advocacy. This implies guarding patient rights, preserving patient values, championing social justice in health care, and serving as the conservator of the patient's best interests (Sines, 1994). Reeducating nurses and other providers to enhance the advocate role may improve care within a health care agency and empower individuals.

Ask Yourself

How Does Language Reflect One's Values?

How do the values reflected in the language of the following statements imply victim blaming?

- Most young, single, poor women get pregnant to increase their welfare benefits.
- If poor, homeless people would take more responsibility for themselves, they could improve their situation. There are jobs out there for people who want to work.
- The highest calling for a woman is to be the family nurturer.

(Continued)

- If an abused woman wanted help, she would just leave the abusive relationship.
- An important part of assessing for intimate-partner violence is to ask what the woman was doing or if she was drinking right before she was hit.
- Resistance to change is a normal part of aging.
- Loss is a normal part of aging.
- All five senses tend to decline as a person ages.
- How did they get HIV? Are they innocent victims, acquiring it through a blood transfusion?
- She should have known better. If you don't use condoms, you'll be at risk for STI's.
- Since most low-income women do not comply with therapies, it is not cost-effective to spend too much time with them on health education.
- What did you expect? Look at how her mother behaved.
- People can get ahead if they take advantage of life's opportunities.

Language of Violence

Another possible impediment to intervention, specifically with the social situation of violence, is the violence mode that colours speech and actions. Ewing (1987) describes how the health care system uses metaphors of violence such as "attacking" germs, "battling" disease, "plotting strategies" against or "defeating" invasive cells and unwanted organisms, and, ultimately, "suffering defeat" or "achieving victory." The prevailing mindset behind this strategy of confrontation is the antithesis of a needed compassionate approach that values nonviolence. This is especially true for persons experiencing intimate-partner violence. Language that supports violence can inadvertently lead to victim blaming, or covertly encourage futile and dangerous retaliation. Additionally, use of such language may prevent the creation of a safe environment for women or victims of abuse in the health care setting. Indeed a first step in effective intervention with those experiencing violence is to create a milieu that emphasizes nonviolence. The message has to be clear that violence of any form is wrong and, generally, illegal. This may necessitate a change in how health care providers approach and work therapeutically with people experiencing violence.

SOCIAL ISSUES AND SCHOLARSHIP

Many health care interventions are based, properly, on research; however, nurses need to ask if the underlying research, may create problems based on classism, sexism, and racism. For example, growth and development knowledge has traditionally been based largely on studies of the experiences of white heterosexual men (Gilligan, 1982). Thus, application of growth and development theory to both genders and to other races requires prudence. Campbell (1993) provides excellent data that knowledge of the abuser in intimate-partner violence situations is based on sex-role socialization in many families and therefore does not explain the violence in families of other cultures, for example. Demi and Warren (1995) and Vasquez and Eldridge (1994) explore the issues of valid research for vulnerable populations, pointing out that the way family is defined and the systems for recruiting and retaining families contribute to the inability to generalize research findings. In addition, many of the research instruments in use are not designed for diverse and vulnerable populations.

Some research has viewed women as inferior to men and nonwhite groups as inferior to whites (Vasquez & Eldridge, 1994). These historical roots have contributed to a dearth of scholarly studies on women and visible minorities. This means that classroom teachings and clinical knowledge may be based on inadequate research for minority populations.

There is an ethical responsibility to teach how to provide nursing care to diverse cultural groups. Thus, faculty and students must be cognizant of the benefits of selected interventions for all population groups. In addition, they must be vigilant in avoiding generalizations of research findings to diverse population groups. Research on vulnerable populations needs to be done to ensure an adequate data base for working with those growing populations that are experiencing social issues such as poverty, homelessness, intimate-partner violence, unhealthy aging, and racism.

SUMMARY

This chapter focused on ethical dilemmas that emerge when health care is considered for vulnerable population groups. Ethical decisions related to health care for vulnerable populations confront nurses who work with those experiencing the social conditions of poverty, homelessness, domestic violence, unhealthy aging, and racism on a daily basis. Since values affect professional behaviour, nurses must analyze personally held values as well as those of the health care agency where they are employed for appropriate consideration of justice, beneficence, nonmaleficence, and autonomy. Nurses who work with vulnerable groups need to utilize these principles in ethical decision making. Nurses must consider the impact and validity of health care interventions and research on vulnerable populations, and ensure that what nurses teach both in the classroom and to patients is based on research applicable to the populations being served and studied.

CHAPTER HIGHLIGHTS

- Poverty, homelessness, intimate-partner, being elderly, and racism can affect health in a negative fashion. Limited choices and inappropriate treatment options often interfere with the best health care for these vulnerable populations.

- Applying the concept of justice to vulnerable populations can change the way society and the health care system provide health care. Addressing the social conditions of the individual with an illness or disease is basic to health care.

- Nonmaleficence and beneficence may clash with autonomy when providing care for vulnerable populations.
- Victim blaming, evident in covert or overt beliefs that all people are accountable for their own situations and responsible for solutions, interferes with health care delivery for vulnerable populations and is evidence of sexism, classism, or racism.
- Advocacy and caring, which are ways to avoid delivering health care that is grounded in sexism, classism, and racism, require letting go of the power relationships that often dominate health care delivery.
- Clearing speech patterns and other behaviours of words and actions that are based on violence is a step toward therapeutic interventions with those who experience violence in their lives.
- Findings from research studies may not be applicable to vulnerable populations if the vulnerable are not part of the study population.

DISCUSSION QUESTIONS AND ACTIVITIES

1. Visit a homeless shelter or shelter for abused women. Interview residents about their health and ability to access health care.
2. Spend a few afternoons volunteering in a soup kitchen. Talk with people who come in for free meals about their health problems and ability to access health care.
3. Spend some time with a home health nurse or Meals on Wheels, making contact with the elderly who live at home alone. Explore with them their perceptions of quality of life, health dilemmas, and needs.
4. Work with classmates to develop a "health fair" for the homeless, discussing the value of typical activities and materials made available at traditional fairs, while designing a more relevant approach.
5. How many examples of toys, advertisements, acting roles, literature, childrearing practices, and the like can you identify that continue to perpetuate the woman's role as one of caregiver or sexual object? Discuss how the examples contribute to gender inequity for women.
6. Look at the community in which you live. What are the important social issues in this community? How are vulnerable persons supported?
7. In Canada today, despite our health care system, many people still experience barriers to accessing care. What are the reasons for this? Is health care a right or a privilege? What can nurses do to help remove barriers to care?

REFERENCES

American Medical Association. (1992). *Diagnostic and treatment guidelines on domestic violence.* Chicago: Author.

Arcangelo, V. (1994). Should age be a criterion for rationing health care? *Nursing Forum, 29,* 25–29.

Bohn, D. K. (1990). Domestic violence and pregnancy: Implications for practice. *Journal of Nurse Midwifery, 35,* 86–98.

Breton, J. H. (2000). Treating beyond color: Health issues in minority women. *Advance for Nurse Practitioners,* (November), 65–66, 68, 101.

Brown, L. S. (1991). Antiracism as an ethical imperative: An example from feminist therapy. *Ethics and Behavior, 1,* 113–127.

Burg, M. A. (1994). Health problems of sheltered homeless women and their dependent children. *Health and Social Work, 19,* 125–131.

Butler, S. S., & Weatherley, R. A. (1992). Poor women at midlife and categories of neglect. *Social Work, 37,* 510–515.

Campbell, D. W. (1993). Nursing care of African-American battered women: Afrocentric perspectives. *AWHONNS Clinical Issues in Perinatal and Women's Health Nursing, 4,* 407–415.

Campbell, J. C., Pliska, M. J., Taylor, W., & Sheridan, D. (1994). Battered women's experiences in the emergency department. *Journal of Emergency Nursing, 20,* 280–288.

Canadian Charter of Rights and Freedoms. (1982). Retrieved January 20, 2009, from http://laws.justice.gc.ca/en/charter.

Canadian Council on Social Development. (1996). *Poverty statistics.* Retrieved January 20, 2009, from http://www.ccsd.ca/factsheets/fs_pov96.htm.

Canadian Institute of Child Health. (2000). *The health of Canada's children: A Canadian Institute of Child Health profile* (3rd ed.). Ottawa: Author.

Canadian Institute of Child Health. (2001). *Income inequity: A Canadian Institute of Child Health fact sheet.* Ottawa: Author.

Catley, C. M. (1992). Global considerations affecting the health agenda of the 1990s, *Academic Medicine, 67,* 419–424.

Census of Canada. (2001). Retrieved January 20, 2009, from http://www12.statcan.ca/english/census01/home/index.cfm.

Commission on the Future of Health Care in Canada. (2002). *Building on values: The future of health care in Canada*—Final Report. Retrieved January 20, 2009, from http://www.hc-sc.gc.ca/hcs-sss/hhr-rhs/strateg/romanow-eng.php.

Council on Ethical and Judicial Affairs, American Medical Association. (1992). Physicians and domestic violence. *Journal of the American Medical Association, 267,* 3190–3193.

Davis, L. A., & Winkleby, M. A. (1993). Socio-demographic and health related risk factors among African American, Caucasian, and Hispanic homeless men: A comparative study. *Journal of Social Distress and the Homeless, 2,* 83–101.

Demi, A. S., & Warren, N. A. (1995). Issues in conducting research with vulnerable families. *Western Journal of Nursing Research, 17,* 188–202.

Diehm, C., & Ross, M. (1988). Battered women. In S. Rix, ed., *The American woman, 1988–1989* (pp. 292–302). New York: Norton.

Eisler, R. (1987). *The chalice and the blade.* San Francisco: Harper & Row.

Esposito, C. N. (1993). Abuse: Breaking the cycle of violence: The victim's perspective. *Trends in Health Care, Law, and Ethics, 8,* 7–11.

Ewing, W. A. (1987). Domestic violence and community health care ethics: Reflections on systemic intervention. *Family and Community Health, 10,* 54–62.

Fishwick, N. (1995). Getting to the heart of the matter: Nursing assessment and intervention with battered women in psychiatric mental health settings. *Journal of the American Psychiatric Nurses Association, 1,* 48–54.

Fowler, B. A., & Risner, P. B. (1994). A health promotion program evaluation in a minority industry. *ABNF Journal, 5*, 72–76.

Funkhouser, S. W., & Moser, D. K. (1990). Is health care racist? *Advances in Nursing Science, 12*, 47–55.

Gilligan, C. (1982). *In a different voice.* Cambridge, MA: Harvard University Press.

Goodman, L. A. (1991). The prevalence of abuse among homeless and housed poor mothers: A comparison study. *American Journal of Ortho Psychiatry, 61*, 489–500.

Hall, C. (1993). Long term care and the minority elderly. *Pride Institute Journal of Long Term Health Care, 12*, 3–8.

Hogue, C. J. R., & Hargroves, M. A. (1993). Class, race and infant mortality in the United States. *American Journal of Public Health, 83*, 20–33.

Kanna, M., Singh, N., Nemil, M., & Best, A. (1992). Homeless women and their families: Characteristics, life circumstances, and needs. *Journal of Child and Family Studies, 1*, 155–165.

Kernic, M. A., Wolf, M. E., & Holt, V. L. (2000). Rates and relative risk of hospital admission among women in violent intimate partner relationships. *American Journal Of Public Health, 90*(9), 1416–1420.

Limandri, B. J., & Tilden, V. P. (1993). Domestic violence: Ethical issues in the health care system. *AWHONNS Clinical Issues in Perinatal and Women's Health Nursing, 4*, 493–502.

Little, M. (2000). Introduction to the ethics of care. Presentation at *New century, new challenges: Intensive bioethics course XXVI,* Kennedy Institute of Ethics, Georgetown University, Washington, DC, June 10, 2000.

MMWR morbidity and mortality weekly report (2000). Prevalence of intimate partner violence and injuries—Washington, 1998. (July 7, 2000), 49 (26), 589–592.

Melville, M. B. (1988). Hispanics: Race, class, or ethnicity? *The Journal of Ethnic Studies, 16*(1), 67–83.

Minister of Public Works and Government Services, Canada. (2005). *A Canada for all: Canada's action plan against racism—An overview.* Ottawa: Government of Canada. Retrieved January 20, 2009, from http://www.cic.gc.ca/multi/pln/pdf/action-eng.pdf.

Mondragon, D. (1993). No more "Let them eat admonitions": The Clinton administration's emerging approach to minority health. *Journal of Health Care for the Poor and Underserved, 4*, 77–82.

Murphy, B. (2000). *On the street: How we created homelessness.* Winnipeg: Shillingford Publishing.

Price, J. H., Desmond, S. M., & Eoff, T. A. (1989). Nurses' perceptions regarding health care and the poor. *Psychological Reports, 65*, 1043–1052.

Raphael, D. (2001). From increasing poverty to societal disintegration: How economic inequality affects the health of individuals and communities. In P. Armstrong (Ed.), *Unhealthy Times* (pp. 223–246). Don Mills: Oxford University Press.

Roberts, D. (2000). Race, gender, justice, and reproductive health policy. Presentation at *New century, new challenges: intensive bioethics course XXVI,* Kennedy Institute of Ethics, Georgetown University, Washington, DC, June 9, 2000.

Sines, D. (1994). The arrogance of power. A reflection on contemporary mental health nursing practice. *Journal of Advanced Nursing, 20*, 894–903.

Skaff, M. M., & Pearlin, L. J. (1992). Caregiving: Role engulfment and the loss of self. *Gerontologist, 32*, 656–664.

Spigner, C. (1994). Black participation in health research: A functionalist overview. *Journal of Health Education, 25,* 210–214.

Stark, P. L. (1991). Health care under seige: Challenge for change. *Nursing and Health Care, 12,* 26–30.

Statistics Canada. (2002). *Ethnic diversity survey: Portrait of a multicultural society.* Retrieved January 20, 2009, from http://dsp-psd.communication.gc.ca/collection/statcan/89-593-X/89-593-XIE.html.

Tebb, S. (1995). An aid to empowerment: A caregiver well-being scale. *Health and Social Work, 20,* 87–92.

Vasquez, M. J. T., & Eldridge, N. S. (1994). Bringing ethics alive: Training practitioners about gender, ethnicity, and sexual orientation issues. *Women & Therapy, 15,* 1–6.

Wallerstein, N. (1992). Powerlessness, empowerment, and health: Implications for health promotion programs. *American Journal of Health Promotion 6*(3):197–205.

Wessell, M. L. (1992). Said another way: An ethical issue for a profession for all seasons. *Nursing Forum, 27,* 29–33.

Windom, E. (1988). An aging nation presents new challenges to the health care system. *Public Health Reports, 103,* 1–2.

WEBSITES

The Canadian Charter of Rights and Freedoms
http://laws.justice.gc.ca/en/charter/

A Canada for All: Canada's Action Plan Against Racism
http://www.pch.gc.ca/multi/plan_action_plan/index_e.cfm

The *Canadian Human Rights Act*
http://laws.justice.gc.ca/en/H-6/index.html

The *Canadian Bill of Rights*
http://laws.justice.gc.ca/en/C-12.3/index.html

The *Employment Equity Act*
http://laws.justice.gc.ca/en/E-5.401/

The *Official Languages Act*
http://laws.justice.gc.ca/en/O-3.01

The *Canadian Multiculturalism Act*
http://www.canadianheritage.gc.ca/progs/multi/policy/act_e.cfm

The *Immigration and Refugee Protection Act*
http://www.irb-cisr.gc.ca/en/about/publications/irpa/index_e.htm

The *Citizenship Act*
http://laws.justice.gc.ca/en/C-29/index.html

CHAPTER 17

Gender Issues

By Sandra L. Cotton

OBJECTIVES

After completing this chapter, the reader should be able to:

1. Describe historical bases of gender issues in nursing.
2. Describe factors associated with and the impact of sex discrimination in nursing.
3. Discuss sexual harassment within a nursing context.
4. Discuss communication issues related to gender.
5. Describe nursing issues related to modern sexism.

INTRODUCTION

In a perfect world, people would consistently relate to each other with mutual respect and empathy. Unfortunately, the reality of our lives is that our interactions are sometimes clouded by prejudice or lack of understanding. The workplace is a common arena for many societal issues to manifest. Issues such as employment equity, employment opportunities, sexual harassment, and role strain are but a few examples of gender-influenced conflicts that may be encountered in professional relationships. There are two basic approaches to dealing with these social justice issues. We can simply pretend that these issues do not exist. This approach may result in increased frustration as unresolved feelings and issues play out on the job. Alternatively, we can become aware of the issues and define ways to deal with the realities of our society in a straightforward and genuinely thoughtful way. This chapter focuses on the latter approach and explores issues concerning gender in the nursing workplace.

HISTORICAL PERSPECTIVES AND OVERVIEW OF GENDER-BASED ISSUES

Recently, in 2005, the legalization of same-sex marriage in Canada in 2005 was met with both jubilation as well as vocal opposition, mostly from various church and conservative groups; some, like the Catholic church, organized formal protests of the Chrétien government. With over 40 percent of the Canadian population noting an affiliation with the Catholic church (Statistics Canada, 2005), it was important that two things happened. First, it was critical to hear both sides of the argument and differentiate between deep-seated religious beliefs and homophobia. Second, it was, and remains, important to not assume that all those who list themselves as having an affiliation with the Catholic church share the same views as those in the Church with the most power, who are also most vocal in the public sphere.

In the United States, the passing of the California ballot proposition known as Proposition 8 restricted the state's Constitution so that it limited the definition of marriage to being between only a man and a women. Campaigns against the passing of Proposition 8 were widespread and continuing as the state put the Proposition into immediate effect the day after the 2008 election.

These two events demonstrate that there is still significant discrimination against lesbians and gay men, whether in the workplace or in their efforts to seek, ensure, and enjoy the same kinds of rights that everyone in society is due.

While some authors contend that most have come to accept the term *"nurse"* as "a person who cares for or tends to the needs of the sick" (Ellis and Hartley, 1995, p. 6), controversy remains concerning exactly what a person who provides nursing care should be called, and how, if at all, this relates to the gender of the person providing the care (Bernardi, 1996).

In her comprehensive work, *Woman as Healer,* Achterberg chronicles the journey of women in healing professions. Citing the masculinization of medicine as one of many issues that challenge nurses, Achterberg states that, although nursing has gained professional status, it suffers in some contexts because of issues of "nurses' functioning subordinate to multiple layers of authority" (1990, p. 177).

Lewenson (1996) notes that nurses have had to struggle with paternalistic ideology that continues to permeate the profession. **Paternalism** has been defined as "the system, principle, or practice of managing or governing individuals, businesses, or nations, etc. . . . in the manner of a father dealing benevolently and often intrusively with his children" (*Webster*'s, 1995). Lewenson contends that paternalism coupled with **nursism**, "a form of sexism that specifically maligns the caring role in society [has led to] discrimination in nursing by virtue of the role undertaken, regardless of gender" (1996, pp. 226, 228).

Societal Expectations

As nursing continues to be a predominantly female profession, societal issues that have affected women have also been reflected in nursing. In a nineteenth-century commentary entitled *The Hospital Hotel*, nurses were noted for being "well-bred, well-educated specimens of womanhood" (JAMA, 1996, p. 324). Women have been socialized to achieve or be less than they are capable of becoming. This reluctance to achieve is evident in the lack of women in positions of power, especially in the political arena (Hamilton, 1996). Although more recent societal influences have had a positive impact in this regard, nursing is still a female-dominated profession, which unfortunately has a history of oppression that many believe it has yet to overcome.

Ask Yourself

Is There Gender Stereotyping in Nursing?

One American-based survey indicates that many families would approve of nursing as a career choice for their sons (Begany, 1994). Of those opposed to having their sons in nursing, "a nurse should be a woman" was cited as the most frequent response for opposition to the profession.

- In what ways do you think nurses can help dispel this declining but continuing stereotype?

- How would you respond if your son or daughter chose nursing as a profession? Would you encourage him or her? Why or why not?

Authors such as Achterberg (1990), Baldwin (1995), Kane & Thomas (2000), Kavanagh (1996), Lewenson (1996), and Stromberg (1988) believe that nurses have been forced to work within a framework that focuses on societal expectations of women and what is considered women's work. In what has been termed the medicalization of North American society, nursing has been forced to overcome the prejudices of a society that has historically embraced the biomedical curative model of health care. As diversified "consumers" of health care are demanding more sophisticated and culturally congruent care, nurses are in a prime position to provide, high-quality, relevant, and individualized care. If nursing is to be successful in this and other arenas, it must concomitantly address issues of territoriality, power, and authority within its own ranks as well as with other health care professionals. A model of interdependence that seeks to create a positive situation for all providers and "consumers" of care may be most desirable (Baldwin, 1995).

GENDER DISCRIMINATION IN NURSING

Historically, women have worked for lower pay than their male counterparts. Employment equity is generally protected by federal and provincial legislation. Over the past thirty years, many initiatives have been undertaken to address pay inequity on the basis of gender. The United Nations Convention on the Elimination of All Forms of Discrimination Against Women, adopted in 1979 and now under the auspices of the Office of the High Commissioner for Human Rights in Geneva, attempted to define discrimination and facilitate the elimination of such at national levels in all UN countries (Office of the United Nations High Commissioner for Human Rights, 1979). There are laws governing employment equity in provinces across Canada, and equal pay for equal work is a right protected by the *Canadian Human Rights Act*, specifically the Equal Wages Guidelines (1986). Additionally, in 2001, a pay equity task force was formed by the federal government to find ways to address employment equity and implement changes necessary to ensure pay equity and to keep pace with the changes of a modern society and the dynamic nature of the workplace (Department of Justice Canada, 2001). Despite these and more legislation and activism, women, on average, still earn less than men for the same work. In fact, one source notes that, as of 2005, a woman gets paid, on average, 70 percent of what a man earns in a similar position (Canadian Labour Congress, 2005). Salaries in nursing remain low compared with other professions that require comparably high levels of skill, education, and responsibility. Some suspect that the increasing presence of men in nursing is helping to raise salaries; however, other economic considerations, such as nursing shortages, fair-labour-related legislation, and collective bargaining, may be responsible (Ellis & Hartley, 2001). Although a disparity in earnings, known as a *pay gap*, exists between men and women of many occupations, the gap is considerably narrower for nurses (Reskin & Padavic, 1994). When compared to other occupations, the fact that nurses have historically earned less may account for this lack of difference (Stromberg, 1988). However, the fact that a gap exists at all is striking in that men comprise only a small percentage of the nursing profession (Benokraitis & Feagin, 1995). As Gilloran (1995) notes, the development of a patriarchal structure within nursing, with fewer women in senior management positions, may account for this gap. However, this trend is also changing.

According to sociologist Christine Williams (1995), issues of comparable worth are a real concern for nurses. Williams identifies several hidden advantages to being a man in nursing, particularly related to hiring and promotion. Williams's work supports Gilloran's (1995) assertions of gender disequity, as men are typically *tracked* into higher paying and more prestigious positions. Even in a predominantly female profession, women may be experiencing a form of economic gender discrimination.

Gender Issues in Women's Health

Although men *may* have hidden advantages in nursing, some areas, primarily in women's health, have remained closed (Ketter, 1994); in an interesting case from the U.S., California exempts labour and delivery rooms from state job discrimination laws by upholding a hospital's ban on employing nurses who are men in these areas (Letizia, 1994). California's Fair Employment and Housing Commission cited "invasion of a woman's privacy" as justification for the exemption, but one nurse called it "the most outlandish ruling" she had ever encountered (Thompson, 1995, p. 9).

In court proceedings that addressed this issue, the fact that most obstetricians are male was not deemed analogous to the situation of the nurse who is male (Ketter, 1994). Most courts cited that the doctor was chosen by the patient, while the nurse was not. Several state courts addressed this aspect of gender discrimination; however, none sided with the nurse. Section 703(e)(1) of the *Civil Rights Act* in the U.S. allows for gender-based discrimination if gender "is a bona fide occupational qualification reasonably necessary to the normal operation of that particular business or enterprise" (Ketter, p. 24). Many men in nursing believe this form of discrimination is reinforced in educational settings when faculty members seek the permission for male student nurses to observe or participate in procedures with female patients, but do not seek the permission of male patients when female students are involved. Some postulate that women are more universally accepted by patients because they are viewed as nurturers (Ellis & Hartley, 2001). Although no data support these assumptions, institutions continue to promote this form of gender discrimination when they proactively provide for the modesty and privacy of their female patients. Some nurses agree with this position, while others do not (Spancraft, 1995; Thompson, 1995).

Expanding Numbers of Men in the Profession

Although the number of men in nursing has increased steadily, men still comprise a relatively small number of all practising RNs in Canada and the United States (National League of Nursing, 1995). Sullivan (2000) stresses the value of gender diversity in nursing, noting that men play an important role in the profession. Citing societal stereotyping as one of the major limiting factors for men in nursing, Squires (1995) may be categorizing men further when he asserts that health care reform that increases responsibility and autonomy will attract more men to the nursing profession. Perhaps what Williams (1995) perceives as hidden advantages for men in nursing adds some credence to Squires's assertions. Despite these and other stereotypes, Squires considers the lure of nursing to be universal regardless of gender. Noting the challenge, variety, and excitement of nursing, Squires is quick to acknowledge that the road men in nursing have travelled thus far has not been without controversy. One professional organization formed in 1974, in the U.S., the American Assembly for Men in Nursing (AAMN), addresses these issues, with a goal to "encourage men to become nurses, support those men already in nursing, and educate society as to the benefits of male nurses" (AAMN, 2001).

Gender and Caring

In 2005, the total number of nurses in Canada exceeded 268,000 with only 5.6 percent or approximately 1400 of those nurses male (Canadian Nurses Association, 2006). Canada is lagging behind other countries such as the United Kingdom, where over 25 percent of all nurses are male. This number, according to a 2007 *Canadian Nurse* article, is rapidly increasing in the United Kingdom.

Even rates of attrition from nursing programs are higher for male students than female, with rates of almost 50 percent, compared to an average attrition rate of 20 percent for their female colleagues (Tosh-Kennedy, 2007). Nursing graduate degree programs report a steady increase in the number of male students entering their programs (NLN). As the number of men in nursing increases, research directed toward gender-related issues in the profession has begun to emerge (Ekstrom, 1999; Fisher, 1999; Gilloran, 1995; Paterson, Crawford, Saydak, Venkatesh, Tschikota, & Aronowitz, 1995). For example, many authors have focused nursing research on caring as it relates to gender. Although much of this work is in its infancy, research questions related to possible differences in the learning or expression of caring as it relates to the gender of the student, educator, or recipient of care demonstrate the attention these and other issues in nursing have commanded. Recognition of the need to explore gender became evident for Peter and Gallop (1994) in their comparative study designed to examine whether caring uniquely reflected the moral orientation of nursing students. They discovered that differences in caring noted between medical and nursing students appeared to be related to gender differences. A study exploring the relationship between nurse gender and both nurse and patient perceptions of caring found no significant difference in actual caring according to nurse gender (Ekstrom, 1999). However, from both nurse and patient perspectives, expectations of certain nurse caring behaviours were lower for male nurses.

Ironically, a gender bias may already exist in the literature that focuses on caring. Reverby (1987) offers an historical perspective of caring as it relates to women, but does not address any possible implications in relation to the addition of men to the profession. Chinn (1991) devoted an entire anthology to caring, but did not explore gender in relation to caring, except as it related to economic gains (or lack thereof) for male faculty members in male-dominated academic centres. The exclusion of men by Grigsby and Megel (1995) as they explored the caring experiences of nursing faculty is another example of current nursing research that does not include men.

Despite an increased interest in the caring aspect of nursing, Begany (1994) perpetuates a nursing stereotype by equating the positive attribute of caring to images of nurturer or handmaiden. Some men in nursing may already experience a form of gender discrimination with regard to the stereotypical belief that all men in nursing are homosexuals. This stereotype is rooted in gender-based role assumptions, such as Begany's, related to the caring attributes that many perceive as feminine. Because nursing has historically been viewed as "woman's work," men in nursing have been stereotyped as feminine. Often, assumptions are made that male nurses must be homosexual. Even though Williams (1995) found there were hidden advantages in nursing for men, she also discovered that, ironically, these "opportunities . . . may extend only to those who exhibit conventional masculine characteristics, including a heterosexual orientation" (p. 65).

❓ Think About It

Do Men and Women Express Caring in Different Ways?

- What do you think of Begany's (1994) images of caring? What does caring mean to you?

- Williams (1995) believes that organizations are gender biased in how they regard masculine behaviours versus feminine ones. She suggests the development of gender-sensitive evaluation tools that would acknowledge women's contributions to the profession. If you were appointed to develop such an evaluation tool, what attributes would your tool reward and recognize as unique to women? What justice issues may be involved in using gender-sensitive evaluation processes?

- Goals of the American Assembly for Men in Nursing include supporting men already in nursing and educating society about the benefits of male nurses. What do you think are the benefits of nurses who are men? How do these differ from the benefits of nurses who are women?

As more men enter the profession, additional gender issues may be identified. According to one author, some areas of nursing have more male nurses than others, including mental health, intensive care, and the operating and emergency rooms (Vere-Jones, 2008). Why some areas attract and retain male nurses more than others is an area for further research and discussion. For example, once in the workforce, men in nursing may experience difficulty when cross-gender mentoring relationships exist (Feist-Price, 1994). Feist-Price notes several potential adversities in cross-gender mentoring relationships, mainly related to communication differences between men and women (Tannen, 1990). Feist-Price further notes that cross-gender mentoring relationships have successful outcomes, especially when formal mechanisms are in place to deal with issues as they arise. One final implication for nursing may be in the area of caring. If differences in the development or expression of caring in male nurses indeed exist, these and other differences need to be explored and further utilized to improve the practice of nursing and optimize gender differences. However, there is a persistent lack of strong male role models in nursing along with few positive or realistic media representations of male nurses (Meadus & Creina Twomey, 2007). Add to that almost no targeted recruitment strategies for young males seeking career counselling in high school or university to even suggest nursing as a viable, fulfilling, and challenging career. This implies that, certainly, unless these issues are explored and strategies put in place to recruit, attract, and retain more men in the profession, we will continue to have small numbers of male nurses in Canada.

SEXUAL HARASSMENT IN NURSING

Bullough (1990) describes Florence Nightingale's encounters with harassment and the prevailing strategy of the day "to gain respect" through being a lady (Nightingale, 1859). Bullough contends that sexual harassment has been a recurring theme in Western nursing. The Supreme Court of Canada defines sexual harassment as "unwelcome conduct of a sexual nature that detrimentally affects the work environment or leads to adverse job-related consequences for the victims." (*Marinaki v. Human Resources Development Canada*, 2000). The Ontario Human Rights Commission notes that sexual harassment is unwanted words or actions that are related to gender or of a sexual nature. Often referred to under the umbrella of workplace harassment, sexual harassment may include them touching in a way that is inappropriate or uninvited; staring or making comments in a sexual way; being verbally abusive because of gender; making sexual requests, jokes, or remarks about a person or about a specific gender or displaying sexually offensive images of any kind to others (Ontario Human Rights Commission, 2008). There are two important things to note about sexual harassment. First, it may not be overtly sexual in nature, despite its label. It may refer to being bothered or harassed simply because of gender. Second, sexual harassment doesn't only happen to women; it can happen to anyone, in any situation (Ontario Human Rights Commission, 2008). Nurses may not immediately recognize or label behaviours as sexual harassment, and often have difficulty finding appropriate words to describe the experience concisely (Madison & Minichiello, 2000). Indicators of sexual harassment by individuals identified by these authors include:

- A feeling of having your space invaded or being cornered;
- A feeling of being disrespected;
- Noting behaviour that feels forced or too friendly.

According to the same authors, indicators of an environment or workplace in which sexual harassment might happen more readily may include:

- Other persons confirming that they have been harassed;

- Power or administrative structures that support or protect the harasser while providing limited options for the harassed;

- A workplace in which sexual innuendo, images, or humour is common or tolerated.

Bullough suggests that nurses need to employ specific strategies to combat sexual harassment. The National Organization for Women (NOW) recommends being assertive, seeking support from other workers, keeping a diary to document each incident, filing a complaint or grievance, keeping performance documents, seeking counselling, initiating legal action, and seeking a new job as strategies to deal with sexual harassment on the job (NOW, 1993). In addition to these recommendations, NOW recommends being active and vocal advocates for safe workplaces for all (NOW, 2000).

Ask Yourself

Discrimination and Inequality in Nursing

When we talk about issues of women's rights or sexual discrimination (which can affect both genders), we need to be attentive to the fact that many forms of discrimination can occur. Section 15 of Canada's *Charter of Rights and Freedoms* (1982) clearly precludes any form of discrimination or practised inequality, with the exception of affirmative action for the purpose of ameliorating marginalized individuals or groups.

15. (1) Every individual is equal before and under the law and has the right to the equal protection and equal benefit of the law without discrimination and, in particular, without discrimination based on race, national or ethnic origin, colour, religion, sex, age or mental or physical disability.

(2) Subsection (1) does not preclude any law, program or activity that has as its object the amelioration of conditions of disadvantaged individuals or groups including those that are disadvantaged because of race, national or ethnic origin, colour, religion, sex, age or mental or physical disability.

- Do issues of discrimination affect nurses in a unique way?

- As advocates for others, discuss what responsibility you think nurses have in relation to marginalized or vulnerable populations, such as the homeless or persons without legalized status.

- Reflect on experiences you have had, in which you might have felt discriminated against, by virtue of your gender, abilities, religion, age or ethnic origin. How did you feel? What did you do? How would you approach a situation like this again, if you encountered it?

We do not need to venture far to find images that reinforce the view that nurses are sexual objects. A quick tour of the *get well* section at your local greeting card shop graphically illustrates this point. Although sexual harassment does not recognize gender boundaries, clearly sexual harassment has historically been the bane of women. As more men enter the nursing profession, issues concerning sexual harassment directed toward them or from them may emerge. Research is needed that is directed toward understanding issues concerning sexual harassment in nursing, how best to address the needs of men in nursing, and implications for the women with whom they work.

COMMUNICATION ISSUES RELATED TO GENDER

How nurses communicate with each other, their patients, and their colleagues has long been discussed in the nursing literature (Campbell-Heider & Hart, 1993; Sweet & Norman, 1995; Corser, 1998). Nurses need to address how changing societal roles and expectations relate to the practice of nursing, and what research is needed to promote and bring about positive change.

"The Doctor–Nurse Game"

A gender division of labour has been a significant factor in how nurses, who are primarily women, and physicians, a traditionally male dominated profession, relate to each other in health care settings. Initially described as the *doctor–nurse game* (Stein, 1967), issues regarding communication with physicians remain an area of primary concern for many nurses (Anderson, Maloney, Oliver, Brown, & Hardy, 1996). Favourable patient outcomes have been positively associated with successful nurse–physician communication (Shortell, Zimmerman, Rousseau, Gillies, Wagner, Draper, Knaus, & Duffy, 1994; Zimmerman, Shortell, Rousseau, Duffy, Gillies, Knaus, Devers, Wagner, & Draper, 1993).

Many nurses still use less than straightforward methods to manage conflict among themselves or between nurses and physician colleagues (Valentine, 1995). Valentine indicates that staff nurses are most comfortable using avoidance, while nurse managers tend to use compromise as their primary method of conflict management. These methods may be reinforced by nursing educators, whom Valentine found also employed avoidance as their primary conflict management tool. According to Tannen (1990), the primary reason for these and other communication conflicts relates to identifying and understanding gender differences in communication. Previously linked to societal roles and expectations of women, the "doctor–nurse game" was re-examined by Stein, Watts, and Howell (1990). The authors found that a more humanistic public image of physicians and the increasing numbers of female physicians and male nurses have generally improved physician–nurse relations.

Think About It

Do Men and Women Communicate Differently?

Tannen (1990) asserts that men and women communicate from such differing frames of reference that their communication could be considered a cultural clash of sorts.

- What has your experience been in this area?
- What communication concerns with fellow students, faculty, patients, or physicians have you experienced in your program of study?
- How would you rate the nurse–physician communication in your clinical agencies? Describe why.
- Describe potential gender-based differences in communication.

With females comprising nearly 50 percent of students entering medicine, and a slowly increasing percentage of males entering nursing school, perhaps the patriarchal system of health care will shift. The implications this may have for nursing remain unknown.

Communicating with Patients

Today, one trend that has permeated health care from the street is the casual nature of attire and approach to work (Twenge, 2006). In nursing, uniform policies and requirements have changed to reflect a more casual society, with a concern for comfort over formality. Starched white dresses, hats, and polished shoes have been replaced by scrubs, T-shirts, and casual wear. While this has advantages—making nurses appear to be more friendly and accessible, it also has a downside. Many people find that it is difficult to tell what roles people play in health care environments as their dress does not help to identify them as unique, skilled professionals. Furthermore, the casual comfortable nature of dress is seen by many as unprofessional and indicative of a casual approach to work, as well as appearance. While it would be foolhardy and impractical to return to the formal traditional dress of nurses as noted above, it is worth giving thought to what you look like when you approach patients—remembering that you are there as a trusted, capable, and highly skilled professional. To some degree, your appearance should reflect that. For example, scrubs with teddy bears on them may be appropriate for a pediatric unit, but would not be appropriate for an adult setting and might inadvertently communicate to patients a message of incompetence or immaturity.

Through informal dress and communications, nurses may in fact be sending powerful negative messages to their patients and medical colleagues (Campbell-Heider & Hart, 1993). The bedside manner of nurses is discussed by these authors, who note that the tone of familiarity expressed by nurses who use their first names with patients may translate sociologically into persistent stereotypic themes and become a mechanism of social control. While superior nursing care may reduce these stereotypes, Campbell-Heider and Hart discuss the role of deliberative communication strategies, both verbal and nonverbal, in accelerating professional recognition.

Successful interpersonal communication with patients is central to the practice of nursing. In relation to sensitive issues and sexuality, Propst (1996) found that registered nurses' communication practices are lacking. Only half of the respondents in her sample of women's health nurses discussed issues concerning sexuality with their patients. Even in a specialty practice area, such as women's health, nurses are not immune to communication issues when sensitive topics are involved.

MODERN SEXISM

Even though women have made tremendous inroads in the workplace, Benokraitis and Feagin (1995) report that sex inequality is still a major problem. In fact, it may be on the rise in some areas. **Sexism** is "the assumption that members of one sex are superior to those of the other" (Kavanagh, 1996, p. 296). In our predominantly male-oriented health care system, issues concerning sexism may evidence themselves in power struggles for reimbursement, as nurses take on advanced practice roles (Baldwin, 1995). Unfortunately, even within the nursing profession, issues of sexism related to men in nursing are present. An example of this is the male colleague who feels he has a hiring edge over women in nursing, because he never needs to be off for maternity leave or stay home from work to care for sick children.

Ask Yourself

Are Male Nurses Perceived as More Competent?

Benokraitis and Feagin (1995) interviewed male nurses. The authors report that physicians view male nurses as more competent than their female counterparts. They also found that female nurses were often ignored, whereas male nurses' opinions were valued.

- Have you observed this behaviour in your clinical or classroom settings?
- How could you best deal with this form of modern sexism?

SEXUAL ORIENTATION

Heterosexism is "the assumption that everyone is or should be heterosexual, and that heterosexuality is superior and expectable" (Kavanagh, 1996, p. 296). We must be alert for this form of sexism directed toward patients and some nurses (Stevens, 1995; Williams, 1995). Van Ooijen and Charnock (1995) note that very little attention is given to addressing this and other gender issues within the nursing curriculum, despite the belief that developing an understanding of these issues may have a tremendous effect upon nursing care.

Lesbians and gay men may be the largest minority group in nursing. These nurses are practising in every province and working in every hospital. Fearing sexual harassment or discrimination from coworkers, superiors, and bureaucratic systems, many remain reluctant to have their sexual orientation known.

Sexual harassment and bigotry is a fact of life for many lesbians and gay men. Twenty-five years after the birth of the modern gay rights movement, a poll in *Time* magazine revealed that 52 percent of respondents consider same-gender relationships between consenting adults to be morally wrong (Henry, 1994). This culturally prevalent attitude can range from prejudice to homophobia. Prejudice that is operationalized on the institutional level leads to discrimination. More extreme forms of bigotry include harassment and physical violence. Zurlinden (1997) writes, "Unmasked, homophobia is really hatred, willful ignorance, mean-spiritedness, and narrow-mindedness. People suffering from homophobia do not run screaming in terror when they encounter a lesbian or gay man. Instead, they assume they are justified to be cruel; to discriminate in housing, employment, and education; and to pass laws to prevent gay men and lesbians from enjoying the civil liberties that other Americans take for granted" (p. 11).

Within institutions, hidden *bigotry* can be insidious, damaging, and difficult to change and prove. Some employers systematically discriminate against lesbians and gay men through hiring, promotion, and disciplinary practices. This may be the result of institutional policy (as in the military), discriminatory administrative practice, punitive supervisors, or discrimination by coworkers (Zurlinden, 1997). Discrimination may also take the form of absence of employment benefits available to heterosexuals. Though a few university hospitals have agreed to extend spousal benefits such as health insurance, life insurance, and maternity leave to same-gender couples, these may not be available in most institutions. The International Council of Nurses Position Statement on Ethical Nurse Recruitment cites freedom from discrimination as a guiding principle, stating that "Nurses have the right to expect fair treatment such as working conditions, promotion and continuing education" (ICN, 2007).

While there has been progress in recognizing and dealing with issues of discrimination against persons for their sexual orientation, much remains to be done. Tolerance for behaviours, language, or practice that discriminates against persons for their gender or sexual orientation, in any context or institution, is difficult to understand or endorse in any way. Federal and provincial position statements and legislation exist for supporting non-discriminatory practices and having zero tolerance for anything otherwise. However, leading organizations such as the Canadian Nurses Association and provincial nursing regulatory bodies should take stronger stances on this issue in a public way.

SUMMARY

Nursing has been faced with gender issues since the early days of the profession. Nursing's role and status has been coloured by societal expectations of women and paternalistic ideology permeating the health care arena. Considerations of gender can be related to lower salaries for nurses compared with primarily male professions, communication patterns with physicians and patients, perceptions of abilities to carry out nursing's caring imperative, and stereotypical expectations of how nurses should look and act. While men in the profession face the challenge of dealing with societal stereotypes, they are also often tracked into higher-paying and more prestigious positions. Issues concerning discrimination based on sexual orientation occur on many fronts and may be underrecognized. Awareness of these issues enables nurses of both genders to be alert for inequities and to develop strategies for change.

CHAPTER HIGHLIGHTS

- Controversy exists regarding how the title of the person caring for the sick relates to the gender of the person providing care. Both women and men in nursing must deal with social stereotyping regarding expected roles and behaviours.

- Societal expectations of women and paternalistic ideology throughout history have led to discrimination in nursing, though gender discrimination may exist for both women and men in different nursing settings.

- Issues of comparable worth relative to gender are of concern in nursing, particularly in areas of salary and positions of prestige and responsibility.

- Nurses need to be alert to and employ strategies to combat sexual harassment.

- Gender-based differences in styles and patterns of communication can affect all areas of nursing practice, requiring attentiveness to effective communication with patients and colleagues in order to foster better patient outcomes.

- Sexism, occurring in both subtle and overt ways, continues to be an issue in nursing, and harassment and discrimination based on sexual orientation may be underrecognized.

DISCUSSION QUESTIONS AND ACTIVITIES

1. One frequently cited political action strategy is to build coalitions with "powerful persons of like mind" (Hamilton, 1996). If nurses in your community are to become empowered, with whom would they build coalitions?

2. Paterson et al. (1995) discuss ways in which nursing students who are males learn to care. Read an article on how nursing students learn to care. Do men learn about, or express caring, differently than women? How does this relate to your experiences as a student nurse? How does this relate to Begany's (1994) images of nurturer or handmaiden?

3. What stereotypes of nurses are present in your community or national media? What types of *get well* cards are in your local card shop? What do you think it will take to change these and other stereotypes about nurses?

4. What is the gender makeup of your local nursing administration? How many women are in positions of authority or power within your health care setting?

5. Observe gender-based communication patterns between nurses and physicians. Consider your own style of communication with same-gender and other-gender friends and colleagues. What patterns do you identify? How might these patterns affect your professional interactions? Are there areas that need to be modified in order to promote more effective communication?

6. Explore various web sites to determine guidelines regarding sexual harassment that are offered by the American Nurse's Association, the Canadian Nurses Association, and other professional organizations. http://www.cna-nurses.ca and http://www.nursingworld.org.

REFERENCES

Achterberg, J. (1990). *Woman as healer*. Boston, MA: Shambhala.

American Assembly for Men in Nursing. (2001). *Membership* [Brochure]. Pensacola, FL: Author.

American Nurses Association. (1995). *Nursing's social policy statement* [Brochure]. Washington, DC: Author.

American Nurses Association. (2001). *Code of ethics for nurses*. Kansas City, MO: Author.

Amott, T., & Matthaei, J. (1996). *Race, gender, and work; A multicultural economic history of women in the United States* (2nd ed.). Boston: South End Press.

Anderson, F., Maloney, J., Oliver, D., Brown, D., & Hardy, M. (1996). Nurse-physician communication: Perceptions of nurses at an army medical center. *Military Medicine, 161,* 411–415.

Baldwin, D. (1995). Territoriality and power in the health professions. In final report of the Council on Graduate Medical Education, National Advisory Council on Nurse Education and Practice, *Report on primary care workforce projections* (pp. 1–36). Washington, DC: U.S. Department of Health and Human Services.

Begany, T. (1994). Your image is brighter than ever. *RN, 57,* 28–35.

Benokraitis, N. V., & Feagin, J. R. (1995). *Modern sexism: Blatant, subtle, and covert discrimination* (2nd ed.). Englewood Cliffs, NJ: Prentice-Hall.

Bernardi, A. (1996, Winter). Untitled. [Letter to the editor]. Interaction, *Newsletter of the American Assembly for Men in Nursing*, p. 3.

Bullough, V. (1990). Nightingale, nursing, and harassment. *Image, 22,* 4–7.

California bans prices based on gender. (1995, October 14). *The Dominion Post*, p. A2.

Campbell-Heider, N., & Hart, C. (1993). Updating the nurse's bedside manner. *Image, 25,* 133–139.

Canadian Labour Congress. (2005). *Pay equity*. Retrieved August 15, 2008, from http://canadianlabour.ca/en/pay-equity.

Canadian Nurses Association. (2006). *2005 Workplace profile of registered nurses in Canada*. Ottawa: Author.

Chinn, P. L. (1991). *Anthology on caring*. New York: National League of Nursing Press.

Corser, W. D. (1998). A conceptual model of collaborative nurse-physician interactions: The management of traditional influences and personal tendencies. *Scholarly Inquiry for Nursing Practice, 12*(4), 343–346.

Department of Justice Canada. (2001). Canadian Human Rights Act (R.S., 1985, c. H-6). Government of Canada: Ottawa. Retrieved August 15, 2008, from http://laws.justice.gc.ca/en/showdoc/cs/H-6///en?page=1.

Department of Justice, Government of Canada. (1982). Charter of Rights and Freedoms. Schedule B. Constitution Act, 1982. Retrieved August 17, 2008, from http://laws.justice.gc.ca/en/const/annex_e.html#I.

Ekstrom, D. N. (1999). Gender and perceived caring in nurse-patient dyads. *Journal of Advanced Nursing, 29*(6), 1393–1401.

Ellis, J., & Hartley, C. (2001). *Nursing in today's world* (7th ed.). Philadelphia, PA: Lippincott.

Feist-Price, S. (1994). Cross-gender mentoring relationships: Critical issues. *Journal of Rehabilitation, 60*, 13–17.

Fisher, M. (1999). Sex role characteristics of males in nursing. *Contemporary Nursing, 8*(3), 65–71.

Foolchand, M. (1995). Promoting racial equality in the nursing curriculum. *Nurse Education Today, 15*, 101–105.

Gilloran, A. (1995). Gender differences in care delivery and supervisory relationship: The case of psychogeriatric nursing. *Journal of Advanced Nursing, 21*, 652–658.

Grigsby, K., & Megel, M. (1995). Caring experiences of nurse educators. *Journal of Nursing Education, 34*, 411–418.

Hamilton, P. (1996). *Realities of contemporary nursing*. Menlo Park, CA: Addison-Wesley.

Henry, W. (1994, June 17). Pride and prejudice. *Time, 143*(26), 57–59.

International Council of Nurses. (2007). Position statement on ethical nurse recruitment. Geneva: ICN. Retrieved January 19, 2009, from http://www.icn.ch/psrecruit01.htm.

International Council of Nurses. (2008). *The ICN definition of nursing*. Retrieved January 2, 2009, from http://www.icn.ch/abouticn.htm.

JAMA (1996). The hospital hotel. *Journal of the American Medical Association, 275*, 324.

Kane, D., & Thomas, B. (2000). Nursing and the "F" word. *Nursing Forum, 35*(2), 17–24.

Kavanagh, K. (1996). Social and cultural dimensions of health and health care. In J. Creasia & B. Parker, eds., *Conceptual foundations of nursing practice* (pp. 285–308). St. Louis, MO: Mosby.

Ketter, J. (1994, April). Sex discrimination targets men in some hospitals. *The American Nurse, 26*, 1, 24.

Letizia, B. (1994, December). Ban on male nurses in labor and delivery is upheld. *RN, 57*, 16.

Lewenson. (1996). *Taking charge: Nursing suffrage & feminism in America, 1873–1920*. New York: National League of Nursing Press.

Madison, J & Minichiello, V. (2000). Recognizing and labeling sex-based and sexual harassment in the health care workplace. *Journal of Nursing Scholarship, 32*(4), 405–410.

Marinaki v. Human Resources Development Canada (2000), TD 3/00 (C.H.R.T.).

Meadus, R. J., Creina Twomey., J. (2007). Men in nursing: Making the right choice. *The Canadian Nurse, 103*(2), 13–6.

National League of Nursing. (1995). 1995 *Nursing data review; NLN division of research*. New York: Author.

National Organization for Women. (1993). *Sexual harassment survival skills* [Brochure]. Morgantown, WV: Author.

National Organization for Women. (2000). *Stamp out workplace harassment and discrimination.* Washington, DC: NOW.

Nightingale, F. (1859/1992). *Notes on nursing: What it is, and what it is not.* London: Harrison & Sons.

Office of the United Nations High Commissioner for Human Rights. (1979). Convention on the Elimination of all Forms of Discrimination against women: New York: UN.

Ontario Human Rights Commission. (2008). *Sexual harassment. Your rights and responsibilities.* Retrieved January 2, 2009, from http://www.ohrc.on.ca/en/issues/sexual_harassment.

Paterson, B., Crawford, M., Saydak, M., Venkatesh, P., Tschikota, S., & Aronowitz, T. (1995). How male nursing students learn to care. *Journal of Advanced Nursing, 22,* 600–609.

Peter, E., & Gallop, R. (1994). The ethic of care: A comparison of nursing and medical students. *Image, 26,* 47–51.

Propst, M. (1996). Registered nurses' practice and perspective toward sexuality in women's health. *Southern Nursing Research Society Abstracts,* 83.

Reskin, B., & Padavic, I. (1994). *Women and men at work.* Thousand Oaks, CA: Pine Forge Press.

Reverby, S. (1987). A caring dilemma: Womanhood and nursing in historical perspective. *Nursing Research, 36,* 5–10.

Shortell, S., Zimmerman, J., Rousseau, D., Gillies, R., Wagner, D., Draper, E., Knaus, W., & Duffy, J. (1994). The performance of intensive care units: Does good management make a difference? *Medical Care, 32,* 508–525.

Spancraft, E. (1995, February). Banning male RNs from L & D is blatantly unfair [Letter to the editor]. *RN, 58,* 9.

Squires, T. (1995). Men in nursing. *RN, 58,* 26–28.

Statistics Canada. (2005). *Population by religion, by provinces and territories.* Retrieved January 19, 2009, from http://www40.statcan.gc.ca/l01/cst01/demo30a-eng.htm.

Stein, L. (1967). The nurse-doctor game. *Archives of General Psychiatry, 16,* 699–703.

Stein, L., Watts, D., & Howell, T. (1990). The doctor-nurse game revisited. *New England Journal of Medicine, 322,* 546–549.

Stevens, P. (1995). Structural and interpersonal impact of heterosexual assumptions on lesbian health care clients. *Nursing Research, 44,* 25–30.

Stromberg, A. (1988). Women in female-dominated professions. In A. Stromberg & S. Harkess, eds., *Women working: Theories, and facts in perspective* (pp. 206–224). Mountain View, CA: Mayfield.

Sullivan, E. J. (2000). Men in nursing: The importance of gender diversity. *Journal of Professional Nursing, 16*(5), 253–254.

Sweet, S., & Norman, I. (1995). The nurse-doctor relationship: A selective literature review. *Journal of Advanced Nursing, 22,* 165–170.

Tannen, D. (1990). *You just don't understand: Women and men in conversation.* New York: Ballantine.

Thompson, J. (1995, February). Banning male RNs from L & D is blatantly unfair [Letter to the editor]. *RN, 58,* 9.

Tosh-Kennedy, T. (2007). Increasing the numbers. *The Canadian Nurse, 103*(2), 17.

Twenge, J. (2006). *Generation Me: Why today's young Americans are more confident, assertive, entitled—and more miserable than ever before.* New York: Free Press.

United Nations. (1979). Convention on the Elimination of Discrimination of all Forms Against Women. United Nations Division for the Advancement of Women: Department of Economic and Social Affairs.

van Ooijen, E., & Charnock, A. (1995). How men and women view the world: A sexual perspective. *Nursing Times, 91*, 38–39.

Vere-Jones, E. (2008). Why are there so few men in nursing? *Nursing Times, 104*(9), 18.

Webster's college dictionary. (1995). New York: Random House.

Williams, C. (1995). Hidden advantages for men in nursing. *Nursing Administration Quarterly, 19*, 63–70.

Zimmerman, J., Shortell, S., Rousseau, D., Duffy, J., Gillies, R., Knaus, W., Devers, K., Wagner, D., & Draper, E. (1993). Improving intensive care: Observations based on organizational case studies in nine intensive care units. *Critical Care Medicine, 21*, 1443–1451.

Zurlinden, J. (1997). *Lesbian and gay nurses.* Albany, NY: Delmar.

CHAPTER 18

Transcultural and Spiritual Issues

Written in collaboration with Mary Gail Nagai-Jacobson

OBJECTIVES

At the end of this chapter, the reader should be able to:

1. Describe factors associated with cultural sensitivity within nursing.
2. Discuss the influence of culture on health and health care decisions.
3. Identify approaches for dealing with transcultural issues in nursing.
4. Discuss issues related to the use of complementary therapies by patients.
5. Identify legal considerations related to transcultural issues.

6. Discuss the relationship between spirituality and health.

7. Identify the nursing role in addressing patients' spiritual concerns.

8. Discuss considerations regarding nurturing one's spirit.

INTRODUCTION

The influence of culture and spirituality are major factors in the development of values. Because nurses deal with people from varied cultural and spiritual backgrounds, they must be alert for issues relating to these areas. This chapter presents general considerations regarding culture and spirituality and discusses related issues that may arise when caring for patients.

TRANSCULTURAL ISSUES

We live in a multicultural society, alive with diversity. Such diversity of people and backgrounds provides a richness to our lives, yet challenges our abilities to appreciate, rather than judge or fear, differences. **Diversity** is encountered wherever there are differences, whether these be gender, age, socioeconomic position, sexual orientation, health status, ethnicity, race, or culture (Kavanagh, 1993). Dealing with diversity is an essential component of nursing care. Nurses need competence in providing culturally appropriate care. **Cultural competence** (Waters, 1996; Engebretson & Headley, 2000) includes **cultural awareness**—knowledge about values, beliefs, behaviours, and the like of cultures other than one's own—and **cultural sensitivity**—the ability to incorporate the patient's cultural perspective into nursing assessments and to modify nursing care in order to be as congruent as possible with the patient's cultural perspective.

The same phenomenon may be viewed differently by people from different cultures, because culture teaches us to understand a perception of reality. For example, the *man in the moon* that most people in this country have been taught to "see" is identified in other cultures as a *frog in the moon, a woman in the moon,* or a *rabbit in the moon* (Tafoya, 1996). Another way of appreciating different perspectives is to consider what we see when we are in the valley, compared with what we see from halfway up the mountain or the view from the top of the mountain. Different perceptions of the same reality derive from the perspectives from which it is viewed. One view of reality is not more correct than the other; the different views merely come from different perspectives.

The most recent Canadian census notes that one-fifth of the total population of Canada comprises persons who identify themselves as immigrants, i.e., persons who are, or have ever been, landed immigrants (Statistics Canada, 2006). Of the over six million persons who identify as immigrants in Canada, over 1.1 million immigrated between 2001 and 2006. What is not captured in the census, of course, are those persons who may be in Canada as refugees, or with no legal status.

Undocumented evidence supports that these numbers may be increasing and that the needs of persons in such groups to maintain health and well-being is of the utmost importance to bring to the attention of the public. Many of the lives of persons without legal status are precarious, invisible to others, and highly dangerous, both in their place of origin and here in Canada. Persons living without legal status may not have access to health care, child care, social services, or other important supports. In cities and communities across Canada, attention must be given to the plight of such persons and how best to accommodate and meet their needs, in a holistic and compassionate manner, given the diverse contexts of each story and situation.

The Canadian Nurses Association (2000) notes that cultural diversity is not merely an issue for large urban areas, as trends demonstrate that increasing numbers of immigrants are moving from cities into smaller communities and rural areas.

The census also notes that of the total population of Canada, only half of all persons identify English as the first language used at home in childhood and still understood (Statistics Canada, 2006). This has a tremendous impact on communication and education within the therapeutic nursing relationship.

Other changes in the demographics of Canadians, have an effect on how health care should be provided in a holistic and relevant manner. Approximately 45 000 persons identified as being in a same-sex relationship, living in the same household. This is likely not only an underestimation of reality, but additionally, not reflective of many same-sex relationships in which persons do not cohabitate. Of the 45 000 persons, 7000 identify as married. Again, while these are underestimations and mere glimpses of Canadian demographics, it is clear that the faces of Canadian identity and the notion of family in Canada have been and are, rapidly, changing. In turn, nursing as a profession must not only reflect these kinds of changes by ensuring access to the profession for persons of diverse cultures, races, genders, abilities and sexual orientation but also openly discuss, reflect upon, and educate nurses about diversity and the notion of comprehensive cultural competence (Leininger, 2002).

Ask Yourself

How Do You Deal with Diversity?

Consider a situation in which you judged someone you did not know because she or he was different from you.

- What about the person or situation triggered your judgment?
- Why do you think you reacted to the person or situation the way you did?
- How and from whom did you learn to react in this way?
- What has helped you to understand diversity?
- How can nurses learn to appreciate rather than fear diversity among colleagues and patients?

Understanding Culture

Self-awareness is a key factor in dealing with transcultural issues. The best starting point for becoming sensitive to the culture of another is to understand our own culture and its influence on our perceptions and behaviours. **Culture** refers to the total lifeways of a group of interacting individuals, consisting of learned patterns of values, beliefs, behaviours, and customs shared by that group (Tripp-Reimer, 1987; Engebretson & Headley, 2000; Hopkins, 1997). These *learned patterns* are passed from one generation to the next in formal ways, such as through educational settings, and in informal ways, such as through role modelling. Unique cultural expressions can be observed within many groups of interacting individuals—for example, the culture of the deaf community, prison culture, or the culture of health care. We need to recognize that each of us is part of a culture and to identify values, beliefs, and behaviours that we hold dear, as these reflect our own cultural perspective. In this process we each must be alert to our own **ethnocentrism,** reflected in the tendency to judge behaviours of someone from another culture by the standards of our own culture.

Nurses must develop cultural sensitivity, which implies understanding behaviours and values of another culture within the context of that culture, without imposing our own cultural values on others. In this process we must avoid **stereotyping,** which is expecting all persons from a particular group to behave, think, or respond in a certain way based on preconceived ideas. Every culture contains variation, and some people within the group may not ascribe to all beliefs and values attributed to that culture.

Understanding Diversity

Culturally competent nurses, writes Maier-Lorentz (2008), are those who are not only sensitive to issues and differences "related to culture, race, ethnicity, gender and sexual orientation" (p. 37), but also willing and eager to engage, on a continual basis, in achieving a seamless ability to work with persons without having cultural differences constrain or confine the therapeutic relationship.

Leininger (2002) notes that cultural competence, at its best, implies a strong awareness of diversity, skills in transcultural knowledge developed over time, and a strong personal and professional respect for those from varying cultures or contexts.

For many, the notion of cultural competence means having an awareness of the varying values and beliefs others may hold, as a result of their culture, race, birth place, or ethnicity. However, in today's world, cultural competence implies that we also understand that the values and beliefs of others are due to factors related to gender, sexual orientation, family structure, political stance, and socioeconomic status. Differences in approaches to health and illness may arise not only from one's culture. As care providers to a wide variety of diverse persons, in terms of factors other than simply culture, nurses need to be aware that, for all of us, our worldview and value system are developed out of other kinds of experiences and personal characteristics. Developing cultural competence, as Leininger and others characterize it, means exploring more than simply culture, in order to provide holistic care.

Furthermore, in today's multicultural societies, especially in urban centres, such as Toronto, Montreal, and Vancouver, many cultures and ethnicities overlap and have far less defined boundaries than in the past. Many persons are born in other countries but identify as Canadian, having immigrated to this country. Identifying persons or assuming values and beliefs based on a person's accent or skin colour is highly problematic. Naively, nurses may not expect that someone who is originally from the Indian subcontinent would not embrace the practices of Ayurvedic medicine to treat and heal illness. Or they may be surprised that a person who is not Chinese adopts practices from Chinese medicine to maintain health or manage chronic illness. Certainly, nurses must attend to their own stereotypes and programmed expectations in order to achieve true cultural competence.

Cultural Safety

The notion of cultural safety (University of Victoria, 2008) goes beyond the three concepts of cultural awareness, cultural sensitivity, and cultural competence, while acknowledging their importance. Cultural safety "involves the recognition that we are all bearers of culture and we need to be aware of and challenge unequal power relations at the individual, family, community, and societal level" (University of Victoria, 2008, p. 1). This concept challenges us, in discussions of culture and diversity, to be more open about issues of oppression, unequal power, and social and political contexts that underlie beliefs, practices, and language.

Ask Yourself

How Might Ethnocentrism Affect Nursing Care?

Consider the varied meanings the following behaviours may have depending upon the cultural context in which they occur: direct eye contact may connote honesty or intrusion; a firm handshake may be viewed as confidence or hostility.

- How might behaviours such as these be judged by people within the dominant culture in this country?

- How do practices and expectations within health care settings reflect ethnocentrism regarding behaviours such as these?

- How might ethnocentrism or stereotyping affect interaction with others, especially within a nursing setting?

Cultural Values and Beliefs

Because culture is one of the key organizing concepts of nursing, nurses need to be actively learning about:

> the health beliefs and values of clients. [This kind of active learning] include [exploring] how these influence their response to health care

and beliefs about self-care in health and illness, the role of health care providers and hospitalization, birth practices, death and dying, family involvement, spirituality, customs, rituals, food and alternative or traditional therapies. This encourages respectful and open exploration of client attitudes, beliefs, perceptions and goals." (CNA, 2000)

Cultural values and beliefs guide our thinking, being, and doing in patterned ways. Beliefs about health and practices related to health and healing are some of the patterns influenced by culture that are significant in providing health care. Such beliefs and practices manifest in both direct and subtle ways, and sensitivity to them can affect patient outcomes and satisfaction with care. It is helpful to recognize a distinction between **disease**, which is the biomedical explanation of sickness, and **illness**, which is a personal response to the disease flowing from how our culture teaches us to be sick (Burkhardt, 1985; Tafoya, 1996). Transcultural issues are often present in nursing situations, but may not be identified as such. Instead, patients may be labelled as stoic, uncooperative, noncompliant, strange, or "crazy" because of choices they make, and their health and care may be compromised. Leininger (1991) has delineated principles of transcultural care, human rights, and ethical considerations that offer guidance for nurses in dealing with transcultural issues, which are listed in Figure 18–1. Although she offers these principles as a guide particularly for transcultural nurses, they apply as well to other nurses. In light of these principles, many nursing practices derived from the Western biomedical model may benefit from reevaluation.

Figure 18–1 **Transcultural Care Principles, Human Rights, and Ethical Considerations**

1. Human beings of any culture in the world have a right to have their cultural care values known, respected and appropriately used in nursing and other health care services.

2. Human cultures have diverse and universal modes of caring and healing practices that need to be recognized and used by professional nurses to function effectively and therapeutically with people of different cultures.

3. Care is the essence of nursing and a basic human need for growth, healing, well-being, recovery, and survival.

4. Cultural care is a critical component influencing human health, well-being, and recovery from illnesses or disabilities.

5. Every culture has at least two major types of health care systems namely, the *folk (generic, lay or indigenous) care system* and the *professional care system* which influences their health outcomes, and the transcultural nurse is challenged to use this knowledge to guide nursing care decisions and actions.

6. All professional nurses are challenged to respect common human needs and humanistic aspects of people care worldwide, and also the divergent care expressions, meaning, and practices.

(Continued)

7. Transcultural nurses are expected to respect Western and non-Western cultures who often have different values, beliefs, and norms to assess and understand human beings.

8. Transcultural nursing principles and practices are the arching framework for all nursing care practices which differ from nursing practices that rely on traditional medical symptoms, diseases and treatment regimes.

9. Since transcultural nursing focuses upon *comparative cultural care* values, beliefs and practices of cultures, the nurse is expected to work with individuals, families, groups, cultures, subcultures and institutions that reflect cultural care variabilities.

10. Nurses with transcultural knowledge are expected to respond appropriately to *culture care differences* and *similarities* in order to ease or ameliorate a human condition or lifeway, and to help clients face death.

11. Ethical and moral differences and similarities exist among human cultures which necessitates that nurses recognize, respect and respond appropriately to such variabilities.

12. It is essential that transcultural nurses be open-minded and willing to learn from cultural informants about their human values, beliefs, needs and practices in order to make appropriate nursing care plans, judgments and actions.

13. The ability of the nurse to listen, use silence and envision the client's or family's human condition or cultural circumstance with its positive or less positive features is important in transcultural nursing.

14. Transcultural nursing often requires that nurses communicate with clients in their native language to know, learn and understand individuals, families and groups of different cultures.

15. Transcultural nurses are challenged to identify what constitutes ethical or moral principles and norms of cultures and not assume that all cultures are alike.

16. Transcultural nurses are expected to guide other nurses who have not been prepared in transcultural nursing in order to prevent marked ethnocentrism, cultural imposition practices, and inappropriate ethical and moral judgments about clients.

17. Transcultural nursing reflects that an individual or group of a designated culture are active participants and decision-makers in culture care practices in order to develop and maintain creative and effective professional care practices.

18. Clients of diverse or similar cultures have a right to have their caring life styles and expressions known and used in transcultural nursing in order to promote client health or well-being.

19. Transcultural nursing takes into account the world view, environmental context, ethnohistory, social structure features (including the religious, kinship, philosophic, economic, political, technological and cultural values), language, expressions, gender and age difference of people.

20. Transcultural nursing is concerned with the assessment of caregiver and carereceiver [sic] expressions, beliefs and lifeways that often go beyond nurse-client dyadic relationship to that of care relationships with families, groups, institutions and communities in order to facilitate congruent care practices and to avoid unfavorable culture care conflicts, stress and negligent care practices.

21. Since ethical, moral and legal systems of human values [sic] and rights exist in all cultures, it is the task and responsibility of transcultural nurses to discover these dimensions with key and general informants and in diverse cultural contexts.

22. Human care rights tend to be covert and embedded in social structure, cultural values and world view of clients, and so the transcultural nurse is challenged to discover these dimensions mainly through qualitative research methods.

23. Transcultural nurses recognize that cultures are complex, dynamic and change over time and in varying ways.

24. Transcultural nurses recognize that many cultures and subcultures in the world have not been studied and yet nurses are expected to care for all peoples including minorities.

25. Transcultural nursing is a major breakthrough for new nursing knowledge and practices that do not follow the traditional nursing or medical disease, symptom and illness models.

Leininger, M. (1991) *Journal of Transcultural Nursing*, 3, 21–23. Reproduced with permission.

Incorporating cultural assessment into care with patients is an important part of a comprehensive nursing assessment. This assessment facilitates better understanding of sometimes overlooked factors that influence health behaviours and decisions. Cultural assessment helps nurses to appropriately identify and understand the meaning of behaviours that might otherwise be judged negatively or be confusing to the nurse (Giger & Davidhizar, 1995; Engebretson & Headley, 2000; Breton, 2000). We must recognize that each person is culturally unique, and that not all persons in a particular cultural group believe or respond the same way. Cultural assessment includes exploration of six cultural phenomena that are evident in all cultural groups: communication, space, social organization, time, environmental control, and biological variation (Giger & Davidhizar, 1999; Engebretson & Headley, 2000). Such exploration enables nurses to identify areas where modifications in care can be incorporated so that care is more culturally congruent. Although the process may also reveal divergent beliefs that are difficult to accommodate within the current health care system, acknowledging differences may help the patient and family to feel more comfortable within the system. For example, when assessing eating patterns and food preferences, the nurse might discover that the patient commonly eats only two meals a day, consisting of burritos in the morning and rice and beans in the evening. Typical hospital food and a three-meals-a-day pattern might not be appetizing for this patient. The patient's nutrition may suffer, and she may perceive that she is not being fed. By arranging for the patient to have culturally similar foods at similar times, the nurse provides more culturally congruent care.

Because Canadian nurses are expected to learn about cultural diversity, knowledge, skills and attitudes about culture are included in the 1999 CNA Blueprint for the Registered Nurse Examination. These competencies are: demonstrating consideration for client diversity; providing culturally sensitive care (e.g., openness, sensitivity, recognizing culturally based practices and values); and, incorporating cultural practices into health promotion activities.

In order to be able to begin to provide culturally relevant and competent care, the CNA (2000) articulates four nursing responsibilities: to perform cultural assessments, use cultural knowledge, understand communication, and form partnerships. As noted below, from a 2000 article in *Canadian Nurse*, these four responsibilities, alongside strategies to improve responsiveness and awareness at a personal and professional level, are key to developing cultural competence.

Cultural assessment challenges nurses to examine personal attitudes and values about health, illness, and health care. When nurses understand the differences between personal values and beliefs and those of their clients, they appreciate the strength of both. The plan of care can then become mutually respectful and effective.

Cultural knowledge includes learning about the health beliefs and values of clients. It includes how these influence their response to health care and beliefs about self-care in health and illness, the role of health care providers and hospitalization, birth practices, death and dying, family involvement, spirituality, customs, rituals, food, and alternative or traditional therapies. This encourages respectful and open exploration of client attitudes, beliefs, perceptions, and goals.

Verbal and nonverbal communication between client and provider can be a barrier to accessibility of services. The use of facial expressions, body language, and norms related to eye contact are examples of nonverbal communication differences that need to be understood. Listening, respecting, and being open are essential. Specialized health care interpreters can be more effective than volunteer translators in interpreting both the words and the meaning of health information in a culturally accurate context.

Partnership among clients, providers, and funding agencies is essential to develop a system that incorporates culturally diverse practices into health care services while optimizing health outcomes for the client. Partners can establish health care needs and, mutual goals for individuals and communities, and facilitate client choice. [Canadian Nurses Association (2000). Cultural Diversity: Changes and Challenges. *The Canadian Nurse*. 96.2. Reprinted with Permission from the Canadian Nurses Association.]

CASE PRESENTATION

Cultural Differences

Angie is a home care nurse in Manitoba. She has been working with a family of a newborn child with complex needs. The family have lived in Canada all their lives and are practising Muslims. The child is now at home, with significant supports for the complex technology and therapy that the child requires on a daily basis. However, the parents, both well-educated professionals, have learned quickly how to provide the complexity of care that their child requires.

Today Angie is called on an emergent basis by her manager to attend to the family. This morning the child died at home. When Angie arrives, the emergency services are already there and they have called the medical examiner, as is the practice with deaths of unknown causes. The family are distraught and Angie tries to comfort them.

The paramedics inform the family that an autopsy will have to be performed and that the medical examiner will come to collect the child's body for this purpose. The family agree. The child's mother asks the paramedic when the autopsy might be performed. He replies that he is unsure, but likely within 72 hours.

Both parents turn to Angie for help. They tell her that their religious traditions require burial rituals to be performed, if at all possible, within 24 hours of death at their mosque. The paramedic, overhearing, says gently to the family that this is almost impossible, with the volume of cases to which the medical examiner must attend. He goes on to say that this is not unusual, and it is "always" the case that people have to wait this long.

Think About It

How Can Nurses Develop Cultural Competence?

- In what way is there a demonstrable lack of cultural competence?
- How can Angie help to make the care, from all, at this point, to be more culturally sensitive?
- In this case, what strategies do you see as an important step in helping to avoid this situation recurring?
- For now, if you were Angie, what would you do to advocate for your clients?

Culture and the Health Care System

Concepts of health and healing, of right and wrong, of what is proper and what is not, are rooted in culture. Cultures have different explanatory models regarding health and illness that reflect their beliefs about the causes, symptoms, and treatments of illness, and response to dying and death. Our explanatory model helps us to recognize, respond to, interpret, cope with, and make sense of illness and other life experiences (Engebretson & Headley, 2000).

Transcultural issues arise when nurses, patients, and families hold differing views of what is important or necessary regarding health, recovery, illness, or the dying process. The contemporary health care system is not user-friendly when it comes to incorporating diversity. By virtue of its history, the system reflects predominantly middle-class, European American, Judeo-Christian, paternalistic values and perspectives (Kavanagh, 1993). This system includes the attitude that the health care provider knows what is "best for the patient," as viewed from the health provider's perspective.

The health provider's perspective generally derives from a combination of two cultural orientations. The primary cultural orientation is the biomedical model, and the secondary cultural orientation is the provider's personal cultural background. If the patient's perspective is different from this model and is not considered, dilemmas may emerge. Consider, for example, a situation in which the physician, who is schooled in the Western biomedical model, views death as "the enemy" to be overcome at all costs. The patient, who comes from an Aboriginal culture, views death as a part of life that one prepares for by being in harmony with one's surroundings. Medical or surgical interventions that may prolong the patient's life a few weeks, which would be very important in the physician's world view, may be very low on the list of considerations for the patient. A patient who believes the suffering from his illness is a way of atoning for his sins may resist taking pain medication that health professionals deem important for his recovery.

We must be aware that the health care system is a different culture from that of most of the patients served by the system. The language, values, norms, behaviours, rituals, and environment are generally unfamiliar to those who seek its services. Even people who belong to the same dominant culture in society as their health care providers are often strangers when they enter the institutions of the system. For those who do not belong to the dominant culture, negotiating the system can be a formidable task. Lack of understanding of language, procedures, expectations, and other elements of the culture can lead to miscommunication, unclear decisions, and a sense of powerlessness or lack of control. Ethical dilemmas may arise due to misunderstandings. Consider the case of a mentally alert ninety-year-old woman who, after her doctor of thirty-five years retired, sought care from a new young physician. After a few visits she stopped going to see him, even though she was having serious health problems, because, in her perception, he did not do anything for her. Essentially, he did not talk with her nor spend the kind of time with her that her former physician had, and instead gave her medicines that she felt made her sick and that she did not need.

In turn, the physician may have also felt that he was providing thorough and holistic care. He may have decided that the priority of care was not to have long discussions, but to carefully and thoroughly treat the elderly woman's medical problems. In examining common problems such as these, we often discover that while the problem appears to be an issue of diverse or conflicting values and practices, usually it is simply a matter of miscommunication, lack of effective communication, or a lack of the time to understand the priorities of the other.

When we speak of values such as autonomy, beneficence, justice, or the right to self-determination, we must ask from whose perspective these values are understood—that of the nurse or that of the patient. This same question is appropriate regarding definitions of health. For example, many cultures place a higher emphasis on loyalty to the group than on the self-reliance and autonomy valued within the broader North American Culture (Andrews, 1999; Davis, 1999; Ludwick & Silva, 2000). Health care decisions in these cultures are often made by a group such as the family, community, or society, rather than by the individual.

As Ellis and Early note (2006), Aboriginal persons define themselves as part of a collective and a community. Their identity is rooted within a community and a deep sense of the shared is part of their culture and everyday decision making processes. This paradigm can be contrasted to that of what we consider to be mainstream North American culture, in which great worth is placed on the individual; therefore, individual decision making in matters related to health care is valued, and even cherished, above all. For Aboriginal persons, health is maintained by a connection to not only the environment, but also the community around oneself (University of Victoria, 2008). These ideas are not new, as fundamental parts of Aboriginal culture. But for some nurses, these ideas and values may not be in "alignment" with the traditional North American biomedical model, which is part of much of our health care system.

Cultural assessment provides insight into the congruence, or lack thereof, between patients' and nurses' values and understandings of health. Consider, for example, a situation in which the nurse believes that health includes being able to be a productive member of society and that health problems provide opportunities for one to grow and become more self-actualized. The patient, on the other hand, believes that his work-related injury is an act of *fate* and focuses on being free of pain and able to "get around." If the differing perceptions of health are not recognized and addressed, efforts to have the patient participate in rehabilitation and job retraining or to utilize nonpharmacological measures for pain control may meet with much resistance and, justifiably, patient dissatisfaction.

Complementary Therapies

Culture guides one's choice of when to go for health care, what kind of care to seek, to whom to go, and how long to participate in care. Many people who utilize conventional health care settings also utilize alternative or complementary therapies (Eisenberg, Kessler, Foster, Norlock, Calkins, & Delbanco, 1993; Eisenberg, Rogers, Ettner, Appel, Wilkey, Van Rompay, & Kessler, 1998). The Tzu Chi Institute, as cited in the Canadian Nursing Association's publication *Nursing Now* (1999), defines complementary therapies as "therapies that are used alongside mainstream medicine, such as massage therapy" while alternative therapies are defined as "independent healing systems or interventions used outside the realm of western theory and practice, such as Ayurvedic medicine and homeopathy." Such therapies may derive from traditions in the patient's own culture, or may be borrowed from traditions of another culture. Complementary therapies include a wide variety of modalities, such as relaxation techniques, healing touch and other energy-based healing techniques, spiritual healing, biofeedback, nutritional practices, herbal treatments, massage and other body work, meditation, prayer, homeopathy, acupuncture, and biofeedback.

Today in Canada, there is a increasing trend toward the use of complementary and alternative therapies, due to a number of possible factors, including increased access and availability of such therapies, an increase in the number of persons living with chronic illnesses and disease, a fear of highly technological interventions, and increased attention to quality of life. (The College of Registered Nurses of Nova Scotia (2005) refers to alternative therapies as treatments that are not widely used, taught, or practised in traditional health care professions and complementary therapies as treatments that are used alongside what might be considered traditional or customary interventions.

These therapies are often used concurrently with what are considered to be more conventional therapies, but they may be chosen in lieu of conventional therapies. In order to have a broad picture of the many factors affecting a patient's health and healing, we need to be aware of various therapies being utilized by the patient. We should incorporate discussion of complementary therapies into nursing assessment in an open way, since patients may be hesitant to bring up the subject. We do not need to ascribe to such therapies in order to become knowledgeable about them. Complementary therapies often derive from paradigms that differ from, and may not make sense when viewed only from the perspective of the conventional medical model, yet may be very useful in the healing process. These types of therapies might be labelled as unorthodox, nontraditional, or questionable in terms of their effectiveness or validity by those who have not taken the time to try to understand or seek further information about them. Hufford (1996) suggests that the patient has the major responsibility for seeking information regarding alternative therapies and making health choices in this regard, but that today's health care providers must have knowledge about risks and benefits involved. When patients are interested in complementary therapies, we must determine whether there are risks associated with their use. If there are significant risks involved, and the patient is committed to utilizing the therapy, we need to work with other health team members to minimize risks and maximize benefits, while respecting the patient's wishes and values. When there is not a strong commitment to the nonconventional modality, we should encourage ongoing discussion of known risks and benefits related to various options (Hufford, 1996). When conventional health care providers can work with traditional systems and their healers, the overall care becomes more culturally congruent.

The principle of patient self-determination directs us to honour the right of persons to use both conventional and complementary therapies to address their health care needs (Burkhardt & Nagai-Jacobson, 1996). Respect for persons calls us to be open to views other than our own, and to appreciate that there are many paths to healing. Complementary modalities should never be discounted merely because they are not understood within the Western biomedical frame of reference. We need to respect convictions that derive from belief systems that are different from our own, and to be open to the contributions to health offered by other explanatory models. A nonjudgmental approach that respects differing values and beliefs and is sensitive to ethnocentric bias enhances the opportunity to explore jointly the efficacy of all options with the patient.

The area of informed consent presents some important questions relative to complementary therapies. Since noting alternative treatments is an important element of an informed consent, we must consider whether it is an ethical duty for practitioners of bioscientific medicine to include discussion of complementary therapies in discussion of therapeutic alternatives. Similarly, we must ask if practitioners of other healing modalities should be sure that their clients are aware of biomedical alternatives. Those who offer complementary therapies should explain the intervention and discuss risks, expected effects and benefits, and treatment options prior to initiating therapy. It is prudent to appraise other health team members of the use of complementary therapies, because they can affect conventional interventions in varying ways. Typical attitudes toward complementary therapies may reflect an assumption that, because they are not traditional biomedical therapies, such as pharmaceuticals, ultrasound, or surgery, they are less "potent" or powerful. This is a dangerous assumption. Many complementary therapies not only interact significantly with biomedical therapies, but also have significant or notable effects on patients. To not acknowledge that is more problematic than simply failing to understand; it can have serious implications for health and illness of patients.

Practitioners of both conventional and complementary therapies need to be alert to potential threats to patient autonomy that flow from practitioner attitudes. When we assume that patient values and thought processes are the same as ours, we may believe that what we suggest is the only reasonable course of action. When patients choose another course of action, we may question their decision-making capacity or label them as unreasonable. In conventional practice, this may show up in referring to nonconventional therapies as quackery or nonscientific, trying to dissuade patients from using them, and even deriding the patient for making such choices. We must remember that a patient's choice of an option that may seem unreasonable from our perspective does not necessarily mean that he or she has not thought it through. Such differences reflect diverse values, beliefs, and paradigms.

Think About It

How Should Nurses Deal with Complementary Therapies?

Conventional medicine and medical practitioners tend to be skeptical of healing modalities that have not been subjected to empirical scientific study; thus, discussion of nonconventional modalities is not included in lists of alternatives for patients, nor are these modalities available in most conventional health care settings.

- What do you think about this attitude toward complementary therapies?
- What experiences have you had with complementary therapies?

(Continued)

- How might attitudes toward complementary therapies affect the ability of nurses to provide culturally congruent care for their patients?

- What are the ethical implications related to limiting a patient's access to complementary therapies and practitioners within conventional health care institutions?

- What is your view of complementary therapies within nursing practice? What, if anything, do you think needs to change?

Factors important for the healing process are often culturally prescribed. For example, the involvement of family in the care of a sick member may be very important in some cultures. It can be quite distressing for nursing staff on a hospital unit when multiple family members "spend long periods of time" in a patient's room or the nearby hallway, or bring food from home that is not on a patient's diet. Providing culturally congruent care in such situations may include relaxing visiting regulations and collaborating with the family regarding appropriate foods from home. If the needs of one patient are different from those of the roommate, dilemmas may arise that require diplomatic and sensitive interventions by the nurse.

Legal Considerations Related to Transcultural Issues

Cultural misunderstandings can provide fertile ground for litigation. Communication—verbal, nonverbal, and written—is always of utmost importance. When a patient's first language is different from that of the nurse, we must determine the extent of the patient's understanding of the nurse's language. When the patient uses another language (including sign language), having an interpreter fluent in the patient's language is essential. If the interpreter is a member of the patient's family, the translation may be filtered through the perspective of the family member. Consider, for example, an elderly Cambodian man who is in the hospital and not doing well. His grandson serves as interpreter. The grandson was born in this country and is embarrassed by his grandfather's "old" ways. When the man says that he needs a particular traditional herbal tea each afternoon in order to get well (which is available in a local ethnic store), the grandson translates this generically as "tea." Even though the nurse responds by making sure that the patient has tea each afternoon, the patient's needs are not met.

The language in which we explain procedures and consent forms presents other issues. Be sure that the patient or family member is able to read the language in which the form is written, and that all terms used are understood. If the form needs to be interpreted for the patient, it is essential that the interpreter understands the procedure and that an appropriate person is available to clarify any areas of uncertainty. Many hospitals and health care agencies have translators available. Additionally, many health care practitioners and staff speak languages other than English, and can assist. People may indicate that they understand when they do not, in order to avoid offending the nurse or being considered ignorant. One way of dealing with this is having patients describe in their own words what they have been told. Most importantly, adequate time must be put aside to explain procedures and consent processes to those who may require additional time or the services of a translator.

ISSUES RELATED TO SPIRITUALITY

Spirituality is a universal human experience that transcends culture, although it may be coloured and shaped by cultural experiences. Nurses at all levels of practice must be attentive to spirituality and recognize the individual as a body-mind-spirit being who experiences health concerns in all these dimensions. In the midst of advances in technology and scientific discoveries, which have increased our understanding of the nature of illness and disease, attunement to the role of spirituality in health and healing has diminished in many areas of health care. In the past, limited scientific knowledge may have compelled people to believe that health and illness, death, and dying were beyond their control. Many persons were cared for in their homes, even in the case of serious illness. Touching, praying, and presence were a natural part of such environments. Historically, institutions such as hospitals were often staffed by religious orders concerned for both spiritual and physical needs.

Healing and health care has long been connected with the spirituality of a people. Within some communities such as Aboriginal peoples, healing rituals frequently are spiritual in nature (University of Victoria, 2008). People seeking medical care continue to incorporate spiritual and religious rituals and practices into their care for self and others. It is noteworthy that the words "health," "holy," and "whole" all derive from the same old Saxon, *Hal*, and Greek, *Holos*, which mean "whole." By their nature, then, health and healing are associated with that which is holy and whole. A question to ponder is whether contemporary health care culture, now vested in technology, managed care, mergers, and the like, can once again incorporate spirituality within its vision of healing.

Approaching Spirituality

Many definitions of health do not include any notion of spiritual well-being. Most notably, the definition of health, according to the World Health Organization, includes "physical, mental and social well being" (WHO, 1948, p. 100) but does not refer to spirituality of holism in any way.

Spirituality can be defined as "an inner sense of something greater than oneself. Recognition of a meaning to existence that transcends one's immediate circumstances." (Goldrosen and Straus, 2004, p. 918). It is differentiated from religiousness and notions of secularity. However, it is still often discussed alongside religious beliefs and practices in many contexts.

When discussing spirituality in the context of health, we may refer to concepts of quality of life and holism. The National Council on Ageing refers to spirituality as contrasting "fragmentation and isolation" (National Council on Ageing, 2004, p. 1). In the nursing literature, spirituality is often discussed alongside holistic care of persons and attention to spiritual well-being in addition to providing physical care and meeting psychosocial needs (Canadian Nurses Association, 2008). In describing health on a continuum, Neuman consistently refers to persons as having contextual variables that affect where they might be on this continuum, which may include developmental, sociocultural, psychological, physiological and spiritual (Neuman, 1989). According to Watson, health is characterized by a sense of focused harmony within the body, mind, and soul (Watson, 1988). Each of these nursing theorists acknowledges that the spiritual needs of persons must be addressed in order to provide holistic and relevant care. It is evident that, as a profession, nursing has consistently attended to spirituality as part of the holistic care of patients in a variety of settings and contexts. From Nightingale to Neuman and Watson, many nurse theorists and frameworks address the person as having physical, psychological, contextual, and spiritual needs in health and illness. In her *Notes on Nursing,* a fundamental nursing text, Florence Nightingale states that the spiritual needs of persons are equally important as the physical needs of their bodies in all health and illness states (Nightingale, 1969).

The International Council of Nurses' *Code of Ethics for Nurses* directly addresses nurses as having a responsibility to address the spiritual needs of persons in the context of the therapeutic relationship and in order to create an environment of respect (International Council of Nurses, 2006). The American Holistic Nurses' Association states that, "Nursing care should be given within a context mindful of the holistic nature of humans, understanding the body-mind-spirit connection" (AHNA, 2008). Recognizing that spirituality is basic to health, but highly variable between persons and communities, is an important part of holistic nursing care.

Nurturing Spirit

Caregiving is influenced by a nurse's spiritual, as well as physical and emotional, well-being. The ability to attend to spirituality with another requires that nurses first attend to their own spirits (Burkhardt & Nagai-Jacobson, 1997; 2000; 2002). Self-awareness, which includes appreciation of ourself as a unique body-mind-spirit being, underlies our recognition of this same wholeness in others.

Just as sustenance and care are necessary for the health of body and mind, so too does the spirit require nurture. Caring for our spirit includes mindfulness and taking time to attend to our inner being. The spirit can be nurtured in many ways, and we must each discover what our own spirit needs in order to thrive. The spirit may be nurtured through special time with friends or family, or by giving ourself alone time at home, in nature, or in some other sacred space. Attending to our need for rest, play, or creative activity are other ways to care for spirit. The spirit can be nurtured in a very profound way through sharing our story. As we become more adept at nurturing our spirits, we are better able to recognize and support this process with patients and families.

SUMMARY

Attentiveness to spiritual and cultural aspects of care with patients is an important part of holistic nursing care. The diversity of cultures and spiritual expressions within our society requires that nurses be able to identify concerns and issues in these areas and address them competently and confidently. Familiarity with values, beliefs, and practices of various cultures and religions is a useful adjunct to careful cultural and spiritual assessments with patients. Self-awareness regarding our own cultural and spiritual values, beliefs, and expressions is necessary in order to address these areas with patients. Such awareness allows us to act from our own spiritual or cultural perspectives, while taking care not to impose these views on others. In this way care planning can more readily flow from assessments that identify issues and needs regarding the patient's cultural and spiritual expressions and experiences.

CHAPTER HIGHLIGHTS

- Since culture influences beliefs and behaviours regarding health and healing, cultural assessment is integral to a comprehensive nursing assessment.

- Providing effective nursing care within the diversity of our multicultural society requires cultural competence on the part of nurses. Cultural competence can help prevent dilemmas from arising when there are differences in cultural perspective between patient and nurse.

- Complementary therapies are used by many people encountered in conventional health care settings. Nursing care is enhanced when nurses are aware of various therapies being utilized by patients. Knowledge of and working with traditional healing systems and healers can help nurses promote more culturally congruent care.

- Communication is a key factor in providing culturally congruent and spiritually sensitive care and in averting associated legal and other dilemmas.

- Health and healing are associated with that which is holy and whole. Spirituality has long been a component of healing and health care, since by nature, humans are body-mind-spirit beings.

- Grounded in a holistic view of persons, nursing care must include spirituality assessment and interventions addressing spiritual needs, recognizing that religious or spiritual perspective may influence health care choices.

- Expressions of spirituality are many and varied and may include, but are not limited to, the context of religion.

- Providing spiritual care requires that nurses be attentive to their own spirits and the spiritual concerns of patients and create an environment that is open to a variety of spiritual expressions. Nurses need to be aware of acting from their own cultural, spiritual, or religious perspectives, while not imposing these views on others.

DISCUSSION QUESTIONS AND ACTIVITIES

1. Consider how your cultural, spiritual, or religious values affect personal choices regarding health and healing. Discuss this with other students, noting similarities and differences.

2. What aspects of the culture of the health care system are difficult for you as a nurse? Identify personal conflicts and the beliefs and values underlying them.

3. Recall a time when you or someone you know experienced a conflict with persons within the health care system. What values, beliefs, or understandings contributed to this conflict?

4. Discuss with other students nonconventional therapies, or folk remedies, that you or someone you know have used. Why was the therapy used? How did you know about the therapy? Was it used in place of or along with conventional therapies? What was the outcome? What are some implications of using these kinds of therapies? Research the ethical and legal issues surrounding the use of alternative and complementary therapies through Health Canada's website: http://www.hc-sc.gc.ca/index-eng.php.

5. List ten things that nurture you spiritually. Consider how often you have done these in the past day, week, or month. Make a plan to include at least one each day for the next week.

6. Choose a religious tradition or a nonconventional therapy with which you are unfamiliar. Explore this tradition or therapy through readings and discussions with members, practitioners, or persons who have practised the religion or utilized the therapy. Share your findings with classmates.

7. Discuss how nurses can create sacred space within health care settings.

8. Discuss patient health care choices or behaviours which are based on religious beliefs that might present a dilemma for you. Consider how you would approach the situation in a professional manner and describe the ethical stance that would guide your decisions.

REFERENCES

Andrews, M. M. (1999). Cultural diversity in the health care workforce. In M. M. Andrews & J. S. Broyle, *Transcultural concepts in nursing care* (3rd ed., pp. 471–506).

Breton, J. H. (2000). Treating beyond color: Health issues for minority women. *Advance for Nurse Practitioners,* (November), 65–68, 101.

Burkhardt, M. A. (1985). Nursing, health, and wholeness. *Journal of Holistic Nursing, 3,* 35–36.

Burkhardt, M. A., & Nagai-Jacobson, M. G. (1996). Patient self-determination and complementary therapies. *Bioethics Forum, 12*(4), 24–29.

Burkhardt, M. A., & Nagai-Jacobson, M. G. (1997). Spirituality and healing. In B. M. Dossey, ed., *AHNA core curriculum for holistic nursing* (pp. 42–51). Gaithersburg, MD: Aspen.

Burkhardt, M. A., & Nagai-Jacobson, M. G. (2000). Spirituality and health. In B. M. Dossey, L. Keegan, & C. E. Guzzetta, *Holistic nursing: A handbook for practice* (3rd ed., pp. 91–122). Gaithersburg, MD: Aspen.

Burkhardt, M. A., & Nagai-Jacobson, M. G. (2002). *Spirituality and healing: Living our connectedness.* Albany, NY: Delmar Publishers.

Canadian Nurses Association. (1999). Complementary therapies—Finding the right balance. *Nursing Now* (July 1999). Retrieved July 11, 2008, from http://www.cna-nurses.ca/CNA/documents/pdf/publications/ComplimentaryTherapies_July1999_e.pdf.

Canadian Nurses Association. (2000). Cultural diversity: Changes and challenges. The Canadian Nurse. 96:2.

Canadian Nursing Association. (2008). *Code of ethics for Registered Nurses*. Ottawa: CNA.

College of Registered Nurses of Nova Scotia. (2005). *Complementary and alternative therapies: A guide for Registered Nurses*. Nova Scotia: College of Registered Nurses of Nova Scotia.

Davis, A. J. (1999). Global influence of American nursing: Some ethical issues. *Nursing Ethics: An International Journal for Health Care Professionals, 6*(2), 118–125.

Eisenberg, D. M., Kessler, R. C., Foster, C., Norlock, F. E., Calkins, D. R., & Delbanco, T. L. (1993). Unconventional medicine in the United States. *New England Journal of Medicine, 328*, 246–252.

Eisenberg, D. M., Rogers, B. D., Ettner, S., Appel, S., Wilkey, S., Van Rompay, M., & Kessler, R. C. (1998). Trends in alternative medicine use in the United States, 1990–1997. *Journal of the American Medical Association, 280*(18), 1569–1575.

Ellis, J. B., & Early, M. A. (2006). Reciprocity and constructions of informed consent: Researching with indigenous populations. *International Journal of Qualitative Methods, 5*(4), Article 1. Retrieved July 11, 2008, from http://www.ejournals.library.ualberta.ca/index.php/IJQM/article/view/4356/3803.

Engebretson, J. C., & Headley, J. A. (2000). Cultural diversity and care. In B. M. Dossey, L. Keegan, & C. E. Guzzetta, *Holistic nursing: A handbook for practice* (3rd ed., pp. 283–310). Gaithersburg, MD: Aspen.

Giger, J. N., & Davidhizar, R. E. (1995). *Transcultural nursing: Assessment and intervention* (2nd ed.). St. Louis, MO: Mosby.

_____. (1999). *Transcultural nursing: Assessment and intervention* (5th ed.). St. Louis, MD: Mosby.

Goldrosen, M. H., & Straus, S. E. (2004). Complementary and alternative medicine: Assessing the evidence for immunological benefits. *Nature Reviews Immunology, 4*(11): 912–922.

Hopkins, W. E. (1997). *Ethical dimensions of diversity*. Thousand Oaks, CA: Sage.

Hufford, D. J. (1996, January 18–21). *Ethical dimensions of alternative medicine*. Presentation at the First Annual Alternative Therapies Symposium: Creating Integrated Healthcare, San Diego, CA.

International Council of Nurses. (2006). *The ICN code of Ethics for nursing*, Geneva, Switzerland: Imprimerie Fornara.

Kavanagh, K. H. (1993). Transcultural nursing: Facing the challenges of advocacy and diversity/universality. *Journal of Transcultural Nursing, 5*, 4–13.

Leininger, M. (1991). Transcultural care principles, human rights, and ethical considerations. *Journal of Transcultural Nursing, 3*, 21–22.

Leininger, M. (2002). Culture care theory: A major contribution to advance transcultural nursing knowledge and practice. *Journal of Transcultural Nursing, 13*(3), 189–192.

Ludwick, R. & Silva, M. C. (August 14, 2000). Nursing around the world: Cultural values and ethical conflicts. *Online journal of issues in nursing*. Retrieved January 8, 2001, from http://www.nursingworld.org/ojin/ethicol/ethics_4.html.

Maier-Lorentz, M. M. (2008). Transcultural nursing: Its importance in nursing practice. *Journal of Cultural Diversity, 15*(1): 37–44.

National Council on Ageing. (2004). Definition of spiritual well-being. Retrieved July 20, 2008, from http://www.ncoa.org/content.cfm?sectionID=383&detail=394. Electronic Citation.

Neuman, B. (1989). *The Neuman systems model* (2nd ed.) Norwalk, CT: Appleton and Lange.

Nightingale, F. (1860/1969). *Notes on nursing: What it is, and what it is not.* New York: Dover Publications.

Statistics Canada. 2006 Census. Retrieved July 11, 2008, from http://www.12.statcan.ca/census-recensement/index-eng.cfm.

Tafoya, T. (1996, May). *Embracing the shadow: Mending the sacred hoop.* Paper presented at the South Texas AIDS Training (STAT) for Mental Health Providers: The Human, Transcultural, and Spiritual Dimensions of HIV/AIDS, San Antonio, TX.

Tripp-Reimer, T. (1987). Cultural assessment. In J. P. Bellak & P. A. Bamford, eds., *Nursing assessment: A multidimensional approach.* Boston: Jones & Bartlett.

University of Victoria. (2008). Cultural safety: Peoples' experiences of colonization in relation to health care. Modules 1, 2 and 3.

Waters, C. (1996). Professional development in nursing—A culturally diverse postdoctoral experience. *Image, 28,* 47–50.

Watson, J. (1988). *Nursing: Human science and human caring. A theory of nursing.* New York: National League for Nursing.

World Health Organization. (1948). Preamble to the Constitution of the World Health Organization. New York: Author.

THE POWER TO MAKE A DIFFERENCE

Part V discusses the importance of empowerment of nurses and patients. To deal with the complex issues facing nursing today, nurses are required to exercise integrity, accountability, and courage. Nurses have the responsibility, authority, and power to make principled choices. Additionally, empowerment of patients is an important element of nursing care that derives from an appreciation that patients have the ability to discern their needs and make decisions about their lives and health. Being an enabler of empowerment requires nurses to relinquish power and embrace the patient as an equal partner. Nurses can facilitate empowerment by working directly with patients and through addressing social, political, and environmental factors affecting empowerment of individuals and communities. In the midst of an ever-changing and challenging health care environment in which issues of power and control continue to affect patient care, it is imperative that nurses be both empowered and competent enablers of patient empowerment.

CHAPTER 19

Empowerment
for Nurses

Written in collaboration with Barbara C. Banonis

OBJECTIVES

After completing this chapter, the reader should be able to:

1. Describe metaphors for nursing and discuss their impact on nursing ethics.
2. Explain the impact on nursing practice of perceptions about nursing from within and outside the profession.
3. Describe the concepts of power and empowerment.

4. Discuss personal empowerment and its importance within nursing.

5. Discuss the relationship among professional empowerment, principled behaviour, and nursing practice.

6. Describe the role of diversity in empowerment.

7. Discuss the notion of whistleblowing.

INTRODUCTION

Dealing in a principled way with issues facing nursing requires integrity, accountability, and courage. Discussion of issues in this book are grounded in the belief that (1) nurses have the power to make choices and to act in responsible and principled ways, and (2) nurses have authority to make decisions and recommendations regarding activities that are within the scope of their practice. The parameters of nursing's power and authority, however, are not always clear. Many nurses feel constrained by the systems within which they work and by attitudes that promote disempowerment. They also often can feel a lack of support from within their own profession. This chapter discusses the concept of empowerment as a process through which nurses are enabled to clarify and claim their ability to make decisions regarding issues related to nursing practice. Elements of personal empowerment are addressed, and factors associated with professional empowerment are considered. The principles regarding empowerment for nurses that are discussed in this chapter apply as well to empowering patients, which is the focus of Chapter 20.

INFLUENCES ON NURSING'S PERCEPTIONS OF PRINCIPLED PRACTICE

Nurses, patients, and other health care providers may vary greatly in their perceptions of ideals for nursing and nursing practice. These perceptions influence expectations and decisions regarding care, authority, and accountability. Expectations regarding good nursing care or taking an ethical stance flow from such perceptions. We recognize that factors in our internal and external environments affect both personal and professional decision making. External environment factors include norms, ideals, and expectations of patients, families, other health care providers, and the professional and social systems within which we interact. The internal environment includes our *mind set* or our personal beliefs and perceptions.

Influence of Mindsets

Aroskar suggests that our mindsets, that is, our views and beliefs about the health care system, influence how we identify and respond to ethical issues and dilemmas in practice. For example, when nurses view health care in terms of medical cases focused on the cure of disease, the physician may be seen as the dominant authority. Following physician's orders (whether or not the nurse agrees with them) and blind loyalty to the physician and institution are considered legitimate and ethical focus of nursing activities in this kind of a model. Aroskar states that "this mind set may well impede efforts to achieve more ethical practice which requires critical, reflective thinking and challenges the decision-making structure of the present system" (1982, p. 26). If nurses view health care as a commodity in which nursing and medical care are "consumed" by clients or consumers of health care, the nurse's primary responsibility is to the employing institution. Within this view, needs of individual patients may be subordinated to the utilitarian goal focused on the good of the greatest number of people or the institutional goal of making a profit or meeting targets. Nurses who hold this view may not challenge the rightness or wrongness of nursing actions, provided they are congruent with goals and policies of the institution. When nurses view health care as a basic human need and a right for each person, the nurse's primary responsibility is to the patient. The legitimate and ethical focus of nursing activities within this mindset must include attention to patient rights, safety, and overall well-being.

Metaphors of Nursing

Metaphors help us to understand a concept by comparing two things that are different yet share common characteristics. People often use *metaphors* to focus attention on particular aspects of reality in order to enhance understandings of roles, events, and experiences. Metaphors may also influence our perceptions of these events and experiences. For example, likening nurses to *angels in white* calls attention to nursing roles of caring, protecting, and serving; yet viewing nurses as angels may set up the expectation that they be somewhat distant and above human frailties. Metaphors that have been associated with nursing reflect different ideas about nursing roles and responsibilities in health care. These metaphors also suggest different approaches to determining an appropriate ethical stance for nursing care delivery.

Winslow discusses the impact on nursing ethics of a shift from a military metaphor for nursing, which stresses loyalty, to a legal metaphor for nursing as advocate for patient rights. The military metaphor is associated with obedience to higher authority, a view of disease as the enemy, discipline, respect for those of higher rank, uniform dress, and, above all, loyalty. Winslow notes that "loyalty meant refusal to criticize the nurse's hospital or training school, fellow nurses, and most importantly, the physician under whom the nurse worked . . . being loyal to the physician by preserving the patient's confidence was the same as being loyal to the patient" (1984, p. 33). Ethical imperatives that flow from this metaphor include following physician orders, even if the nurse questions their appropriateness; upholding the patient's faith in the physician, even if the nurse questions the doctor's competence; and being loyal to health care colleagues, even at the expense of the patient.

In the early history of nursing, following the physician's order without question would have absolved the nurse from guilt, even in the event of a harmful outcome for the patient. Today, however, this is not the case. Nursing's move from vocation to profession requires that nurses be accountable for their actions. Court rulings have held nurses legally responsible for their decisions and actions. Legal decisions, changes in the health care delivery system, and feminist awarenesses within the nursing profession have encouraged the transition from the metaphor of loyal soldier to that of patient advocate. Winslow (1984) notes that a significant revision in nursing's self-image began in the 1960s and 1970s. Greater emphasis on consumerism and patient rights, coupled with growing dissatisfaction with increased costs and depersonalization of health care, helped to open the door for nurses to expand their roles as patient advocates. As advocates for patient rights, nurses are responsible to those who require nursing care. Current nursing codes and standards that stress responsibility to patients through collegial membership in the health team reflect ethical imperatives flowing from the metaphor of advocacy.

Loyalty remains a valued virtue for nurses within the advocacy metaphor. Although ideally the nurse's first loyalty is to the patient, circumstances of conflicting loyalty may occur. Loyalty to colleagues and to employers is also important, and nurses may at times be faced with making difficult decisions between advocacy for patients or loyalty to colleagues. Such situations require personal integrity, knowledge, and courage on the part of the nurse.

How nurses picture nursing and the vision they hold of their role in health care influences their ability to practise in a holistic, patient-focused way. Nursing's self-image is evident in metaphors nurses use to describe their roles and their practice. In studying metaphors nurses use to capture their experience of nursing, Hartrick and Schreiber (1998) discovered a wide variety of images reflecting the tasks and responsibilities of nursing; the pivotal role nurses play in the system; the experience of empowerment and powerlessness; personal development and discovery; and the relational and caring nature of nursing. They note that the images of nursing reflected in these metaphors illuminate the complexities and ambiguities of nursing practice. These images highlight as well the influence of social, organizational, and cultural constraints on nurses. These constraints often prompt nurses to feel unable to practise nursing in a way that is consistent with their values.

❓ Think About It

Two years after completing her degree, Tonisha is a young charge nurse on a busy cardiac surgery unit. Tonight one of the postoperative patients, Mr. M, is having difficulty with producing urine—a common problem after cardiac surgery. Sonam, the new graduate nurse looking after Mr. M, upon examination, notes that his bladder is full. She calls the resident, who is in the operating room. Over the phone, the resident tells Sonam to insert a foley catheter and do an in-and-out catheterization to empty the patient's bladder. Sonam carefully takes the order down and checks it with Tonisha.

Five minutes later, Sonam is at the unit desk, nearly in tears. She tells Tonisha that Mr. M refused to have her catheterize him. He insisted that only a physician could do that and said to Sonam that nurses aren't smart or skilled enough to insert a foley catheter. He also insisted that she was "too young of a nurse" to do skilled

(Continued)

work. Sonam explained that catheterization is in fact a nursing skill, that she has had a great deal of experience with foley catheterization, and that the resident was unavailable. Even if available, the resident would not carry out a routine catheterization. The patient still refused, insisting that nurses should be only "giving out pills that the doctor orders, taking blood pressures, and giving bed baths."

- How can Tonisha best support Sonam at this point?
- Should the physician be called to insert the catheter? Why or why not?
- What should Sonam do next? What should Tonisha do next?
- What kinds of things might be influencing Mr. M's perceptions about nursing?
- What is the most realistic outcome in this situation? What about the most ideal outcome?

How Nursing Is Perceived by Others

Factors such as mindsets and metaphors influence our perceptions of and choices regarding principled behaviour. Perceptions of others also affect our considerations regarding appropriate or ethical nursing actions. Although nursing as a profession has claimed the metaphor of advocate in lieu of that of loyal soldier, many nurses within the profession have not fully embraced the change. As well, awareness of nursing's current professional imperatives is often lacking among patients, families, physicians, and health care administrators. The role of nursing as perceived by many outside the profession remains embedded in the loyal soldier metaphor, and health care as medical cases or commodity mindsets. The hierarchical, patriarchal system remains the norm in many health care institutions. Since physicians are perceived to be of higher rank, their influence often holds more sway than that of nurses who may challenge them. Although patients and families often have more continual and direct contact with nurses, they may not fully understand that the nurse is their advocate. Instead, they often function from the mindset that the physician is the captain of a ship in which the nurse is a member of the crew. Images in the media that depict nurses in ancillary, subordinate roles also affect perceptions of patients and others regarding expectations of nurses.

Kalisch and Kalisch (1982) surveyed various media outlets for images of nurses portrayed over a century. From the collection of references and images that they collected, they categorized the images of nurses into five distinct groups which reflect five successive time periods: "The Angel of Mercy," "The Girl Friday," "The Heroine," "The Mother," and "The Sex Object."

The "Angel of Mercy" (mid-1800s until early 1900s) refers to an image that is noble, virtuous, and based strongly in religion. This image persisted through the First World War, in which nurses were first portrayed as heroic, noble, and strongly rooted in service to others. The "Girl Friday" (~1920–1930) was an image of nursing with less emphasis on the nobility and strength of a professional nurse and more attention to the nurse's role as subservient, dedicated, and highly cooperative. This image was reflective of the lack of nursing education standards, the strong link between hospitals and schools of nursing, and the use of nurses and nursing students as simply labour to staff hospitals.

With the rise of the motion picture industry in the 1930s and 1940s, the image of nursing was glamorized and nurses were portrayed in the movies as the adventurous and independent "Heroine." As the Second World War progressed, the image of the nurse as a heroine was intensified by positive images of nurses on recruitment posters and propaganda. With the end of the war, North American culture experienced a strongly conservative trend, valuing the traditional family and the return of married women and mothers to the home. At this time, the image of nurses reflected this, as nurses were portrayed as "The Mother": Maternal, domestic, and more passive.

With the 1960s came the sexual revolution and the civil rights movement. Images of women across all contexts were changing and so were images of nurses, portrayed as more sexual objects at this time. This image has persisted as many negative and highly sexualized images of nurses still exist today.

Kalisch and Kalisch, however, go one step further. While noting both the positive and negative aspects of the five images they describe, they also note a more ideal image, that, to some degree, captures elements of the images they identified. This image, also known as the "Careerist" is embraced by many professional groups in Canada. The image of the nurse as career professional, embodying accountability, empathy, intelligence, and progressiveness is one that many nurse educators strive to communicate to the public at large and to student nurses, who often are struggling with their own self-image against the stereotypical images of nursing that persist.

UNDERSTANDING POWER AND EMPOWERMENT

Nurses have the power to make a difference by acting in principled ways in all areas of their lives and practice. However, as has been evident throughout the discussions in this book, many factors mitigate against nurses claiming this power. Gordon and Buresh (2000) note that nursing, as a profession, although the largest group of health care professionals, is still markedly invisible and silent. In health care forums across the country, the voice of nursing is largely unheard. A larger and related concern is the lack of public knowledge about just what it is nurses do in their work. While the public continues to hold nursing in high esteem, deeming nurses as some of the most trusted professionals, members of the public have little knowledge about the kind of work that nurses do. Furthermore, as a profession, we have only begun to understand how to publicize our work and attend to our image as a profession. Nurses need to develop skills in communication, empowerment, and acting collectively in order to function fully in their legitimate roles within health care and optimize their professional capabilities and roles. Nurses must be aware of values, beliefs, and other factors affecting personal decision making, and expand their knowledge of ethical principles, legal considerations, and issues facing nursing. Understanding **power** and **empowerment** can help in developing strategies for action in this regard.

Although the word *"power"* is often understood in terms of strength, force, or control, a primary dictionary definition of the term, derived from its Latin root "potere," is "the ability to do or act, capability of doing or accomplishing something" (*The Random House Dictionary of the English Language*, 1987). To have power, then, implies having the ability to do or act; and to *"empower"* would be to facilitate the ability of another person to do or to act.

Rodwell suggests that empowerment is a "helping process whereby groups of individuals are enabled to change a situation, given skills, resources, opportunities and authority to do so. It is a partnership which respects and values self and others—aiming to develop positive beliefs in self and the future" (1996, p. 309). Similarly, Ellis-Stoll and Popkess-Vawter (1998) describe empowerment as a participative process, or partnership between a nurse and patient, which is designed to assist in changing unhealthy behaviours. This partnership is viewed by some as a social process of recognizing, promoting, and enhancing patients' abilities to meet their own needs, solve their own problems, and mobilize the necessary resources in order to feel in control of their own lives (Connelly, Keele, Kleinbeck, Schneider, & Cobb, 1993; Fulton, 1997). Bolton & Brookings (1998) describe empowerment as the capacity of disenfranchised people to understand and become active participants in the matters that affect their lives, suggesting that a personal attitude that change is possible is important for empowerment to occur. Gurka (1995) reflects that empowerment is a philosophy or world view flowing from belief in each person's inherent worth and process of self-discovery that involves creating a vision, taking risks, making choices, and behaving in authentic ways. Empowerment requires respect for an individual's personal beliefs and goals and trust in the person's ability to make decisions, take action, and be accountable for the actions. Although sharing of knowledge through education is important for empowerment, the literature clearly indicates that emotional and social support is essential as well.

In-depth analyses of the concept suggests that empowerment is both process and outcome, taking different forms within different people and contexts (Gibson, 1991; Hawks, 1992; Rodwell, 1996; Ellis-Stoll & Popkess-Vawter, 1998; Ryles, 1999). Because of this, empowerment needs to be defined by the people concerned. Empowerment is a transactional process involving relationship with others. This relationship includes mutually beneficial interactions aimed at strengthening rather than weakening; power sharing through mutual sharing of knowledge, resources, and opportunities; and respect for self and others. Empowerment is nurtured by collaborative efforts that focus on solutions rather than problems, and on strengths, rights, and abilities rather than deficits. Empowerment derives from a feminine perspective of *power with* or *power to*, which implies sharing responsibility, knowledge, and resources; collaboration for goal achievement; incorporating diversity; valuing the contributions of each person; and valuing the process. In contrast is the masculine view of *power over* that incorporates a sense of paternalistic control, struggle for and protection of limited resources, separation of leaders and followers, expediency, and results even at the expense of persons (Chinn, 1995).

Empowerment can seem like a rather abstract term, and you may be wondering what being empowered looks and feels like. Certainly, two people in the same circumstances can have different experiences of empowerment. Nurse scholars use a variety of descriptive terms when discussing people who are empowered. These include *positive self-concept, personal satisfaction, self-efficacy, sense of mastery regarding self and the environment, sense of control, sense of connectedness, self-development, feeling of hope, the ability to make changes, self-determination, action orientation, authority, autonomy, capability of social intercourse, caring, choosing, self-confidence, courage, decision-making ability, emancipatory power, endurance, expertise, freedom, influence, instrumental exercise of power, participation, resilience, rights, self-control, solidarity, strength, sturdiness, taking a position, assertiveness, coercion, enabling,* and *freedom to make choices* (Bolton & Brookings, 1998; Byrne, 1999; Chavasse, 1992; Connelly, Keele, Kleinbeck, Schneider, & Cobb, 1993; Ellis-Stoll & Popkess-Vawter, 1998; Fulton, 1997; Hartrick & Schreiber, 1998; Hawks, 1992; Jones, O'Toole, Hoa, Chau, & Muc, 2000; Klakovich, 1995; Kuokkanen & Leino-Kilpi, 2000; Laschinger, Wong, McMahon, & Kaufmann, 1999; Rodwell, 1996; Ryles, 1999; Wallerstein & Bernstein, 1988). Although not all of these attributes are necessarily part of every experience of empowerment, they provide markers that help us identify the process and presence of empowerment.

Empowerment implies choice on the part of those being empowered. We cannot empower another, because to presume to do so removes the element of choice. Individuals and groups must ultimately motivate and empower themselves. This process requires self-awareness, positive self-esteem, commitment to self and others, and the desire and ability to make decisions. Responsibility and accountability for our actions and having the authority to act are implicit in the ability to choose.

Through the empowerment process, we can enable others to develop awareness of areas that need change, foster a desire to take action, and share resources, skills, and opportunities that support the change. Rodwell (1996) notes that it is self-awareness and resources, rather than the services provided to persons, that self-empower. Enhanced self-esteem, personal satisfaction, sense of connectedness, the ability to set and reach goals, a sense of control over life and change processes, and a sense of hope and direction are outcomes of empowerment.

Ask Yourself

What Makes You Feel Empowered?

- Consider a situation in which you felt empowered. Describe factors contributing to your sense of empowerment.

- Recall a time when you felt disempowered. What contributed to this sense? How might you have felt more empowered in the situation?

(Continued)

- Nursing students often feel disempowered by virtue of their position relative to instructors, faculty members, and Registered Nurses with whom they work. Reflect on your own experience as a student nurse. What made you feel disempowered? What helped you to feel better supported and empowered?

- Patients often describe feelings of disempowerment as a result of feeling that health care practitioners are acting in a paternalistic or overly protective manner, or as a result of feeling uninformed or left out of decision-making processes. Reflect on the way in which you interact with patients. Do you approach patients in a way that includes them in decisions, keeps them informed, and allows them the freedom to articulate and explore what they consider to be their best interests?

- Reflect on a patient care situation in which a patient required extra time and information from you in order to help make a decision regarding their care and you were rushed, impatient, and unable to take the time to spend with the patient. How do you think the patient felt?

- Look at your own work conditions. Do you have input into the environment and milieu of the unit or agency in which you work? Are you able to provide feedback about decisions that will affect patient care or your own satisfaction with your practice? Are you allowed some degree of autonomy in how you choose to approach day-to-day situations as well as more significant issues?

PERSONAL EMPOWERMENT

Nursing's power to make a difference in care with patients derives from many factors. In order to serve as credible models of empowerment for others, we must demonstrate congruence between values and behaviours in our own lives. Personal integrity implies an ability to be honest with and care for ourselves, as well as respond to the needs of others. Often nurses, and especially women, have learned to value care for others before or instead of care for self. A true value for human life must include value for our own life as well. We must attend to ourselves and treat ourselves with the same respect and dignity as we treat others. Personal empowerment begins with actions that support the meeting of our own needs and self-actualization. It is from our personal stores of creativity, empowerment, and health that we are able to inspire, teach, and assist others in achieving their potential.

In principle many nurses would agree with the concept of care for self; however, actions often conflict with this acknowledged belief. Nurses often agree to work additional hours even when they are exhausted; consume large amounts of caffeine and sugar to boost waning energy; go home to care for children, spouse, and friends; and collapse into bed only to get up and do it all again the next day because they feel limited power to do otherwise. What causes a person to behave in a way that conflicts with their stated values? Often the person has learned conflicting messages. A belief in caring for ourselves may conflict with a learned belief that caring for others is more admirable or important than caring for ourselves. Many people find that they have feelings of guilt if they are not putting others ahead of themselves. We emphasize the idea of a fiduciary duty for health care professionals who are caring for patients. This duty, when considered in the context of health care, encompasses the notion of putting others' needs ahead of our own. Many nurses, women, and men are socialized to put others' needs before their own needs. While it is notably admirable to care for others ahead of oneself, doing so disproportionately or while neglecting oneself is neither constructive nor healthy and will ultimately result in an inability to provide competent or thoughtful care to others.

Some people feel very little control over any area of their lives. Others may feel empowered to make decisions in some situations but not in others—for example, a person may actively make decisions in the home environment while feeling like a pawn of the system at work. The sense of power that nurses have in their personal lives may affect their perception of empowerment in the professional arena and vice versa. Burnout, job dissatisfaction, and limited professional commitment affect the quality of patient care, and are often associated with feelings of powerlessness (Moss, 1995). Attributes of empowerment noted in the previous section reflect important considerations for self-empowerment on both personal and professional levels.

The ability to facilitate empowerment in others requires us to attend to personal empowerment. This means valuing ourselves and "listening inwardly to your own senses as well as listening intently and actively to others, consciously taking in and forming strength" (Chinn, 1995, p. 3). Self-awareness is necessary, since self-perception has a direct link to quality of patient care (Moss, 1995). Such awareness requires attentiveness to factors that influence our thoughts, feelings, actions, and reactions in the present circumstance and reflective considerations of such influences on past experiences as well as an ability to critically look toward the future.

Self-awareness of this kind involves recognizing old or repetitive thought patterns and changing those that are no longer supporting a creative, actualizing life. Extreme self-criticism, being overly judgmental of self or others, and engaging in consistent negative thinking can be particularly confining or limiting, in terms of self actualization. Old thinking can be updated with new knowledge. Questioning the origin of particular thoughts can reveal ideas that were true at one time but are no longer true. For example, a child who was always told that she did not know enough to make a decision, and that mother knew best, may become an adult who still consults her mother before making decisions. Seeking alternative views of situations, and learning logical or critical thinking skills, are other ways to restructure thought patterns.

Feelings are transient signals that alert us to what is positive or objectionable in a situation. Owning our feelings means acknowledging and exploring the reasons that we might be reacting in a particular way, rather than blaming other persons or situations for our feelings. People may experience different feelings in similar situations. For example, a grave diagnosis may elicit a variety of feelings in different persons. Some reactions might include fear, panic, trepidation, or extreme anxiety. Others may elicit feelings of despair or disbelief. Some may describe feelings of resignation, powerlessness, or anger. Still others may even demonstrate feelings of hope, relief, or feeling a sense of direction in their life. Feelings and reactions are as diverse as the persons who have them. While events may be triggers of certain feelings, it is important to note that feelings are elicited *within the person* and not *within the event*.

It is important to try to articulate and take ownership of personal values and, in doing so, claim our ability to make choices. When experiencing a lack of control in life, we should identify both internal and external barriers to having control, consider the degree of control we wish to have, and explore what we need to do and are willing to risk in order to exercise some degree of control. Consciously acting based upon clear evaluation of the current situation, rather than acting automatically, is one way to own our behaviour. Taking ownership of behaviour requires being able to see options and being realistic about those options. Believing there are no viable options can result in feeling powerless, trapped, or victimized. Even when we do not believe we can change a current unacceptable situation immediately, we can make a plan for change and set that plan into motion one step at a time. A *victim* waits and hopes something or someone else will change; makes excuses for not taking action (time, cost, fatigue, and the like); blames people, places, or things for the situation; and is trapped and unaware of options. An *empowered person* decides to be accountable for personal responses, makes plans, considers options, develops strategies for change, and acts on plans by doing what is necessary to succeed. Even in a situation in which it may be impossible to exercise control or have access to realistic options, empowered persons are able to reflect on what they have learned from a situation or event and prospectively consider how such a situation might be approached differently in the future.

Personal empowerment "is growth of personal strength, power, and ability to enact one's own will and love for self in the context of love and respect for others . . . [and] is only possible when individuals express respect and reverence for all other forms of life and ground the energy of the Self as one with the earth" (Chinn, 1995, p. 3). A commitment to personal growth and self-care, developing a positive sense of self, awareness of strengths and abilities as well as limitations, and drawing on our supports and sources of connectedness foster this process. It is essential that we trust ourselves and our knowledge and abilities and are courageous in taking risks. Empathy with others, appreciation of diversity, tolerance, flexibility, and willingness to compromise empower a person. Empowerment requires being true to ourselves and our values while respecting the diverse choices of others.

PROFESSIONAL EMPOWERMENT

Professional empowerment is built upon the foundational elements of personal accountability and support of nursing colleagues. In order to deal in a principled way with issues and dilemmas arising within health care settings, nurses must feel personally and professionally empowered to act on sometimes difficult choices. Many factors affect nursing actions in the professional arena, including personal attitudes and self-concept; the structural and functional interrelatedness of health care systems; political, economic, and social forces; and interactions with patients and colleagues.

Barriers to empowerment exist within the community of nursing and are also imposed from external sources. Curtin reminds us that "many nurses are unwilling to assume responsibility for decision making and that nursing has failed to develop an adequate support system for nurses" (1982, p. 10).

Empowerment requires nurses to become knowledgeable about and address system issues as well as interpersonal issues. Such issues include recognizing the need for changing the power base within the current health care system, moving from a paternalistic, hierarchical model of control toward one that values collaboration, and the power of the collective. Nurses must become involved in shared decision making and in being involved in the formation of institutional policies as part of this process (Chandler, 1991; Gaul, 1995; Moss, 1995).

The effect of nurses' empowerment in the health care environment can have personal, institutional, and patient care implications. In terms of nursing management and health systems, some authors view empowerment as a method for delegating authority and sharing power and a strategy for improving productivity of nurses. Laschinger and colleagues (1999) report that empowered nurses are more likely to initiate and sustain independent behaviours to accomplish task objectives in the face of difficulty, thereby increasing work effectiveness. One study suggests a link between staff nurses' perceptions of their work effectiveness and workplace empowerment (Laschinger and Wong, 1999). The authors identify three factors that have a positive impact on empowerment: access to the structures of information, support, and resource. Moss (1995) relates empowerment to increased efficiency, job satisfaction, and better patient care. In contrast, Moss notes that feelings of powerlessness are associated with job dissatisfaction and low levels of professional commitment, which are barriers to quality patient care. This author links nurses' perceptions of themselves to quality of patient care, reflecting that nurses who are burned out and dissatisfied are more inclined to give only the most routine care. Klakovich (1995) proposes that only an empowered work force can be effective in today's recent innovations of patient-focused care and shared governance. Inherent in this perspective is a sense that each person is free to make choices, and that those who are empowered, both internally and by the system, feel more in control of their lives, are able to act in appropriate, meaningful ways and to do what they truly want to do.

A related concept is the notion of emancipation actions in nursing, described by Kendall (1992). Some feel that this is an extension of the concept of empowerment. Derived from work by Habermas and others, the notion of emancipatory nursing refers to not just helping those who might be oppressed, marginalized, or disenfranchised to cope with the difficulties or challenges in their lives, but to fight back against the socially constructed barriers that oppress them. Acting in an advocacy role by simply facilitating coping with difficulties is not enough, according to Kendall. Instead, this new type of empowered caring involves "living, teaching, encouraging and activating emancipatory behaviors, rather than relying heavily on the concepts of coping and adaptation" (Kendall, p. 2).

Nevertheless, nurses can and do feel disempowered in their work settings, and instead of feeling empowered or enacting emancipatory nursing actions, they may choose the *victim* stance, which relinquishes power to the system, or they can challenge the system. Dealing with the system requires skills in conflict management, negotiation, and effective communication. Challenging the system can take many forms. Being a change agent begins with the nurse's personal presence and attitude. For example, one nurse described how her commitment to caring for the whole person was challenged when she began working in a level III trauma centre. Feeling constantly criticized by co-workers as she incorporated emotional and spiritual support into her care, she made the choice to act out of her values as a holistic nurse and return a loving spirit to the injustice of their criticism. She noted that this choice came as a great challenge, and that it was often difficult to go to work under the scrutiny focused in her direction. However, she used each opportunity of conversation to suggest that they work together to unite the staff with an attitude of mutual caring, support, and nurturance. Her presence was reflected in her choice to stand in her power and speak her truth. Although this was not easy, living her values contributed to a change in attitude within the whole staff, particularly regarding how they supported and cared for each other.

Nurses can address social and economic constraints on nursing and health care through their involvement in professional organizations and through becoming politically active. Participation on institution boards or committees that focus on patient care and professional practice concerns is another way to challenge the system, as is speaking out about unsafe or questionable practices. Speaking out is sometimes referred to as **whistleblowing**. However, speaking out or challenging the status quo is not always the same as whistle-blowing. The term "whistleblowing" comes from the image of someone blowing a shrill whistle, loud enough to jolt others away from the "false harmony" (Ray, 2006, p. 438) of the status quo, to attend to perceived inequities, incompetence, abuse or danger, usually within or from outside an organization or hierarchy.

Whistleblowing should always be a last resort when looking at ways to deal with unsafe, unethical, illegal, or challenging practices in the workplace i.e., when all other legitimate ways of approaching a problem have failed. Whistleblowing is not without risks, as well as significant physical and emotional side effects for those who may choose this method to speak out. In one nursing study, stress-induced effects were noted in both nurses who chose to blow the whistle as well as those who did not choose to do so in dealing with a difficult situation (McDonald, 2002). It is not surprising that simply being involved in a situation in which one identifies as potentially dangerous or unethical can induce feelings similar to any stressful situation; however, these things and others must be taken into account before one decides to "blow the whistle."

The Canadian Nurses Association notes that whistleblowing should be considered only after all other ways of addressing a problem have been tried. They continue, stating that there might be a moral right on behalf of nurses to disclose cases of public harm and, in some cases, even a moral obligation to do so. The association also notes that having a right to speak up does not imply that one ought to then engage in whistleblowing (Baker, 1988). Three things must be explored prior to making the decision to engage in whistleblowing. First, there must be serious harm or potential harm to the public involved. Second, one must have reported the problem, issue, or events appropriately through the hierarchy of one's organization. Finally, and most importantly, perhaps, the whistleblower must be convinced or have evidence that the act of speaking out in this manner will likely result in positive or desired change (Baker, 1988).

Empowerment incorporates divergent and conflicting solutions to problems based on value in support of others rather than in divisiveness (Chinn, 1995; Gibson, 1991). It implies embracing diversity and moving from fear of that which is different to appreciation of the strength derived from and unity contained in diversity. Nurses need to recognize that systems exert control, in part, by fostering divisiveness among workers in order to deter unity of opposition to system policies. When nurses unite with and support colleagues who challenge harmful or potentially harmful practices, they are personally and professionally empowered.

Challenging unjust, unprofessional, or unethical practices is not an easy decision, and may entail risk for nurses. Feeling empowered to take a stand requires personal integrity and support from others. Before whistleblowing, consider the following:

- Determine if you are ready, both personally and professionally, to take action through personal reflection and consultation with others.

- Consult a lawyer or your professional association for legal advice.

- Use a journal to document instances that give you concern and that compromise care, creating a paper trail that includes dates, times, and outcomes of unsafe or inappropriate care. Make a copy of all documentation and keep all electronic communication.

- Remember when communicating by email to never make any statements you would not want attributed to you on the front page of any newspaper.

- Speak only the truth, state only the facts, and follow the institution's chain of command to the letter before contacting an outside agency.

- Build leadership skills and unity among your colleagues.

- Most of all, contribute to developing a strong sense of ethical integrity in your nursing community. Pay attention to issues of inequity or threats to others' integrity, find places to initiate discussions about ethical and practical challenges, and create safe places to voice concerns.

Nurses need to be willing to struggle with difficult questions and arrive at decisions that flow from their internal values and perspective, rather than looking for the *right* answer from an external source. Empowerment implies accountability for our own choices and actions. Jameton (1984) reflects that people pretend they are forced to do things when they are not. He gives the example of a nurse who instructs a patient to take a medication because the physician ordered it, noting that both patient and nurse pretend that they must act because of the physician's order, although each could make another choice. Reflecting that nurses who choose to work in systems such as hospitals are accountable for their actions despite the existence of systemic problems affecting health care, Jameton writes,

> If one fails to resist exploitation, incompetence, and corrupt practices, one becomes responsible for them. If one resists them, one enters

into conflict with conventional conceptions of behavior for employees and thereby risks reprisals. One has to choose between complic-
ity and self-sacrifice, or enter the uncomfortable middle ground of
irony. Ethics does not give a clear answer as to which one must
choose. Instead, one is free to move in the direction of the kind of
world one personally desires to create. (1984, p. 289)

We must decide whether we prefer a world in which we are empowered in the professional arena, or one in which we are controlled by others. The choices we make
influence the outcome.

SUMMARY

Empowerment is a multifaceted concept. Awareness of attitudes about nursing's role
in health care and factors that shape these attitudes enables nurses to identify more
effectively that which supports or diminishes both personal and professional empowerment. Attentiveness to personal empowerment, which includes integrity, accountability, and courage, is foundational for addressing empowerment issues within the
profession. No one can empower another. However, we can facilitate the inner process
of empowerment when knowledge and resources are offered within an environment
of mutual respect and support. Empowerment for nurses requires remembering *who*
we are, recognizing that *knowing* must be the same as *doing*, and following our own
vision of nursing.

CHAPTER HIGHLIGHTS

- Mindsets regarding health care influence how nurses identify and respond to
  ethical issues and dilemmas in practice settings.
- Nursing's contemporary self-perception reflects the legal metaphor of patient
  advocate rather than the military metaphor of loyal soldier. Each of these
  metaphors implies different ethical imperatives for nursing.
- Current nursing codes and standards of practice reflect ethical imperatives that
  flow from the advocacy metaphor.
- Empowerment, which is both process and outcome, derives from a feminine perspective of *power to* or *power with*, reflecting a supportive partnership based on
  mutual love and respect that enables people to change situations given necessary resources, knowledge, skills, and opportunities. Empowerment comes from
  within a person and involves choice; we cannot empower another.
- The ability to deal with health care issues and dilemmas in a principled way
  derives from personal and professional empowerment and requires attentiveness
  to intrapersonal, interpersonal, and systems issues.
- Personal empowerment requires self-awareness and is characterized by maintaining personal integrity in the midst of a loving response to the choices of others.
  Self-concept and sense of power in a nurse's personal life affects nursing care
  and a nurse's ability to enable empowerment in others.

- Recognizing unity in diversity and incorporating divergent views and solutions empowers nurses and others.
- Defining nursing according to nursing's own vision is an act of empowerment that implies accountability for our own choices and actions, with awareness that each choice helps create the kind of world and environment within which nurses must practise.

DISCUSSION QUESTIONS AND ACTIVITIES

1. Talk with both retired and practising nurses about ethical imperatives that guide (or guided) their nursing practice. Identify mind sets and metaphors reflective of these imperatives.

2. Where in your life do you feel most or least personally empowered? Discuss the circumstances surrounding your feelings of empowerment with other students.

3. Review Chapters 5 and 6 and reflect on how your values and current phase of development affect your sense of personal empowerment.

4. Describe a situation in which you took responsibility for your own feelings or actions. Describe a time when you found yourself blaming others or assuming a victim stance. Discuss with classmates factors prompting each stance and how you felt in each situation.

5. What aspects of empowerment do you think are most important in nursing practice settings? Support your perspective.

6. Interview practising nurses regarding personal and professional power, including situations where they feel empowered to make decisions, where they derive authority to make decisions, and situations in which they have experienced dilemmas around the issue of power. Ask them to describe their ideal image of nursing and compare that to their current reality.

REFERENCES

Aroskar, M. A. (1982). Are nurses' mind sets compatible with ethical practice? *Topics in Clinical Nursing, 4*, 22–32.

Baker, J. (1988). Confidentiality and when to blow the whistle. As cited in Ethics in Practice. Canadian Nurses Association. November 1999. C.N.A.: Ottawa.

Bolton, B., & Brookings, J. (1998). Development of a measure of intrapersonal empowerment. *Rehabilitation Psychology, 43*(2), 131–142.

Byrne, C. (1999). Facilitating empowerment groups: Dismantling professional boundaries. *Issues in Mental Health Nursing, 19*, 55–71.

Chandler, G. E. (1991). Creating an environment to empower nurses. *Nursing Management, 22*, 20–23.

Chavasse, J. M. (1992). New dimensions of empowerment in nursing—and challenges. *Journal of Advanced nursing, 17*, 1–2.

Chinn, P. (1995). *Peace and power: Building communities for the future.* New York: National League of Nursing Press.

Connelly, L. M., Keele, B. S., Kleinbeck, V. M., Schneider, J. K., & Cobb, A. K. (1993). A place to be yourself: Empowerment from the client's perspective. *IMAGE: Journal of Nursing Scholarship, 25*(4), 297–303.

Curtin, L. (1982). Autonomy, accountability and nursing practice. *Topics in Clinical Nursing, 4*, 7–14.

Curtin, L. (1996). *Nursing into the 21st century.* Springhouse, PA: Springhouse.

Ellis-Stoll, C. C., & Popkess-Vawter, S. (1998). A concept analysis on the process of empowerment. *Advances in Nursing Science, 21*(2), 62–68.

Fulton, Y. (1997). Nurses' views on empowerment: A critical social theory perspective. *Journal of Advanced Nursing, 26*, 529–536.

Gibson, C. H. (1991). A concept analysis of empowerment. *Journal of Advanced Nursing, 16*, 354–361.

Gordon, S., & Buresh, B. (2000). From silence to voice: What nurses know and must communicate to the public. Canadian Nurses Association: Ottawa.

Gurka, A. M. (1995). Transformational leadership: Qualities and strategies for the CNS. *Clinical Nurse Specialist, 9*, 169–174.

Habermas, J. (1971). *Knowledge and Human Interests.* Boston: Beacon Press.

Hartrick, G., & Schreiber, R. (1998). Imaging ourselves: Nurses' metaphors of practice. *Journal of Holistic Nursing, 16*(4), 420–434.

Hawks, J. H. (1992). Empowerment in nursing education: Concept analysis and application to philosophy, learning and instruction. *Journal of Advanced Nursing, 17,* 609–618.

Jameton, A. (1984). *Nursing practice: The ethical issues.* Englewood Cliffs, NJ: Prentice-Hall.

Jones, P. S., O'Toole, M. T., Hoa, N., Chau, T. T., & Muc, P. D. (2000). Empowerment of nursing as a socially significant profession in Vietnam. *Journal of Nursing Scholarship, 32*(3), 317–321.

Kalisch, B., & Kalisch, P. (1982). Anatomy of the image of the nurse: Dissonant and ideal models. In C. Williams (Ed.), Image-making in nursing (pp. 3–23). American Academy of Nursing: Kansas City.

Kendall, J. (1992). Fighting back: Emancipatory nursing actions. *Advances in Nursing Science. 15*(2): 1–15.

Klakovich, M. (1995). Development and psychometric evaluation of the reciprocal empowerment scale. *Journal of Nursing Management, 3*(2), 127–143.

Kuokkanen, L., & Leino-Kilpi, H. (2000). Power and empowerment in nursing: Three theoretical approaches. *Journal of Advanced Nursing, 31*(1), 235–241.

Laschinger, H. K., & Wong, C. (1999). Staff nurse empowerment and collective accountability: Effect on perceived productivity and self-rated work effectiveness. *Nursing Economics, 17*(6), 308–316.

Laschinger, H. K., Wong, C., McMahon, L., & Kaufmann, C. (1999). Leader behavior impact on staff nurse empowerment, job tension, and work effectiveness. *JONA, 29*(5), 28–39.

McDonald, S. (2002). Physical and emotional effects of whistle blowing. *Journal of Psychosocial Nursing & Mental Health Services, 40*(1), 14–27. Retrieved September 6, 2008, from ProQuest Nursing & Allied Health Source database. (Document ID: 103437026).

Moss, M. T. (1995). Foundations of nursing empowerment. *Nursing Economics, 13*, 112–114.

Random House dictionary of the English language, second edition unabridged. (1987). New York: Random House.

Ray. S. (2006). Whistle-blowing and organizational ethics. *Nursing ethics, 13*(4): 438–445.

Rodwell, C. M. (1996). An analysis of the concept of empowerment. *Journal of Advanced Nursing, 23*, 305–313.

Ryles, S. M. (1999). A concept analysis of empowerment: Its relationship to mental health nursing. *Journal of Advanced Nursing, 29*(3), 600–607.

Storch, J. (2006). Ethical dimensions of leadership. In Nursing Leadership and Management in Canada. Hibberd, J. M. and Smith, D. L. (eds.) Elsevier: Toronto.

Wallerstein, N., & Bernstein, E. (1988). Empowerment education: Freire's ideas adapted to health education. *Health Education Quarterly, 15*(4), 379–394.

Winslow, G. R. (1984). From loyalty to advocacy: A new metaphor for nursing. *The Hastings Center Report, 14*, 32–40.

CHAPTER 20

Enabling Patient Empowerment

OBJECTIVES

After completing this chapter, the reader should be able to:

1. Discuss the meaning of patient empowerment.
2. Discuss the nursing role in empowerment of patients.
3. Describe attitudes of nurses that enable empowerment.
4. Identify nursing knowledge and skills basic to empowerment.
5. Describe factors that enhance or block patient empowerment.
6. Discuss approaches to fostering empowerment with patients.

INTRODUCTION

The concept of empowerment relates to the principle of autonomy and to the nursing role of patient advocate. Fostering empowerment in others requires nurses to be attentive to both personal and professional empowerment. This chapter focuses on nursing's role in facilitating empowerment of patients. Understanding of power and empowerment, discussed in Chapter 19, apply to patients as well as nurses. The discussion of empowerment in this chapter flows from these same understandings.

PATIENTS AND EMPOWERMENT

The concept of empowering patients has emerged as nursing has directed its ethical focus to advocacy for patients. Adherence to principles discussed throughout this book, particularly respect for persons, autonomy, justice, and beneficence, makes it incumbent upon nurses to involve patients in making decisions about their health and care. Some patients have both desire and skills to take charge of their lives, some have desire but need assistance or support, while others have limitations in ability and desire. Negotiating within a system that has traditionally placed decision-making authority and power primarily within the hands of physicians requires skill, support, and a strong sense of personal empowerment. Factors discussed in Chapter 19 regarding personal empowerment for nurses apply as well to patients. Patient empowerment is both a process and outcome in which nurses have an active role.

NURSES AND PATIENT EMPOWERMENT

We cannot empower another, as that would strip him or her of the ability to choose. Although empowerment is something that comes from within a person, nurses can serve as enablers of the process. Enabling the empowerment process requires a paradigm shift away from the paternalistic attitude of knowing what is best for the patient. Instead we recognize and accept that patients are essentially responsible for their own health and have the ability to discern what they need, make decisions, and direct their own destinies. In order to make appropriate decisions, however, people may need information and support.

Gibson describes empowerment in the health care arena as "a social process of recognizing, promoting and enhancing people's abilities to meet their own needs, solve their own problems and mobilize the necessary resources in order to feel in control of their own lives . . . a process of helping people to assert control over the factors which affect their health" (1991, p. 339). In light of this description and nursing's focus on patient advocacy, nurses are called to be enablers of the empowerment process with patients, families, and communities. Certain attitudes, knowledge, and skills are basic to fulfilling this role.

Attitudes of Nurses That Enable Empowerment

A view of the nurse as an advocate, facilitator, and resource rather than merely one who provides services for patients is basic to enabling empowerment with patients (Gibson, 1991; Ellis-Stoll & Popkess-Vawter, 1998; Fulton, 1997). Nurses must learn to surrender their need for control, developing instead attitudes of collaboration and mutual participation in decision making. This requires self-reflection on the part of the nurse, through which the nurse confronts personal values and subtle, and not so subtle, benefits gained from being in a position of power. It is essential that nurses make a commitment to being with patients as they struggle with their questions and issues and seek meaning in the process. Relinquishing control also means that nurses need to accept decisions made by patients and families, even when they are different from what the nurse might do or suggest. Respect for persons, which includes valuing others and mutual trust, is key (Gibson, 1991; Rodwell, 1996; Ellis-Stoll & Popkess-Vawter, 1998; Ryles, 1999).

Nursing Knowledge and Skills Necessary for Enabling Empowerment

Information presented throughout this book provides a foundation for facilitating the empowerment process. Attention to ethical principles and processes of decision making fosters empowerment. Awareness of the development of values and their impact on choices allows nurses to be more clear about their own perspectives, so as to foster integrity and avoid imposing personal values on others. Knowledge of social, cultural, political, economic, and other forces affecting a person's options and health choices is essential.

Empowerment is an interactive process. As in many other areas of nursing, effective communication is necessary for facilitating empowerment. The ability to listen with our whole being and to trust intuitive as well as intellectual understanding is important. Reflective listening allows us to help people to recognize their own strengths, abilities, and personal power. Active listening also helps people develop awareness of root causes of problems and to determine their readiness to take action for change. If it is determined that the patient does not want to be empowered, nursing interventions need to be provided in a style of empowerment rather than control (Gibson, 1991). This means approaching patients with an attitude of trust in their abilities to know, at some place within themselves, what they need, and to incorporate behaviours such as offering choices about aspects of care over which they can have control.

Having opportunities and resources necessary for understanding and changing our world is part of the empowerment process. Nurses must have knowledge of factors affecting a patient's health and health care decisions in order to help provide or share the necessary resources. Such knowledge includes awareness of patient and family values and decision-making style; cultural context; social, political, and economic influences on our options; and health care system constraints. We also recognize that individual responsibility for health is necessarily tempered by social and economic factors. Gibson (1991) suggests that nurses need to focus health promotion efforts on the macro social level, attending to conditions that control, influence, and produce health or illness in people. Efforts as individuals, within professional organizations, and within communities, aimed at providing access to health care for all, provide a broad base of support for empowerment.

Nurses must approach patients as equal partners. Skillful collaboration and negotiation, which incorporate power sharing and mutually beneficial interactions, enable empowerment. Relinquishing professional power returns power to the patient.

ENHANCING PATIENT CAPACITY FOR DECISION MAKING

The ability to make decisions regarding our life and destiny requires a basic level of cognitive functioning and sense of control over life and change processes. Empowerment originates in self-esteem; is developed through a sense of connectedness, responsibility, and opportunities for choice; and is supported through perceived meaning and hope in life (Rodwell, 1996).

Helping patients through the process of self-discovery facilitates empowerment by enabling them to decide what they want to do based on appreciation of who they are. Empowerment, according to Purtilo and Meier (1993), arises out of a person's ability to reflect upon and understand oneself. This may require facilitating a patient's self-awareness on many levels, such as identifying personal values, sources of these values, where and with whom they feel connected, and where and how they experience control in life. Utilizing the decision-making process discussed in Chapter 6 can facilitate empowerment with patients.

Determining whether a person functions primarily from a sense of internal or external locus of control can be useful. **Locus of control** refers to beliefs about the ability to control events in our life. People who believe that they are able to influence or control things that happen to them are considered to have an **internal locus of control**. On the other hand, people who feel that forces outside themselves direct or rule their lives, whether these be generalized forces such as fate or other persons who are perceived as more powerful, are considered to have an **external locus of control**. Persons who are internally motivated are more likely to perceive themselves as having power to make choices and control their lives, and to be motivated to make necessary changes. Those who are externally motivated tend to be more fatalistic, expecting their lives to be controlled by powerful others, and less likely to enact personal power (Dawson, 1994; Miller, 1993).

Ask Yourself

How Does Locus of Control Affect Empowerment?

- Reflect on how you have thought through significant decisions in your life. Do you consider that you are more internally or externally motivated? Give specific examples to support your self-assessment.

(Continued)

- In working with patients, what would you consider indications of internal and external locus of control?
- How would your approach to facilitating empowerment be different with persons who exhibit internal locus of control compared to those with external locus of control?

Barriers to Empowerment

Empowerment involves a willingness to take risks, to move beyond that which is known and perhaps comfortable, to the unknown. It often requires a change in self-perception, developing a different vision of who we are. This can stimulate anxiety and fear. Nurses need to recognize such barriers and appreciate that not everyone wants to take the risks and assume the responsibility that empowerment demands. Patients who may be used to the more traditional patriarchal model of the health care professional–patient relationship may have difficulty with or be uncomfortable when given the opportunity to have the "power" to decision make about their own care, preferring to relinquish such decision-making power to physicians or other health care professionals, like nurses. This also arises from a belief that medical or nursing knowledge is of greater value than patients' own knowledge of self. Ideally, both specific physiological, biomedical, and nursing knowledge as well as the particular context and situation of a patient are both important considerations in providing quality care. Paternalistic attitudes within the health care system have fostered reliance on health care providers to determine what patients need for health. Other barriers include patient lack of knowledge of resources or strategies that promote empowerment, dependency, apathy, mistrust, and being labelled by staff (Connelly, Keele, Kleinbeck, Schneider, & Cobb, 1993). Social, cultural, economic, or political factors can present barriers such as limitation of resources, control of knowledge about options, locking people into traditional roles and expectations, social labelling that stereotypes and devalues certain people or behaviours, and restriction of access to resources. Patients may also feel reticent to take part in decision making for fear of making poor decisions or decisions that their medical provider might feel are irresponsible or inappropriate. Often, patients feel that they are being blamed for their decisions, especially those decisions that are made regarding lifestyle habits (e.g., smoking, alcohol use, risky sexual practices, a poor diet) Furthermore, they may feel that the notion of being empowered is, to some degree, an empty and overused concept, as it is invoked so frequently and in such divergent contexts, such as direct-to-consumer advertisements for drugs (only in the United States but frequently viewed on American television channels by Canadians), advocacy groups, policy makers, and politicians, who all quote the best interests of patients and the goal of empowerment, until it loses all meaningfulness (Tomes, 2007). Lack of empowerment of professionals and their inability to relinquish power to patients affect patient empowerment as well. Honouring patient decisions may be very threatening to nurses who do not appreciate that patients know what they need.

One important barrier to the empowerment of patients is a fundamental lack of or inability to practise patient-centred care. In their discussion on patient-centredness, Mead and Bower (2000) talk about the kinds of factors that influence the ability of physicians, specifically, to engage in patient-centred care. While patient-centred care is different from empowerment, it is certainly a pre-requisite at best. This phenomenon, while contextualized in the physician–patient relationship, is also highly relevant to relationships patients have with other health care professionals. The authors identify five categories of factors that influence patient-centred care. These are patient factors, physician (or health care professional) factors; consultation-level influences, professional context influences, and shapers. Patient factors include things like attitudes and expectations, level of knowledge, age, and gender. Health care professional factors include attitudes, values, level of knowledge and expertise, age, gender, and knowledge of patient. Consultation-level influences are things like how frequent interruptions are during a patient-professional interaction, physical barriers, time limitations, communication barriers, and presence of third parties. Professional context influences include professional norms, performance incentives, accreditation, and policies. Finally, shapers include formal and informal learning of patients via the media, personal experience of both the health care professional and the patient, and socioeconomic background (Mead and Bower, 2000). This is interesting, because, before we can, as nurses, begin to think about empowering patients, we must first reflect on whether or not we are facilitating patient-centred care and ensuring that we examine these kinds of influences on our ability to put our patients and their interests first. Only after we do that can we claim to be in a position, both reflectively and practically, to empower others.

FOSTERING PATIENT EMPOWERMENT

We can facilitate empowerment in others by being role models of self-empowerment. As noted previously, belief that patients have the right and ability to make choices regarding their health, and other areas of their lives, is basic to empowerment. Patients need to be given opportunities for choice regarding small as well as major decisions. This means that there needs to be participatory decision making, involving collaboration and negotiation, in what we might consider the "less important" decisions regarding things like all areas of health care. For example, involving patients in making decisions about when they will bathe, what foods to include in their diet, or when to take their medications is as important to empowerment as their participation in decision making regarding life-support measures. Because of social, environmental, and other factors, some people have had limited opportunities for making choices and may need education, practice, and encouragement in this area. Offering options and developing strategies to enhance the patient's ability to set and reach goals are important parts of the nursing role. Connelly et al. (1993) suggest that choosing implies having both the freedom and the courage to choose from different options. Support is an important part of the encouraging process.

Support can take many forms. We provide support by determining what patients identify as empowering to them and encouraging these choices, behaviours, or attitudes.

Caring relationships, in which experiences are shared and patients are accepted for who they are, offer support. Having at least one other person who supports a choice made or a stance that a person takes enhances the likelihood that the person will follow through on the decision.

Considering options and making choices implies having both knowledge and availability of needed resources. Enabling empowerment may require us to provide or help patients discover how to access resources. In some instances this may mean becoming politically and socially active regarding health care issues affecting vulnerable populations. We need to develop strategies that enhance a patient's ability to acquire necessary knowledge. This may mean working with patients and communities to identify both health concerns and socioculturally relevant approaches to dealing with these concerns. We foster empowerment by promoting processes that encourage mutually respectful exchange of ideas and analysis of concerns and potential solutions. Success in achieving goals must be defined from the perspective of the patient or community.

Think About It

Outcomes of Patient Empowerment

Upholding the view that patients know what they need opens nurses to the probability that some patients will make decisions that are not consistent with what the nurse or other health team members think is best. Such decisions may have a relatively minor impact on a patient's or family's health and well-being or may be judged to have potentially serious outcomes for the patient or family.

- What factors need to be considered when dealing with decisions involving differing values between patients and nurses?

- Give examples of situations in which patient empowerment might potentiate an ethical dilemma for you. Reflect on how you would approach such a situation.

- If you feel a patient is making an unwise decision, how would you respond? How should you respond?

- Discuss your view regarding any limits or constraints on patient empowerment.

SUMMARY

Patient empowerment is an important element of nursing care that derives from an appreciation that patients have the ability to discern their needs and make decisions about their lives and health. Being an enabler of empowerment requires that nurses learn to relinquish power and embrace the patient as an equal partner. Self-awareness, respect for others, and effective communication skills serve as foundations for the process. Knowledge about and availability of resources, support, and opportunities for choice are necessary for empowerment. Nurses can facilitate empowerment by working directly with patients and through addressing social, political, and environmental factors affecting empowerment of individuals and communities. In the midst of an ever-changing and challenging health care environment in which issues of power and control continue to affect patient care, nurses must be competent enablers of patient empowerment.

CHAPTER HIGHLIGHTS

- Patient empowerment, which is both a process and an outcome, relates to ethical principles and flows from nursing's focus on patient advocacy.

- Although nurses cannot empower patients, they can be enablers of empowerment, a process that requires recognition and acceptance that patients have the ability to discern what they need, to make decisions, and to direct their own destinies.

- Empowerment is interactive and requires knowledge of personal values and needs for control, mutual trust and respect, effective communication and reflective listening skills, and a willingness to accept patient decisions regardless of whether the nurse thinks they are best.

- Empowerment requires us to first reflect on whether or not we are truly practising "patient-centred" care.

- Fostering patient empowerment requires knowledge of social, political, cultural, economic, and environmental factors affecting a person's options and health choices and may involve addressing health promotion efforts on the macro social level.

- Empowerment is fostered through self-discovery, enhanced self-esteem, a sense of connectedness, support, opportunities for choice, and having needed resources, knowledge, and skills.

- Empowerment strategies that mesh with a person's or community's sociocultural context are more effective.

DISCUSSION QUESTIONS AND ACTIVITIES

1. Describe a personal experience as a patient within the health care system in which you felt that you were empowered. What contributed to the empowerment process for you?

2. Describe a patient or family with whom you have worked who exhibited empowerment. Give specific examples of evidences of empowerment from your perspective.

3. Observe practising nurses in a clinical setting and describe attitudes and behaviours that foster or block empowerment with patients.

4. Discuss factors within the health care system that inhibit patient empowerment.

5. Describe the relationship between patient empowerment and principled behaviour in nursing.

6. Describe a situation in which you believe you fostered empowerment with a patient or family. How did you enable the process? Describe the outcome.

7. What would indicate to you that a patient might not want to be empowered? How would you approach and work with this patient?

REFERENCES

Connelly, L. M., Keele, B. S., Kleinbeck, S. V. M., Schneider, J. K., & Cobb, A. K. (1993). A place to be yourself: Empowerment from the client's perspective. *Image, 25*, 297–303.

Dawson, M. S. (1994). Using locus of control to empower student nurses to be professional. *Nursing Forum, 29*, 10–15.

Ellis-Stoll, C. C., & Popkess-Vawter, S. (1998). A concept analysis on the process of empowerment. *Advances in Nursing Science, 21*(2), 62–68.

Fulton, Y. (1997). Nurses' views on empowerment: A critical social theory perspective. *Journal of Advanced Nursing, 26*, 529–536.

Gibson, C. H. (1991). A concept analysis of empowerment. *Journal of Advanced Nursing, 16*, 354–361.

Mead, N., & Bower, P. (2000). Patient-centredness: A conceptual framework and review of the empirical literature. *Social Science and Medicine, Volume 51*, 1087–1110.

Miller, C. M. (1993). Trajectory and empowerment theory applied to care of patients with multiple sclerosis. *Journal of Neuroscience Nursing, 25*, 343–348.

Purtilo, R. B., & Meier, R. H. (1993). Team challenges: Regulatory constraints and patient empowerment. *American Journal of Physical Medicine & Rehabilitation, 72*, 327–330.

Rodwell, C. M. (1996). An analysis of the concept of empowerment. *Journal of Advanced Nursing, 23*, 305–313.

Ryles, S. M. (1999). A concept analysis of empowerment: Its relationship to mental health nursing. *Journal of Advanced Nursing, 29*(3), 600–607.

Tomes, N. (2007). Patient empowerment and the dilemmas of late-modern medicalisation. *Lancet, 369*, 698–700.

APPENDIX A

The Canadian Nurses Association Code of Ethics for Registered Nurses

PREAMBLE

The Canadian Nurses Association's *Code of Ethics for Registered Nurses*[1] is a statement of the ethical[2] **values**[3] of **nurses** and of nurses' commitments to persons with health-care needs and **persons receiving care**. It is intended for nurses in all contexts and domains of nursing practice[4] and at all levels of decision-making. It is developed by nurses for nurses and can assist nurses in practising ethically and working through ethical challenges that arise in their practice with individuals, **families**, communities and public health systems.

The societal context in which nurses work is constantly changing and can be a significant influence on their practice. The quality of the work environment in which nurses practise is also fundamental to their ability to practise ethically. The code of ethics is revised periodically (see Appendix A [All Appendices refer to those in the *Code of Ethics*. They are not included here.]) to ensure that it is attuned to the needs of nurses by reflecting changes in social values and conditions that affect the public, nurses and other **health-care providers**, and the health-care system (see Appendix B, for a list of societal changes envisioned to affect nursing practice in the coming decade). Periodic revisions also promote lively dialogue and create greater awareness of and engagement with ethical issues among nurses in Canada.

Purpose of the Code

The *Code of Ethics for Registered Nurses* serves as a foundation for nurses' ethical practice. The specific values and ethical responsibilities expected of registered nurses in Canada are set out in part I. Endeavours that nurses may undertake to address social **inequities** as part of ethical practice are outlined in part II.

The code provides guidance for ethical relationships, responsibilities, behaviours and decision-making, and it is to be used in conjunction with the professional standards, laws and regulations that guide practice.

It serves as a means of self-evaluation and self-reflection for ethical nursing practice and provides a basis for feedback and peer review. The code also serves as an ethical basis from which nurses can **advocate** for **quality work environments** that support the delivery of safe, **compassionate**, competent and ethical care.

Nurses recognize the privilege of being part of a self-regulating profession and have a responsibility to merit this privilege. The code informs other health-care professionals as well as members of the public about the ethical commitments of nurses and the responsibilities nurses accept as being part of a self-regulating profession.

Foundation of the Code

Ethical nursing practice involves core ethical responsibilities that nurses are expected to uphold. Nurses are accountable for these ethical responsibilities in their professional relationships with individuals, families, groups, populations, communities and colleagues.

---

[1] In this document, the terms *registered nurse* and *nurse* include nurses who are registered or licensed in extended roles, such as nurse practitioners.

[2] In this document, the terms *moral* and *ethical* are used interchangeably based upon consultation with nurse ethicists and philosophers. We acknowledge that not everyone concurs in this usage.

[3] Words or phrases in bold print are found in the glossary. They are shown in bold only on first appearance.

[4] In this document, *nursing practice* refers to all areas of nursing practice, including direct care (which includes community and public health), education, administration, research and policy development.

As well, nursing **ethics** is concerned with how broad societal issues affect **health** and **well-being**. This means that nurses endeavour to maintain awareness of aspects of **social justice** that affect health and well-being and to advocate for change. Although these endeavours are not part of nurses' core ethical responsibilities, they are part of ethical practice and serve as a helpful motivational and educational tool for all nurses.

http://www.cna-nurses.ca/cna/documents/pdf/publications/ CodeofEthics2002_e.pdf. Reprinted with permission from the Canadian Nurses Association.

The code is organized in two parts:

PART I: Part I, "Nursing Values and Ethical Responsibilities," describes the core responsibilities central to ethical nursing practice. These ethical responsibilities are articulated through seven primary values and accompanying responsibility statements, which are grounded in nurses' professional relationships with individuals, families, groups, populations and communities as well as with students, colleagues and other health-care professionals. The seven primary values are:

1. Providing safe, compassionate, competent and ethical care

2. Promoting health and well-being

3. Promoting and respecting informed decision-making

4. Preserving dignity

5. Maintaining **privacy** and **confidentiality**

6. Promoting **justice**

7. Being accountable

PART II: Ethical nursing practice involves endeavouring to address broad aspects of social justice that are associated with health and well-being. Part II, "Ethical Endeavours," describes endeavours that nurses can undertake to address social inequities.

USING THE CODE IN NURSING PRACTICE

Values are related and overlapping. It is important to work toward keeping in mind all of the values in the code at all times for all persons in order to uphold the dignity of all. In health-care practice, values may be in conflict. Such value conflicts need to be considered carefully in relation to the practice situation. When such conflicts occur, or when nurses need to think through an ethical situation, many find it helpful to use an ethics model for guidance in ethical reflection, questioning and decision-making (see Appendix C).

Nursing practice involves both legal and ethical dimensions. Still, the law and ethics remain distinct. Ideally, a system of law would be completely compatible with the values in this code. However, there may be situations in which nurses need to **collaborate** with others to change a law or policy that is incompatible with ethical practice. When this occurs, the code can guide and support nurses in advocating for changes to law, policy or practice. The code can be a powerful political instrument for nurses when they are concerned about being able to practise ethically.

Nurses are responsible for the ethics of their practice. Given the complexity of ethical situations, the code can only outline nurses' ethical responsibilities and guide nurses in their reflection and decision-making. It cannot ensure ethical practice. For ethical practice, other elements are necessary, such as a commitment to do good; sensitivity and receptiveness to ethical matters; and a willingness to enter into relationships with persons receiving care and with groups, populations and communities that have health-care needs and problems. Practice environments have a significant influence on nurses' ability to be successful in upholding the ethics of their practice. In addition, nurses' self-reflection and dialogue with other nurses and health-care providers are essential components of ethical nursing practice. The importance of the work environment and of reflective practice is highlighted below.

Quality Work Environments

Nurses as individuals and as members of groups advocate for practice settings that maximize the quality of health outcomes for persons receiving care, the health and well-being of nurses, organizational performance and societal outcomes (Registered Nurses' Association of Ontario [RNAO], 2006 [All references refer to those in the *Code of Ethics*. They are not included here.]). Such practice environments have the organizational structures and resources necessary to ensure safety, support and respect for all persons in the work setting. Other health-care providers, organizations and policy-makers at regional, provincial/territorial, national and international levels strongly influence ethical practice.

Nurses' Self-Reflection and Dialogue

Quality work environments are crucial to ethical practice, but they are not enough. Nurses need to recognize that they are **moral agents** in providing care. This means that they have a responsibility to conduct themselves ethically in what they do and how they interact with persons receiving care. Nurses in all facets of the profession need to reflect on their practice, on the quality of their interactions with others and on the resources they need to maintain their own well-being. In particular, there is a pressing need for nurses to work with others (i.e., other nurses, other health-care professionals and the public) to create the **moral communities** that enable the provision of safe, compassionate, competent and ethical care.

Nursing ethics encompasses the breadth of issues involved in health-care ethics, but its primary focus is the ethics of the everyday. How nurses attend to ethics in carrying out their daily interactions, including how they approach their practice and reflect on their ethical commitment to the people they serve, is the substance of **everyday ethics**.

In their practice, nurses experience situations involving ethics. The values and responsibility statements in the code are intended to assist nurses in working through these experiences within the context of their unique practice situations.

Types of Ethical Experiences and Situations

When nurses can name the type of ethical concern they are experiencing, they are better able to discuss it with colleagues and supervisors, take steps to address it at an early stage, and receive support and guidance in dealing with it. Identifying an ethical concern can often be a defining moment that allows positive outcomes to emerge from difficult experiences. There are a number of terms that can assist nurses in identifying and reflecting on their ethical experiences and discussing them with others:[5]

Ethical problems involve situations where there are conflicts between one or more values and uncertainty about the correct course of action. Ethical problems involve questions about what is right or good to do at individual, interpersonal, organizational and even societal levels.

Ethical (or moral) uncertainty occurs when a nurse feels indecision or a lack of clarity, or is unable to even know what the moral problem is, while at the same time feeling uneasy or uncomfortable.

Ethical dilemmas or questions arise when there are equally compelling reasons for and against two or more possible courses of action, and where choosing one course of action means that something else is relinquished or let go. True dilemmas are infrequent in health care. More often, there are complex ethical problems with multiple courses of actions from which to choose.

Ethical (or moral) distress arises in situations where nurses know or believe they know the right thing to do, but for various reasons (including fear or circumstances beyond their control) do not or cannot take the right action or prevent a particular harm. When values and commitments are compromised in this way, nurses' identity and **integrity** as moral agents are affected and they feel moral distress.

---

[5]These situations are derived from CNA, 2004b; Fenton, 1988; Jameton, 1984; and Webster & Baylis, 2000.

Ethical (or moral) residue is what nurses experience when they seriously compromise themselves or allow themselves to be compromised. The moral residue that nurses carry forward from these kinds of situations can help them reflect on what they would do differently in similar situations in the future.

Ethical (or moral) disengagement can occur if nurses begin to see the disregard of their ethical commitments as normal. A nurse may then become apathetic or disengage to the point of being unkind, non-compassionate or even cruel to other health-care workers and to persons receiving care.

Ethical violations involve actions or failures to act that breach fundamental duties to the persons receiving care or to colleagues and other health-care providers.

Ethical (or moral) courage is exercised when a nurse stands firm on a point of moral principle or a particular decision about something in the face of overwhelming fear or threat to himself or herself.

PART I: NURSING VALUES AND ETHICAL RESPONSIBILITIES

Nurses in all domains of practice bear the ethical responsibilities identified under each of the seven primary nursing values.[6] These responsibilities apply to nurses' interactions with individuals, families, groups, populations, communities and society as well as with students, colleagues and other health-care professionals. The responsibilities are intended to help nurses apply the code. They also serve to articulate nursing values to employers, other health-care professionals and the public. Nurses help their colleagues implement the code, and they ensure that student nurses are acquainted with the code.

A. Providing Safe, Compassionate, Competent and Ethical Care

Nurses provide safe, compassionate, competent and ethical care.

Ethical responsibilities:

1. Nurses have a responsibility to conduct themselves according to the ethical responsibilities outlined in this document and in practice standards in what they do and how they interact with persons receiving care as well as with families, communities, groups, populations and other members of the **health-care team**.

2. Nurses engage in compassionate care through their speech and body language and through their efforts to understand and care about others' health-care needs.

3. Nurses build trustworthy relationships as the foundation of meaningful communication, recognizing that building these relationships involves a conscious effort. Such relationships are critical to understanding people's needs and concerns.

---

[6]The value and responsibility statements in the code are numbered and lettered for ease of use, not to indicate prioritization. The values are related and overlapping.

4. Nurses question and intervene to address unsafe, non-compassionate, unethical or incompetent practice or conditions that interfere with their ability to provide safe, compassionate, competent and ethical care to those to whom they are providing care, and they support those who do the same. See Appendix D.

5. Nurses admit mistakes[7] and take all necessary actions to prevent or minimize harm arising from an **adverse event.** They work with others to reduce the potential for future risks and preventable harms. See Appendix D.

6. When resources are not available to provide ideal care, nurses collaborate with others to adjust priorities and minimize harm. Nurses keep persons receiving care, families and employers informed about potential and actual changes to delivery of care. They inform employers about potential threats to safety.

7. Nurses planning to take job action or practising in environments where job action occurs take steps to safeguard the health and safety of people during the course of the job action. See Appendix D.

8. During a natural or human-made disaster, including a communicable disease outbreak, nurses have a **duty to provide care** using appropriate safety precautions. See Appendix D.

9. Nurses support, use and engage in research and other activities that promote safe, competent, compassionate and ethical care, and they use guidelines for ethical research[8] that are in keeping with nursing values.

10. Nurses work to prevent and minimize all forms of **violence** by anticipating and assessing the risk of violent situations and by collaborating with others to establish preventive measures. When violence cannot be anticipated or prevented, nurses take action to minimize risk to protect others and themselves.

B. Promoting Health and Well-Being

Nurses work with people to enable them to attain their highest possible level of health and well-being.

Ethical responsibilities:

1. Nurses provide care directed first and foremost toward the health and well-being of the person, family or community in their care.

---

[7]Provincial and territorial legislation and nursing practice standards may include further direction regarding requirements for disclosure and reporting.

[8]See *Ethical Research Guidelines for Registered Nurses* (CNA, 2002) and the *Tri-Council Policy Statement: Ethical Conduct for Research Involving Humans* (Canadian Institutes of Health Research, Natural Sciences and Engineering Research Council of Canada, & Social Sciences and Humanities Research Council, 1998).

2. When a community health intervention interferes with the individual rights of persons receiving care, nurses use and advocate for the use of the least restrictive measures possible for those in their care.

3. Nurses collaborate with other health-care providers and other interested parties to maximize health benefits to persons receiving care and those with health-care needs, recognizing and respecting the knowledge, skills and perspectives of all.

C. Promoting and Respecting Informed Decision-Making

Nurses recognize, respect and promote a person's right to be informed and make decisions.

Ethical responsibilities:

1. Nurses, to the extent possible, provide persons in their care with the information they need to make informed decisions related to their health and well-being. They also work to ensure that health information is given to individuals, families, groups, populations and communities in their care in an open, accurate and transparent manner.

2. Nurses respect the wishes of **capable** persons to decline to receive information about their health condition.

3. Nurses recognize that capable persons may place a different weight on individualism and may choose to defer to family or community values in decision-making.

4. Nurses ensure that nursing care is provided with the person's **informed consent**. Nurses recognize and support a capable person's right to refuse or withdraw **consent** for care or treatment at anytime.

5. Nurses are sensitive to the inherent power differentials between care providers and those receiving care. They do not misuse that power to influence decision-making.

6. Nurses advocate for persons in their care if they believe that the health of those persons is being compromised by factors beyond their control, including the decision-making of others.

7. When family members disagree with the decisions made by a person with health-care needs, nurses assist families in gaining an understanding of the person's decisions.

8. Nurses respect the informed decision-making of capable persons, including choice of lifestyles or treatment not conducive to good health.

9. When illness or other factors reduce a person's capacity for making choices, nurses assist or support that person's participation in making choices appropriate to their capability.

10. If a person receiving care is clearly **incapable** of consent, the nurse respects the law on capacity assessment and substitute decision-making in his or her jurisdiction (Canadian Nurses Protective Society [CNPS], 2004).

11. Nurses, along with other health-care professionals and with **substitute decision-makers,** consider and respect the best interests of the person receiving care and any previously known wishes or **advance directives** that apply in the situation (CNPS, 2004).

D. Preserving Dignity

Nurses recognize and respect the intrinsic worth of each person.

Ethical responsibilities:

1. Nurses, in their professional capacity, relate to all persons with respect.

2. Nurses support the person, family, group, population or community receiving care in maintaining their dignity and integrity.

3. In health-care decision-making, in treatment and in care, nurses work with persons receiving care, including families, groups, populations and communities, to take into account their unique values, customs and spiritual beliefs, as well as their social and economic circumstances.

4. Nurses intervene, and report when necessary,[9] when others fail to respect the dignity of a person receiving care, recognizing that to be silent and passive is to condone the behaviour. See Appendix D.

5. Nurses respect the physical privacy of persons by providing care in a discreet manner and by minimizing intrusions.

6. When providing care, nurses utilize practice standards, best practice guidelines and policies concerning restraint usage.

7. Nurses maintain appropriate professional **boundaries** and ensure their relationships are always for the benefit of the persons they serve. They recognize the potential vulnerability of persons and do not exploit their trust and dependency in a way that might compromise the therapeutic relationship. They do not abuse their relationship for personal or financial gain, and do not enter into personal relationships (romantic, sexual or other) with persons in their care.

8. In all practice settings, nurses work to relieve pain and suffering, including appropriate and effective symptom and pain management, to allow persons to live with dignity.

9. When a person receiving care is terminally ill or dying, nurses foster comfort, alleviate suffering, advocate for adequate relief of discomfort and pain and

---

[9]See footnote 7.

support a dignified and peaceful death. This includes support for the family during and following the death, and care of the person's body after death.

10. Nurses treat each other, colleagues, students and other health-care workers in a respectful manner, recognizing the power differentials among those in formal leadership positions, staff and students. They work with others to resolve differences in a constructive way. See Appendix D.

E. Maintaining Privacy and Confidentiality

Nurses recognize the importance of privacy and confidentiality and safeguard personal, family and community information obtained in the context of a professional relationship.

Ethical responsibilities:

1. Nurses respect the right of people to have control over the collection, use, access and disclosure of their personal information.

2. When nurses are conversing with persons receiving care, they take reasonable measures to prevent confidential information in the conversation from being overheard.

3. Nurses collect, use and disclose health information on a need-to-know basis with the highest degree of anonymity possible in the circumstances and in accordance with privacy laws.

4. When nurses are required to disclose information for a particular purpose, they disclose only the amount of information necessary for that purpose and inform only those necessary. They attempt to do so in ways that minimize any potential harm to the individual, family or community.

5. When nurses engage in any form of communication, including verbal or electronic, involving a discussion of clinical cases, they ensure that their discussion of persons receiving care is respectful and does not identify those persons unless appropriate.

6. Nurses advocate for persons in their care to receive access to their own health-care records through a timely and affordable process when such access is requested.

7. Nurses respect policies that protect and preserve people's privacy, including security safeguards in information technology.

8. Nurses do not abuse their access to information by accessing health-care records, including their own, a family member's or any other person's, for purposes inconsistent with their professional obligations.

9. Nurses do not use photo or other technology to intrude into the privacy of a person receiving care.

10. Nurses intervene if others inappropriately access or disclose personal or health information of persons receiving care.

F. Promoting Justice

Nurses uphold principles of justice by safeguarding human rights, equity and fairness and by promoting the public good.

Ethical responsibilities:

1. When providing care, nurses do not discriminate on the basis of a person's race, ethnicity, **culture**, political and spiritual beliefs, social or marital status, gender, sexual orientation, age, health status, place of origin, lifestyle, mental or physical ability or socio-economic status or any other attribute.

2. Nurses refrain from judging, labelling, demeaning, stigmatizing and humiliating behaviours toward persons receiving care, other health-care professionals and each other.

3. Nurses do not engage in any form of lying, punishment or torture or any form of unusual treatment or action that is inhumane or degrading. They refuse to be complicit in such behaviours. They intervene, and they report such behaviours.

4. Nurses make fair decisions about the allocation of resources under their control based on the needs of persons, groups or communities to whom they are providing care. They advocate for fair treatment and for fair distribution of resources for those in their care.

5. Nurses support a climate of trust that sponsors openness, encourages questioning the status quo and supports those who speak out to address concerns in good faith (e.g., **whistle-blowing**).

G. Being Accountable

Nurses are accountable for their actions and answerable for their practice.

Ethical responsibilities:

1. Nurses, as members of a self-regulating profession, practise according to the values and responsibilities in the *Code of Ethics for Registered Nurses* and in keeping with the professional standards, laws and regulations supporting ethical practice.

2. Nurses are honest and practise with integrity in all of their professional interactions.

3. Nurses practise within the limits of their competence. When aspects of care are beyond their level of competence, they seek additional information or knowledge, seek help from their supervisor or a competent practitioner and/or request a different work assignment. In the meantime, nurses remain with the person receiving care until another nurse is available.

4. Nurses maintain their **fitness to practise.** If they are aware that they do not have the necessary physical, mental or emotional capacity to practise safely and competently, they withdraw from the provision of care after consulting with their employer or, if they are self-employed, arranging that someone else attend to their clients' health-care needs. Nurses then take the necessary steps to regain their fitness to practise.

5. Nurses are attentive to signs that a colleague is unable, for whatever reason, to perform his or her duties. In such a case, nurses will take the necessary steps to protect the safety of persons receiving care. See Appendix D.

6. Nurses clearly and accurately represent themselves with respect to their name, title and role.

7. If nursing care is requested that is in conflict with the nurse's moral beliefs and values but in keeping with professional practice, the nurse provides safe, compassionate, competent and ethical care until alternative care arrangements are in place to meet the person's needs or desires. If nurses can anticipate a conflict with their conscience, they have an obligation to notify their employers or, if the nurse is self-employed, persons receiving care in advance so that alternative arrangements can be made. See Appendix D.

8. Nurses identify and address conflicts of interest. They disclose actual or potential conflicts of interest that arise in their professional roles and relationships and resolve them in the interest of persons receiving care.

9. Nurses share their knowledge and provide feedback, mentorship and guidance for the professional development of nursing students, novice nurses and other health-care team members. See Appendix D.

PART II: ETHICAL ENDEAVOURS

There are broad aspects of social justice that are associated with health and well-being and that ethical nursing practice addresses. These aspects relate to the need for change in systems and societal structures in order to create greater **equity** for all. Nurses should endeavour as much as possible, individually and collectively, to advocate for and work toward eliminating social inequities by:

i. Utilizing the principles of **primary health care** for the benefit of the public and persons receiving care.

ii. Recognizing and working to address organizational, social, economic and political factors that influence health and well-being within the context of nurses' role in the delivery of care.

iii. In collaboration with other health-care team members and professional organizations, advocating for changes to unethical health and social policies, legislation and regulations.

iv. Advocating for a full continuum of accessible health-care services to be provided at the right time and in the right place. This continuum includes **health promotion,** disease prevention and diagnostic, restorative, rehabilitative and palliative care services in hospitals, nursing homes, home care and the community.

v. Recognizing the significance of **social determinants of health** and advocating for policies and programs that address these determinants.

vi. Supporting environmental preservation and restoration and advocating for initiatives that reduce environmentally harmful practices in order to promote health and well-being.

vii. Working with individuals, families, groups, populations and communities to expand the range of health-care choices available, recognizing that some people have limited choices because of social, economic, geographic or other factors that lead to inequities.

viii. Understanding that some groups in society are systemically disadvantaged, which leads to diminished health and well-being. Nurses work to improve the quality of lives of people who are part of disadvantaged and/or **vulnerable groups** and communities, and they take action to overcome barriers to health care.

ix. Advocating for health-care systems that ensure accessibility, universality and comprehensiveness of necessary health-care services.

x. Maintaining awareness of major health concerns such as poverty, inadequate shelter, food insecurity and violence. Nurses work individually and with others for social justice and to advocate for laws, policies and procedures designed to bring about equity.

xi. Maintaining awareness of broader **global health** concerns such as violations of human rights, war, world hunger, gender inequities and environmental pollution. Nurses work individually and with others to bring about social change.

xii. Advocating for the discussion of ethical issues among health-care team members, persons in their care, families and students. Nurses encourage ethical reflection, and they work to develop their own and others' heightened awareness of ethics in practice. See Appendix C.

xiii. Working collaboratively to develop a moral community. As part of the moral community, all nurses acknowledge their responsibility to contribute to positive, healthy work environments.

GLOSSARY

The glossary is intended to provide nurses with a common language for their reflections and discussions about nursing ethics. It may also be instructive, since nurses who read the glossary terms are more likely to investigate these concepts further, especially if they are unfamiliar. The glossary does not necessarily provide formal definitions of terms, but rather it presents information in a manner and language that is meant to be helpful and accessible. Some terms in the glossary are not included in the main body of the code but are in the appendices, others may not appear exactly as noted in the text, and others may not be included in the text but may be useful to nurses in their ethical reflection and practice.

ADVANCE DIRECTIVES: a person's written wishes about how and what decisions should be made if they become incapable of making decisions for themselves. In decisions about life-sustaining treatment, advance directives are meant to assist with decisions about withholding or withdrawing treatment. Also called living wills or personal directives.

ADVERSE EVENTS: unexpected, undesirable incidents resulting in injury or death that are directly associated with the process of providing health care or health services to a person receiving care (Hebert, Hoffman & Davies, 2003).

ADVOCATE: actively supporting a right and good cause; supporting others in speaking for themselves or speaking on behalf of those who cannot speak for themselves.

BOUNDARIES: a boundary in the nurse-person relationship is the point at which the relationship changes from professional and therapeutic to unprofessional and personal (College and Association of Registered Nurses of Alberta [CARNA], 2005a [All references refer to those in the *Code of Ethics*. They are not provided here]).

CAPABLE: being able to understand and appreciate the consequences of various options and make informed decisions about one's own care and treatment.

COLLABORATE: building consensus and working together on common goals, processes and outcomes (RNAO, 2006).

COMPASSIONATE: the ability to convey in speech and body language the hope and intent to relieve the suffering of another. Compassion must coexist with competence. "Compassion is a relational process that involves noticing another person's pain, experiencing an emotional reaction to his or her pain, and acting in some way to help ease or alleviate the pain" (Dutton, Lilius & Kanov, 2007).

COMPETENCY: the integrated knowledge, skills, judgment and attributes required of a registered nurse to practise safely and ethically in a designated role and setting. (Attributes include, but are not limited to, attitudes, values and beliefs.)

CONFIDENTIALITY: the ethical obligation to keep someone's personal and private information secret or private (Fry & Johnstone, 2002).

CONFLICT OF INTEREST: occurs when a nurse's personal or private interests interfere with the interests of a person receiving care or with the nurse's own professional responsibilities (College of Registered Nurses of British Columbia [CRNBC], 2006c).

CONSENT: *See Informed consent.*

CONSCIENTIOUS OBJECTION: a situation in which a nurse requests permission from his or her employer to refrain from providing care because a practice or procedure conflicts with the nurse's moral or religious beliefs (CRNBC, 2007).

CULTURES: the processes that happen between individuals and groups within organizations and society, and that confer meaning and significance; the health-care system has its own culture(s) (Varcoe & Rodney, 2002).

DETERMINANTS OF HEALTH: these include income and social status, social support, education and literacy, employment and working conditions, physical and social environments, biology, genetic endowment, personal health practices and coping skills, healthy child development, health services, gender and culture (Public Health Agency of Canada, 2003).

DIVERSITY: the variation between people in terms of a range of factors such as ethnicity, national origin, race, gender, ability, age, physical characteristics, religion, values, beliefs, sexual orientation, socio-economic class or life experiences (RNAO, 2007a).

DUTY TO PROVIDE CARE: Nurses have a professional duty and a legal obligation to provide persons receiving care with safe, competent, compassionate and ethical care. There may be some circumstances in which it is acceptable for a nurse to withdraw from care provisions or to refuse to provide care (CRNBC, 2007; College of Registered Nurses of Nova Scotia [CRNNS], 2006a). See Appendix D.

EQUITABLE: determining fairness on the basis of people's needs.

EQUITY: in health care, the fulfillment of each individual's needs as well as the individual's opportunity to reach full potential as a human being (Canadian Nurses Association [CNA], 2006).

ETHICS: the moral practices, beliefs and standards of individuals and/or groups (Fry & Johnstone, 2002).

EVERYDAY ETHICS: how nurses pay attention to ethics in carrying out their common daily interactions, including how they approach their practice and reflect on their ethical commitments to persons receiving care and those with health-care needs.

FAIRNESS: equalizing people's opportunities to participate in and enjoy life, given their circumstances (Caplan, Light & Daniels, 1999), and society's equitable distribution of resources (in health care this means an expectation of equitable treatment).

FAMILY/FAMILIES: In matters of caregiving, family is recognized to be those people identified by the person receiving care or in need of care as providing familial support, whether or not there is a biologic relationship. However, in matters of legal decision-making it must be noted that provincial legislation is not uniform across Canada and may include an obligation to recognize family members in priority according to their biologic relationship (CNA, 1994).

FITNESS TO PRACTISE: all the qualities and capabilities of an individual relevant to his or her capacity to practise as a registered nurse, including, but not limited to, freedom from any cognitive, physical, psychological or emotional condition and dependence on alcohol or drugs that impairs his or her ability to practise nursing (CRNBC, 2006a; CRNNS, 2006b).

GLOBAL HEALTH: the optimal well-being of all humans from the individual and the collective perspective. Health is considered a fundamental right and should be equally accessible by all (CNA, 2003).

HEALTH: a state of complete physical, mental (spiritual) and social well-being, not merely the absence of disease (CNA, 2007; World Health Organization [WHO], 2006).

HEALTH-CARE PROVIDERS: all those who are involved in providing care; they may include professionals, personal care attendants, home support workers and others (CNA, 1994).

HEALTH-CARE TEAM: a number of health-care providers from different disciplines (often including both regulated professionals and unregulated workers) working together to provide care for and with individuals, families, groups, populations or communities.

HEALTH PROMOTION: a continuing process of enabling people to increase their control over and improve their health and well-being.

HUMAN RIGHTS: the rights of people as expressed in the *Canadian Charter of Rights and Freedoms* (1982) and the *United Nations Universal Declaration of Human Rights* (1948), and as recorded in the CNA position statement *Registered Nurses and Human Rights* (CNA, 2004a).

INCAPABLE/INCAPACITY: failing to understand the nature of the treatment decisions to be made, as well as the consequences of consenting to treatment or declining treatment.

INEQUITY: an instance of unjust or unfair treatment of each individual's needs; health inequity means a lack of equitable access and opportunity for all people to meet their health needs and potential (CNA, 2006).

INFORMED CONSENT: the process of giving permission or making choices about care. It is based on both a legal doctrine and an ethical principle of respect for an individual's right to sufficient information to make decisions about care, treatment and involvement in research. In the code, the term *informed decision-making* is primarily used to emphasize the choice involved.

INTEGRITY: (1) for persons receiving care, integrity refers to wholeness, and protecting integrity can mean helping them to become whole and complete again; (2) for health-care providers, showing integrity means consistently following accepted moral norms. Implicit in integrity is soundness, trustworthiness and consistency of convictions, actions and emotions (Burkhart & Nathaniel, 2002).

INTERDISCIPLINARY: the integration of concepts across different disciplines. An interdisciplinary team is a team of people with training in different fields: such teams are common in complex environments such as health care (RNAO, 2007b) and may also be referred to as interprofessional teams.

INTERSECTORAL: all sectors of society (government, community and health).

JUSTICE: includes respecting the rights of others, distributing resources fairly, and preserving and promoting the common good (the good of the community).

MORAL AGENT/AGENCY: the capacity or power of a nurse to direct his or her motives and actions to some ethical end; essentially, doing what is good and right.

MORAL CLIMATE: in health care, the implicit and explicit values that drive health-care delivery and shape the workplaces in which care is delivered (Rodney, Hartrick Doane, Storch & Varcoe, 2006).

MORAL COMMUNITY: a workplace where values are made clear and are shared, where these values direct ethical action and where individuals feel safe to be heard (adapted from Rodney & Street, 2004). Coherence between publicly professed values and the lived reality is necessary for there to be a genuine moral community (Webster & Baylis, 2000).

NURSE(S): in this code, refers to registered nurses, including nurses in extended roles such as nurse practitioners.

PERSON/PERSONS RECEIVING CARE: an individual, family, group, community or population that accesses the services of the registered nurse; may also be referred to as client(s) or patient(s).

PRIMARY HEALTH CARE: "Primary health care is essential health care based on practical, scientifically sound and socially acceptable methods and technology made universally accessible to individuals and families in the community through their full participation and at a cost that the community and country can afford to maintain at every stage of their development in the spirit of self-reliance and self-determination. It forms an integral part both of the country's health system, of which it is the central function and main focus, and of the overall social and economic development of the community. It is the first level of contact of individuals, the family and community with the national health system bringing health care as close a spossible to where people live and work, and constitutes the first element of acontinuing health care process" (WHO, 1978).

PRIVACY: (1) physical privacy is the right or interest in controlling or limiting the access of others to oneself; (2) informational privacy is the right of individuals to determine how, when, with whom and for what purposes any of their personal information will be shared.

PUBLIC GOOD: the good of society or the community, often called the common good.

QUALITY PRACTICE ENVIRONMENTS: practice environments that have the organizational and human support allocations necessary for safe, competent and ethical nursing care (CNA, 2001).

SOCIAL DETERMINANTS OF HEALTH: factors in the social environment, external to the health-care system, that exert a major and potentially modifiable influence on the health of populations (Evans, 1994). See also *Determinants of health*.

SOCIAL JUSTICE: the fair distribution of society's benefits and responsibilities and their consequences. It focuses on the relative position of one social group in relation to others in society as well as on the root causes of disparities and what can be done to eliminate them (CNA, 2006).

SUBSTITUTE DECISION-MAKER: an individual designated by operation of a provincial or territorial statute or in an advance directive of a person in care to make decisions about health care and treatment on the person's behalf (CNA, 1994).

UNREGULATED CARE PROVIDER: paid providers who are neither licensed nor registered by a regulatory body (CRNBC, 2006b).

VALUES: standards or qualities that are esteemed, desired, considered important or have worth or merit (Fry & Johnstone, 2002).

VIOLENCE: includes any abuse of power, manipulation or control of one person over another that could result in mental, emotional, social or physical harm.

VULNERABLE GROUPS: groups disadvantaged by attitudes and systems in society that create inequities.

WELL-BEING: a person's state of being well, content and able to make the most of his or her abilities.

WHISTLE-BLOWING: speaking out about unsafe or questionable practices affecting people receiving care or working conditions. This should be resorted to only after a person has unsuccessfully used all appropriate organizational channels to right a wrong and has a sound moral justification for taking this action (Burkhardt & Nathaniel, 2002).

APPENDIX B

The Canadian Charter of Rights and Freedoms AND The Canadian Bill of Rights

Guarantee of Rights and Freedoms
Fundamental Freedoms
Democratic Rights
Mobility Rights
Legal Rights
Equality Rights

SCHEDULE B

Constitution Act, 1982

Enacted as Schedule B to the *Canada Act 1982* (U.K.) 1982, c. 11, which came into force on April 17, 1982

PART I

CANADIAN CHARTER OF RIGHTS AND FREEDOMS

Whereas Canada is founded upon principles that recognize the supremacy of God and the rule of law:

Guarantee of Rights and Freedoms

Rights and freedoms in Canada

1. The *Canadian Charter of Rights and Freedoms* guarantees the rights and freedoms set out in it subject only to such reasonable limits prescribed by law as can be demonstrably justified in a free and democratic society.

Fundamental Freedoms

Fundamental freedoms

2. Everyone has the following fundamental freedoms:

(a) freedom of conscience and religion;

(b) freedom of thought, belief, opinion and expression, including freedom of the press and other media of communication;

(c) freedom of peaceful assembly; and

(d) freedom of association.

Democratic Rights

Democratic rights of citizens

3. Every citizen of Canada has the right to vote in an election of members of the House of Commons or of a legislative assembly and to be qualified for membership therein.

Maximum duration of legislative bodies

4. (1) No House of Commons and no legislative assembly shall continue for longer than five years from the date fixed for the return of the writs of a general election of its members.

Continuation in special circumstances

(2) In time of real or apprehended war, invasion or insurrection, a House of Commons may be continued by Parliament and a legislative assembly may be continued by the legislature beyond five years if such continuation is not opposed by the votes of more than one-third of the members of the House of Commons or the legislative assembly, as the case may be.

5. There shall be a sitting of Parliament and of each legislature at least once every twelve months.

Mobility Rights

6. (1) Every citizen of Canada has the right to enter, remain in and leave Canada.

   (2) Every citizen of Canada and every person who has the status of a permanent resident of Canada has the right

   (a) to move to and take up residence in any province; and

   (b) to pursue the gaining of a livelihood in any province.

   (3) The rights specified in subsection (2) are subject to

   (a) any laws or practices of general application in force in a province other than those that discriminate among persons primarily on the basis of province of present or previous residence; and

   (b) any laws providing for reasonable residency requirements as a qualification for the receipt of publicly provided social services.

   (4) Subsections (2) and (3) do not preclude any law, program or activity that has as its object the amelioration in a province of conditions of individuals in that province who are socially or economically disadvantaged if the rate of employment in that province is below the rate of employment in Canada.

Legal Rights

7. Everyone has the right to life, liberty and security of the person and the right not to be deprived thereof except in accordance with the principles of fundamental justice.

8. Everyone has the right to be secure against unreasonable search or seizure.

9. Everyone has the right not to be arbitrarily detained or imprisoned.

10. Everyone has the right on arrest or detention

   (a) to be informed promptly of the reasons therefor;

   (b) to retain and instruct counsel without delay and to be informed of that right; and

   (c) to have the validity of the detention determined by way of *habeas corpus* and to be released if the detention is not lawful.

11. Any person charged with an offence has the right

   (a) to be informed without unreasonable delay of the specific offence;

   (b) to be tried within a reasonable time;

   (c) not to be compelled to be a witness in proceedings against that person in respect of the offence;

(d) to be presumed innocent until proven guilty according to law in a fair and public hearing by an independent and impartial tribunal;

(e) not to be denied reasonable bail without just cause;

(f) except in the case of an offence under military law tried before a military tribunal, to the benefit of trial by jury where the maximum punishment for the offence is imprisonment for five years or a more severe punishment;

(g) not to be found guilty on account of any act or omission unless, at the time of the act or omission, it constituted an offence under Canadian or international law or was criminal according to the general principles of law recognized by the community of nations;

(h) if finally acquitted of the offence, not to be tried for it again and, if finally found guilty and punished for the offence, not to be tried or punished for it again; and

(i) if found guilty of the offence and if the punishment for the offence has been varied between the time of commission and the time of sentencing, to the benefit of the lesser punishment.

Treatment or punishment **12.** Everyone has the right not to be subjected to any cruel and unusual treatment or punishment.

Self-crimination **13.** A witness who testifies in any proceedings has the right not to have any incriminating evidence so given used to incriminate that witness in any other proceedings, except in a prosecution for perjury or for the giving of contradictory evidence.

Interpreter **14.** A party or witness in any proceedings who does not understand or speak the language in which the proceedings are conducted or who is deaf has the right to the assistance of an interpreter.

Equality Rights

Equality before and under law and equal protection and benefit of law **15.** (1) Every individual is equal before and under the law and has the right to the equal protection and equal benefit of the law without discrimination and, in particular, without discrimination based on race, national or ethnic origin, colour, religion, sex, age or mental or physical disability.

Affirmative action programs (2) Subsection (1) does not preclude any law, program or activity that has as its object the amelioration of conditions of disadvantaged individuals or groups including those that are disadvantaged because of race, national or ethnic origin, colour, religion, sex, age or mental or physical disability.

Official Languages of Canada

Official languages of Canada **16.** (1) English and French are the official languages of Canada and have equality of status and equal rights and privileges as to their use in all institutions of the Parliament and government of Canada.

(2) English and French are the official languages of New Brunswick and have equality of status and equal rights and privileges as to their use in all institutions of the legislature and government of New Brunswick.

Official languages of New Brunswick

(3) Nothing in this Charter limits the authority of Parliament or a legislature to advance the equality of status or use of English and French.

Advancement of status and use

16.1. (1) The English linguistic community and the French linguistic community in New Brunswick have equality of status and equal rights and privileges, including the right to distinct educational institutions and such distinct cultural institutions as are necessary for the preservation and promotion of those communities.

English and French linguistic communities in New Brunswick

(2) The role of the legislature and government of New Brunswick to preserve and promote the status, rights and privileges referred to in subsection (1) is affirmed.

Role of the legislature and government of New Brunswick

17. (1) Everyone has the right to use English or French in any debates and other proceedings of Parliament.

Proceedings of Parliament

(2) Everyone has the right to use English or French in any debates and other proceedings of the legislature of New Brunswick.

Proceedings of New Brunswick legislature

18. (1) The statutes, records and journals of Parliament shall be printed and published in English and French and both language versions are equally authoritative.

Parliamentary statutes and records

(2) The statutes, records and journals of the legislature of New Brunswick shall be printed and published in English and French and both language versions are equally authoritative.

New Brunswick statutes and records

19. (1) Either English or French may be used by any person in, or in any pleading in or process issuing from, any court established by Parliament.

Proceedings in courts established by Parliament

(2) Either English or French may be used by any person in, or in any pleading in or process issuing from, any court of New Brunswick.

Proceedings in New Brunswick courts

20. (1) Any member of the public in Canada has the right to communicate with, and to receive available services from, any head or central office of an institution of the Parliament or government of Canada in English or French, and has the same right with respect to any other office of any such institution where

Communications by public with federal institutions

(a) there is a significant demand for communications with and services from that office in such language; or

(b) due to the nature of the office, it is reasonable that communications with and services from that office be available in both English and French.

(2) Any member of the public in New Brunswick has the right to communicate with, and to receive available services from, any office of an institution of the legislature or government of New Brunswick in English or French.

Communications by public with New Brunswick institutions

Continuation of existing constitutional provisions

21. Nothing in sections 16 to 20 abrogates or derogates from any right, privilege or obligation with respect to the English and French languages, or either of them, that exists or is continued by virtue of any other provision of the Constitution of Canada.

Rights and privileges preserved

22. Nothing in sections 16 to 20 abrogates or derogates from any legal or customary right or privilege acquired or enjoyed either before or after the coming into force of this Charter with respect to any language that is not English or French.

Minority Language Educational Rights

Language of instruction

23. (1) Citizens of Canada

(a) whose first language learned and still understood is that of the English or French linguistic minority population of the province in which they reside, or

(b) who have received their primary school instruction in Canada in English or French and reside in a province where the language in which they received that instruction is the language of the English or French linguistic minority population of the province, have the right to have their children receive primary and secondary school instruction in that language in that province.

Continuity of language instruction

(2) Citizens of Canada of whom any child has received or is receiving primary or secondary school instruction in English or French in Canada, have the right to have all their children receive primary and secondary school instruction in the same language.

Application where numbers warrant

(3) The right of citizens of Canada under subsections (1) and (2) to have their children receive primary and secondary school instruction in the language of the English or French linguistic minority population of a province

(a) applies wherever in the province the number of children of citizens who have such a right is sufficient to warrant the provision to them out of public funds of minority language instruction; and

(b) includes, where the number of those children so warrants, the right to have them receive that instruction in minority language educational facilities provided out of public funds.

Enforcement

Enforcement of guaranteed rights and freedoms

24. (1) Anyone whose rights or freedoms, as guaranteed by this Charter, have been infringed or denied may apply to a court of competent jurisdiction to obtain such remedy as the court considers appropriate and just in the circumstances.

Exclusion of evidence bringing administration of justice into disrepute

(2) Where, in proceedings under subsection (1), a court concludes that evidence was obtained in a manner that infringed or denied any rights or freedoms guaranteed by this Charter, the evidence shall be excluded if it is established that, having regard to all the circumstances, the admission of it in the proceedings would bring the administration of justice into disrepute.

General

25. The guarantee in this Charter of certain rights and freedoms shall not be construed so as to abrogate or derogate from any aboriginal, treaty or other rights or freedoms that pertain to the aboriginal peoples of Canada including

Aboriginal rights and freedoms not affected by Charter

    (a) any rights or freedoms that have been recognized by the Royal Proclamation of October 7, 1763; and

    (b) any rights or freedoms that now exist by way of land claims agreements or may be so acquired.

26. The guarantee in this Charter of certain rights and freedoms shall not be construed as denying the existence of any other rights or freedoms that exist in Canada.

Other rights and freedoms not affected by Charter

27. This Charter shall be interpreted in a manner consistent with the preservation and enhancement of the multicultural heritage of Canadians.

Multicultural heritage

28. Notwithstanding anything in this Charter, the rights and freedoms referred to in it are guaranteed equally to male and female persons.

Rights guaranteed equally to both sexes

29. Nothing in this Charter abrogates or derogates from any rights or privileges guaranteed by or under the Constitution of Canada in respect of denominational, separate or dissentient schools.

Rights respecting certain schools preserved

30. A reference in this Charter to a Province or to the legislative assembly or legislature of a province shall be deemed to include a reference to the Yukon Territory and the Northwest Territories, or to the appropriate legislative authority thereof, as the case may be.

Application to territories and territorial authorities

31. Nothing in this Charter extends the legislative powers of any body or authority.

Legislative powers not extended

Application of Charter

32. (1) This Charter applies

Application of Charter

    (a) to the Parliament and government of Canada in respect of all matters within the authority of Parliament including all matters relating to the Yukon Territory and Northwest Territories; and

    (b) to the legislature and government of each province in respect of all matters within the authority of the legislature of each province.

    (2) Notwithstanding subsection (1), section 15 shall not have effect until three years after this section comes into force.

Exception

33. (1) Parliament or the legislature of a province may expressly declare in an Act of Parliament or of the legislature, as the case may be, that the Act or a provision thereof shall operate notwithstanding a provision included in section 2 or sections 7 to 15 of this Charter.

Exception where express declaration

    (2) An Act or a provision of an Act in respect of which a declaration made under this section is in effect shall have such operation as it would have but for the provision of this Charter referred to in the declaration.

Operation of exception

Five year
limitation
(3) A declaration made under subsection (1) shall cease to have effect five years after it comes into force or on such earlier date as may be specified in the declaration.

Re-enactment
(4) Parliament or the legislature of a province may re-enact a declaration made under subsection (1).

Five year
limitation
(5) Subsection (3) applies in respect of a re-enactment made under subsection (4).

Citation

Citation
34. This Part may be cited as the *Canadian Charter of Rights and Freedoms*.

CANADIAN BILL OF RIGHTS

1960, c. 44

C-12.3
[Assented to August 10th, 1960]

An Act for the Recognition and Protection of Human Rights and Fundamental Freedoms

Preamble

The Parliament of Canada, affirming that the Canadian Nation is founded upon principles that acknowledge the supremacy of God, the dignity and worth of the human person and the position of the family in a society of free men and free institutions;

Affirming also that men and institutions remain free only when freedom is founded upon respect for moral and spiritual values and the rule of law;

And being desirous of enshrining these principles and the human rights and fundamental freedoms derived from them, in a Bill of Rights which shall reflect the respect of Parliament for its constitutional authority and which shall ensure the protection of these rights and freedoms in Canada:

Therefore Her Majesty, by and with the advice and consent of the Senate and House of Commons of Canada, enacts as follows:

PART I

BILL OF RIGHTS

Recognition and declaration of rights and freedoms

1. It is hereby recognized and declared that in Canada there have existed and shall continue to exist without discrimination by reason of race, national origin, colour, religion or sex, the following human rights and fundamental freedoms, namely,

(a) the right of the individual to life, liberty, security of the person and enjoyment of property, and the right not to be deprived thereof except by due process of law;

(b) the right of the individual to equality before the law and the protection of the law;

(c) freedom of religion;

(d) freedom of speech;

(e) freedom of assembly and association; and

(f) freedom of the press.

Construction of law

2. Every law of Canada shall, unless it is expressly declared by an Act of the Parliament of Canada that it shall operate notwithstanding the *Canadian Bill of Rights*, be so construed and applied as not to abrogate, abridge or infringe or to authorize the abrogation, abridgment or infringement of any of the rights or freedoms herein recognized and declared, and in particular, no law of Canada shall be construed or applied so as to

(a) authorize or effect the arbitrary detention, imprisonment or exile of any person;

(b) impose or authorize the imposition of cruel and unusual treatment or punishment;

(c) deprive a person who has been arrested or detained

    (i) of the right to be informed promptly of the reason for his arrest or detention,

    (ii) of the right to retain and instruct counsel without delay, or

    (iii) of the remedy by way of *habeas corpus* for the determination of the validity of his detention and for his release if the detention is not lawful;

(d) authorize a court, tribunal, commission, board or other authority to compel a person to give evidence if he is denied counsel, protection against self crimination or other constitutional safeguards;

(e) deprive a person of the right to a fair hearing in accordance with the principles of fundamental justice for the determination of his rights and obligations;

(f) deprive a person charged with a criminal offence of the right to be presumed innocent until proved guilty according to law in a fair and public hearing by an independent and impartial tribunal, or of the right to reasonable bail without just cause; or

(g) deprive a person of the right to the assistance of an interpreter in any proceedings in which he is involved or in which he is a party or a witness, before a court, commission, board or other tribunal, if he does not understand or speak the language in which such proceedings are conducted.

Duties of Minister of Justice

3. (1) Subject to subsection (2), the Minister of Justice shall, in accordance with such regulations as may be prescribed by the Governor in Council, examine every regulation transmitted to the Clerk of the Privy Council for registration pursuant to the *Statutory Instruments Act* and every Bill introduced in or presented to the House of Commons by a Minister of the Crown, in order to ascertain whether any of the provisions thereof are inconsistent with the purposes and provisions of this Part and he shall report any such inconsistency to the House of Commons at the first convenient opportunity.

Exception

(2) A regulation need not be examined in accordance with subsection (1) if prior to being made it was examined as a proposed regulation in accordance with section 3 of the *Statutory Instruments Act* to ensure that it was not inconsistent with the purposes and provisions of this Part.

1960, c. 44, s. 3; 1970-71-72, c. 38, s. 29; 1985, c. 26, s. 105; 1992, c. 1, s. 144(F).

Short title

4. The provisions of this Part shall be known as the *Canadian Bill of Rights*.

PART II

Savings

5. (1) Nothing in Part I shall be construed to abrogate or abridge any human right or fundamental freedom not enumerated therein that may have existed in Canada at the commencement of this Act.

"Law of Canada" defined

(2) The expression "law of Canada" in Part I means an Act of the Parliament of Canada enacted before or after the coming into force of this Act, any order, rule or regulation thereunder, and any law in force in Canada or in any part of Canada at the commencement of this Act that is subject to be repealed, abolished or altered by the Parliament of Canada.

Jurisdiction of Parliament

(3) The provisions of Part I shall be construed as extending only to matters coming within the legislative authority of the Parliament of Canada.

APPENDIX C
The American Nursing Association Code of Ethics

PREFACE

Ethics is an integral part of the foundation of nursing. Nursing has a distinguished history of concern for the welfare of the sick, injured and vulnerable and for social justice. This concern is embodied in the provision of nursing care to individuals with the community. Nursing encompasses the prevention of illness, the alleviation of suffering, and the protection, promotion and restoration of health in the care of individuals, families, groups and communities. Nurses act to change those aspects of social structures that detract from health and well-being. Individuals who become nurses are expected not only to adhere to the ideals and moral norms of the profession but also to embrace them as a part of what it means to be a nurse. The ethical tradition of nursing is self-reflective, enduring, and distinctive. A code of ethics makes explicit the primary goals, values, and obligations of the profession.

The Code of Ethics for Nurses serves the following purposes:

- It is a succinct statement of the ethical obligations and duties of every individual who enters the nursing profession.
- It is the profession's nonnegotiable ethical standard.
- It is an expression of nursing's own understanding of its commitment to society.

There are numerous approaches for addressing ethics; these include adopting or ascribing to ethical theories, including humanist, feminist, and social ethics, adhering to ethical principles, and cultivating virtues. The Code of Ethics for Nurses reflects all of these approaches. The words "ethical" and "moral" are used throughout the Code of Ethics. "Ethical" is used to refer to reasons for decisions about how one ought to act, using the above mentioned approaches. In general, the word "moral" overlaps with "ethical" but is more aligned with personal belief and cultural values. Statements that describe activities and attributes of nurses in this Code of Ethics are to be understood as normative or prescriptive statements expressing expectations of ethical behavior.

The Code of Ethics uses the term *patient* to refer to recipients of nursing care. The derivation of this word refers to "one who suffers," reflecting a universal aspect of human existence. Nevertheless, it is recognized that nurses also provide services to those seeking health as well as those responding to illness, to students and to staff, in health care facilities as well as in communities. Similarly, the term *practice* refers to the actions of the nurse in whatever role the nurse fulfills, including direct patient care provider, educator, administrator, researcher, policy developer, or other. Thus, the values and obligations expressed in this Code of Ethics applies to nurses in all roles and settings.

The Code of Ethics for Nurses is a dynamic document. As nursing and its social context change, changes to the Code of Ethics are also necessary. The Code of Ethics consists of two components: the provisions and the accompanying interpretive statements. There are nine provisions. The first three describe the most fundamental values and commitments of the nurse; the next three address boundaries of duty and loyalty, and the last three address aspects of duties beyond individual patient encounters. For each provision, there are interpretive statements that provide greater specificity for practice and are responsive to the contemporary context of nursing. Consequently, the interpretive statements are subject to more frequent revision than are the provisions. Additional ethical guidance and detail can be found in ANA or constituent member association position statements that address clinical, research, administrative, educational or public policy issues.

The Code of Ethics for Nurses with Interpretive Statements provides a framework for nurses to use in ethical analysis and decision-making. The Code of Ethics establishes the ethical standard for the profession. It is not negotiable in any setting nor is it subject to revision or amendment except by formal process of the House of Delegates of the ANA. The Code of Ethics for Nurses is a reflection of the proud ethical heritage of nursing, a guide for nurses now and in the future.

1 **The nurse, in all professional relationships, practices with compassion and respect for the inherent dignity, worth and uniqueness of every individual, unrestricted by considerations of social or economic status, personal attributes, or the nature of health problems.**

1.1 Respect for human dignity

A fundamental principle that underlies all nursing practice is respect for the inherent worth, dignity, and human rights of every individual. Nurses take into account the needs and values of all persons in all professional relationships.

1.2 Relationships to patients

The need for health care is universal, transcending all individual differences. The nurse establishes relationships and delivers nursing services with respect for patient needs and values, and without prejudice. An individual's lifestyle, value system and religious beliefs should be considered in planning health care with and for each patient. Such consideration does not suggest that the nurse necessarily agrees with or condones certain individual choices, but that the nurse respects the patient as a person.

1.3 The nature of health problems

The nurse respects the worth, dignity and rights of all human beings irrespective of the nature of the health problems. The worth of the person is not affected by disease, disability, functional status, or proximity to death. This respect extends to all who require the services of the nurse for the promotion of health, the prevention of illness, the restoration of health, the alleviation of suffering, and the provision of supportive care to those who are dying.

The measures nurses take to care for the patient enable the patient to live with as much physical, emotional, social and spiritual well-being as possible. Nursing care aims to maximize the values that the patient has treasured in life and extends supportive care to the family and significant others. Nursing care is directed toward meeting the comprehensive needs of patients and their families across the continuum of care. This is particularly vital in the care of patients and their families at the end of life to prevent and relieve the cascade of symptoms and suffering that are commonly associated with dying.

Nurses are leaders and vigilant advocates for the delivery of dignified and humane care. Nurses actively participate in assessing and assuring the responsible and appropriate use of interventions in order to minimize unwarranted or unwanted treatment and patient suffering. The acceptability and importance of carefully considered decisions regarding resuscitation status, withholding and withdrawing life-sustaining therapies, forgoing medically provided nutrition and hydration, aggressive pain and symptom management and advance directives are increasingly evident. The nurse should provide interventions to relieve pain and other symptoms in the dying patient even when those interventions entail risks of hastening death. However, nurses may not act with the sole intent of ending a patient's life even though such action may be motivated by compassion, respect for autonomy and quality of life considerations. Nurses have invaluable experience, knowledge and insight into care at the end of life and should be actively involved in related research, education, practice and policy development.

1.4 The right to self-determination

Respect for human dignity requires the recognition of specific patient rights, particularly self-determination. Self-determination, also known as autonomy, is the philosophical basis for informed consent in health care. Patients have the moral and legal right to determine what will be done with their own person; to be given accurate, complete, and understandable information in a manner that facilitates an informed judgment; to be assisted with weighing the benefits, burdens and available options in their treatment, including the choice of no treatment; to accept, refuse or terminate treatment without deceit, undue influence, duress, coercion or penalty; and to be given necessary support throughout the decision-making and treatment process. Such support would include the opportunity to make decisions with family and significant others and the provision of advice and support from knowledgeable nurses and other health professionals. Patients should be involved in planning their own health care to the extent they are able and choose to participate.

Each nurse has an obligation to be knowledgeable about the moral and legal rights of all patients to self-determination. The nurse preserves, protects and supports those interests by assessing the patient's comprehension of both the information presented and the implications of decisions. In situations in which the patient lacks the capacity to make a decision, a designated surrogate decision-maker should be consulted. The role of the surrogate is to make decisions as the patient would based upon the patient's previously expressed wishes and known values. In the absence of a designated surrogate decision-maker, decisions should be made in the best interests of the patient, considering the patient's personal values to the extent they are known. The nurse supports patient self-determination by participating in discussions with surrogates, providing guidance and referral to other resources as necessary, and identifying and addressing problems in the decision-making process. Support of autonomy in the broadest sense also includes recognition that people of some cultures place less weight on individualism and choose to defer to family or community values in decision making. Respect not just for the specific decision but also for the patient's method of decision making is consistent with the principle of autonomy.

Individuals are interdependent members of the community. The nurse recognizes that there are situations in which the right to individual self-determination may be outweighed or limited by the rights, health and welfare of others, particularly in relation to public health considerations. Nonetheless, limitation of individual rights must always be considered a serious deviation from the standard of care, justified only when there are no less restrictive means available to preserve the rights of others and the demands of justice.

1.5 Relationships with colleagues and others

The principle of respect for persons extends to all individuals with whom the nurse interacts. The nurse maintains compassionate and caring relationships with colleagues and others with a commitment to the fair treatment of individuals, to integrity-preserving compromise, and to resolving conflict. Nurses function in many roles, including direct care provider, administrator, educator, researcher and consultant. In each of these roles, the nurse treats colleagues, employees, assistants, and students with respect and compassion. This standard of conduct precludes any and all prejudicial actions, any form of harassment or threatening behavior, or disregard for the effect of one's actions on others. The nurse values the distinctive contribution of individuals or groups, and collaborates to meet the shared goal of providing quality health services.

2 The nurse's primary commitment is to the patient, whether an individual, family, group or community.

2.1 Primacy of the patient's interests

The nurse's primary commitment is to the recipient of nursing and health care services—the patient—whether the recipient is an individual, a family, a group, or a community. Nursing holds a fundamental commitment to the uniqueness of the individual patient; therefore, any plan of care must reflect that uniqueness. The nurse strives to provide patients with opportunities to participate in planning care, assures that patients find the plans acceptable and supports the implementation of the plan. Addressing patient interests requires recognition of the patient's place in the family or other networks of relationship. When the patient's wishes are in conflict with others, the nurse seeks to help resolve the conflict. Where conflict persists, the nurse's commitment remains to the identified patient.

2.2 Conflict of interest for nurses

Nurses are frequently put in situations of conflict arising from competing loyalties in the workplace, including situations of conflicting expectations from patients, families, physicians, colleagues, and in many cases, health care organizations and health plans. Nurses must examine the conflicts arising between their own personal and professional values, the values and interests of others who are also responsible for patient care and health care decisions, as well as those of patients. Nurses strive to resolve such conflicts in ways that ensure patient safety, guard the patient's best interests and preserve the professional integrity of the nurse.

Situations created by changes in health care financing and delivery systems, such as incentive systems to decrease spending, pose new possibilities of conflict between economic self-interest and professional integrity. Bonuses, sanctions, and incentives tied to financial targets are examples of features of health care systems that may present such conflict. Conflicts of interest may arise in any domain of nursing activity including clinical practice, administration, education or research. Advance practice nurses who bill directly for services and nursing executives with budgetary responsibilities must be especially cognizant of the potential for conflicts of interest. Nurses should disclose to all relevant parties (e.g., patients, employers, colleagues) any perceived or actual conflict of interest and in some situations should withdraw from further participation. Nurses in all roles must seek to ensure that employment arrangements are just and fair and do not create an unreasonable conflict between patient care and direct personal gain.

2.3 Collaboration

Collaboration is not just cooperation, but it is the concerted effort of individuals and groups to attain a shared goal. In health care, that goal is to address the health needs of the patient and the public. The complexity of health care delivery systems require a multi-disciplinary approach to the delivery of services that has the strong support and active participation of all the health professions. Within this context, nursing's unique contribution, scope of practice, and relationship with other health professions needs to be clearly articulated, represented and preserved. By its very nature, collaboration requires mutual trust, recognition, and respect among the health care team, shared decision making about patient care, and open dialogue among all parties who have an interest in and a concern for health outcomes. Nurses should work to assure that the relevant parties are involved and have a voice in decision-making about patient care issues. Nurses should see that the questions that need to be addressed are asked and the information needed for informed decision-making is available and provided. Nurses should actively promote the collaborative multi-disciplinary planning required to ensure the availability and accessibility of quality health services to all persons who have needs for health care.

Intra-professional collaboration within nursing is fundamental to effectively address the health needs of patients and the public. Nurses engaged in non-clinical roles such as administration or research, while not providing direct care, nonetheless are collaborating in the provision of care through their influence and direction of those who do. Effective nursing care is accomplished through the interdependence of nurses in differing roles—those who teach the needed skills, set standards, manage the environment of care, or expand the boundaries of knowledge used by the profession. In this sense, nurses in all roles share a responsibility for the outcomes of nursing care.

2.4 Professional boundaries

When acting within the role of a professional, the nurse recognizes and maintains boundaries that establish appropriate limits to relationships. While the nature of nursing work has an inherently personal component, nurse-patient relationships and nurse-colleague relationships have, as their foundation, the purpose of preventing illness, alleviating suffering, and protecting, promoting, and restoring the health of patients. In this way, nurse-patient and nurse-colleague relationships differ from those that are purely personal and unstructured, such as friendship. The intimate nature of nursing care, the involvement of nurses in important and sometimes highly stressful life events, and the mutual dependence of colleagues working in close concert all present the potential for blurring of limits to professional relationships. Maintaining authenticity and expressing oneself as an individual while remaining within the bounds established by the purpose of the relationship can be especially difficult in prolonged or long-term relationships. In all encounters, nurses are responsible for retaining their professional boundaries. When these boundaries are jeopardized, the nurse should seek assistance from peers or supervisors or take appropriate steps to remove herself or himself from the situation.

3 The nurse promotes, advocates for and strives to protect the health, safety and rights of the patient.

3.1 Privacy

The nurse safeguards the patient's right to privacy. The need for health care does not justify unwanted intrusion into the patient's life. The nurse advocates for an environment that provides for sufficient physical privacy, including auditory privacy for discussions of a personal nature and policies and practices that protect the confidentiality of information.

3.2 Confidentiality

Associated with the right to privacy, the nurse has a duty to maintain confidentiality of all patient information. The patient's well-being could be jeopardized and the fundamental trust between patient and nurse destroyed by unnecessary access to data or by the inappropriate disclosure of patient identifiable information. The rights, well-being, and safety of the individual patient should be the primary factors in arriving at any professional judgment concerning the disposition of confidential information received from or about the patient, whether oral, written or electronic. The standard of nursing practice and the nurse's responsibility to provide quality care require that relevant data be shared with those members of the health care team who have a need to know. Only information pertinent to a patient's treatment and welfare is disclosed and only to those directly involved with the patient's care. Duties of confidentiality, however, are not absolute and may need to be modified in order to protect the patient, other innocent parties and in circumstances of mandatory disclosure for public health reasons.

Information used for purposes of peer review, third-party payments, and other quality improvement or risk management mechanisms may be disclosed only under defined policies, mandates, or protocols. These written guidelines must assure that the rights, well-being, and safety of the patient are protected. In general, only that information directly relevant to the task or specific responsibility should be disclosed. When using electronic communications, special effort should be made to maintain data security.

3.3 Protection of participants in research

Stemming from the right to self-determination, each individual has the right to choose whether or not to participate in research. It is imperative that the patient or legally authorized surrogate receive sufficient information that is material to an informed decision, to comprehend that information, and to know how to discontinue participation in research without penalty. Necessary information to achieve an adequately informed consent includes the nature of participation, potential harms and benefits, and available alternatives to taking part in the research. Additionally, the patient should be informed of how the data will be protected. The patient has the right to refuse to participate in research or to withdraw at any time without fear of adverse consequences or reprisal.

Research should be conducted and directed only by qualified persons. Prior to implementation, all research should be approved by a qualified review board to ensure patient protection and the ethical integrity of the research. Nurses should be cognizant of the special concerns raised by research involving vulnerable groups, including children, prisoners, students, the elderly, and the poor. The nurse who participates in research in any capacity should be fully informed about both the subject's and the nurse's rights and obligations in the particular research study and in research in general. Nurses have the duty to question and, if necessary, to report and to refuse to participate in research they deem morally objectionable.

3.4 Standards and review mechanisms

Nursing is responsible and accountable for assuring that only those individuals who have demonstrated the knowledge, skill, practice experiences, commitment and integrity essential to professional practice are allowed to enter into and continue to practice within the profession. Nurse educators have a responsibility to ensure that basic competencies are achieved and to promote a commitment to professional practice prior to entry of an individual into practice. Nurse administrators are responsible for assuring that the knowledge and skills of each nurse in the workplace are assessed prior to the assignment of responsibilities requiring preparation beyond basic academic programs.

The nurse has a responsibility to implement and maintain standards of professional nursing practice. The nurse should participate in planning, establishing, implementing, and evaluating review mechanisms designed to safeguard patients and nurses, such as peer review processes or committees, credentialing processes, quality improvement initiatives, and ethics committees. Nurse administrators must ensure that nurses have access to and inclusion on institutional ethics committees. Nurses must bring forward difficult issues related to patient care and/or institutional constraints upon ethical practice for discussion and review. The nurse acts to promote inclusion of appropriate others in all deliberations related to patient care.

Nurses should also be active participants in the development of policies and review mechanisms designed to promote patient safety, reduce the likelihood of errors, and address both environmental system factors and human factors that present increased risk to patients. In addition, when errors do occur, nurses are expected to follow institutional guidelines in reporting errors committed or observed to the appropriate supervisory personnel and for assuring responsible disclosure of errors to patients. Under no circumstances should the nurse participate in, or condone through silence, either an attempt to hide an error or a punitive response that serves only to fix blame rather than correct the conditions that led to the error.

3.5 Acting on questionable practice

The nurse's primary commitment is to the health, well-being, and safety of the patient across the life span and in all settings in which health care needs are addressed. As an advocate for the patient, the nurse must be alert to and take appropriate action regarding any instances of incompetent, unethical, illegal or impaired practice by any member of the health care team or the health care system or any action on the part of others that places the rights or best interests of the patient in jeopardy. To function effectively in this role, nurses must be knowledgeable about the Code of Ethics, standards of practice of the profession, relevant federal, state and local laws and regulations, and the employing organization's policies and procedures.

When the nurse is aware of inappropriate or questionable practice in the provision or denial of health care, concern should be expressed to the person carrying out the questionable practice. Attention should be called to the possible detrimental effect upon the patient's well-being or best interests as well as the integrity of nursing practice. When factors in the health care delivery system or health care organization threaten the welfare of the patient, similar action should be directed to the responsible administrator. If indicated, the problem should be reported to an appropriate higher authority within the institution or agency, or to an appropriate external authority.

There should be established processes for reporting and handling incompetent, unethical, illegal or impaired practice within the employment settings so that such reporting can go through official channels, thereby reducing the risk of reprisal against the reporting nurse. All nurses have a responsibility to assist those who identify potentially questionable practice. State nurses associations should be prepared to provide assistance and support in the development and evaluation of such processes and reporting procedures. When incompetent, unethical, illegal or impaired practice is not corrected within the employment setting and continues to jeopardize patient well-being and safety, the problem should be reported to other appropriate authorities such as practice committees of the pertinent professional organizations, the legally constituted bodies concerned with licensing of specific categories of health workers and professional practitioners, or the regulatory agencies concerned with evaluating standards of practice. Some situations may warrant the concern and involvement of all such groups. Accurate reporting and factual documentation, and not merely opinion, undergird all such responsible actions. When a nurse chooses to engage in the act of responsible reporting about situations that are perceived as unethical, incompetent, illegal or impaired, the professional organization has a responsibility to provide the nurse with support and assistance and to protect the practice of those nurses who choose to voice their concerns. Reporting unethical, illegal, incompetent or impaired practices, even when done appropriately, may present substantial risks to the nurse; nevertheless, such risks do not eliminate the obligation to address serious threats to patient safety.

3.6 Addressing impaired practice

Nurses must be vigilant to protect the patient, the public and the profession from potential harm when a colleague's practice, in any setting, appears to be impaired. The nurse extends compassion and caring to colleagues who are in recovery from illness or when illness interferes with job performance. In a situation where a nurse suspects another's practice may be impaired, the nurse's duty is to take action designed both to protect patients and to assure that the impaired individual receives assistance in regaining optimal function. Such action should usually begin with consulting supervisory personnel and may also include confronting the individual in a supportive manner and with the assistance of others or helping the individual to access appropriate resources. Nurses are encouraged to follow guidelines outlined by the profession and policies of the employing organization to assist colleagues whose job performance may be adversely affected by mental or physical illness or by personal circumstances. Nurses in all roles should advocate for colleagues whose job performance may be impaired to ensure that they receive appropriate assistance, treatment and access to fair institutional and legal processes. This includes supporting the return to practice of the individual who has sought assistance and is ready to resume professional duties.

If impaired practice poses a threat or danger to self or others, regardless of whether the individual has sought help, the nurse must take action to report the individual to persons authorized to address the problem. Nurses who advocate for others whose job performance creates a risk for harm should be protected from negative consequences. Advocacy may be a difficult process and the nurse is advised to follow workplace policies. If workplace policies do not exist or are inappropriate—that is, they deny the nurse in question access to due legal process or demand resignation—the reporting nurse may obtain guidance from the professional association, state peer assistance programs, employee assistance program or a similar resource.

4 The nurse is responsible and accountable for individual nursing practice, and determines the appropriate delegation of tasks consistent with the nurse's obligation to provide optimum patient care.

4.1 Acceptance of accountability and responsibility

Individual registered nurses bear primary responsibility for the nursing care that their patients receive and are individually accountable for their own practice. Nursing practice includes direct care activities, acts of delegation, and other responsibilities such as teaching, research, and administration. In each instance the nurse retains accountability and responsibility for the quality of practice and for conforming with standards of care.

Nurses are faced with decisions in the context of the increased complexity and changing patterns in the delivery of health care. As the scope of nursing practice changes, the nurse must exercise judgment in accepting responsibilities, seeking consultation, and assigning activities to others who carry out nursing care. For example, some advanced practice nurses have the authority to issue prescription and treatment orders to be carried out by other nurses. These acts are not acts of delegation. Both the advanced practice nurse issuing the order and the nurse accepting the order are responsible for the judgments made and accountable for the actions taken.

4.2 Accountability for nursing judgment and action

Accountability means to be answerable to one's self and others for one's own actions. In order to be accountable, nurses act under a code of ethical conduct that is grounded in the moral principles of fidelity and respect for the dignity, worth, and self-determination of patients. Nurses are accountable for judgments made and actions taken in the course of nursing practice, irrespective of health care organizations' policies or providers' directives.

4.3 Responsibility for nursing judgment and action

Responsibility refers to the specific accountability or liability associated with the performance of duties of a particular role. Nurses accept or reject specific role demands based upon their education, knowledge, competence, and extent of experience. Nurses in administration, education and research also have obligations to the recipients of nursing care. Although nurses in administration, education and research have relationships with patients that are less direct, in assuming the responsibilities of a particular role, they share responsibility for the care provided by those whom they supervise and instruct. The nurse must not engage in practices prohibited by law or delegate activities to others that are prohibited by practice acts of other health care providers.

The individual nurse is responsible for assessing his or her own competence. When the needs of the patient are beyond the qualifications and competencies of the nurse, consultation and collaboration must be sought from qualified nurses, other health professionals, or other appropriate sources. Educational resources should be sought by nurses and provided by institutions to maintain and advance the competence of nurses. Nurse educators act in collaboration with their students to assess the learning needs of the student, the effectiveness of the teaching program, the identification and utilization of appropriate resources, and the support needed for the learning process.

4.4. Delegation of nursing activities

Since the nurse is accountable for the quality of nursing care given to patients, nurses are accountable for the assignment of nursing responsibilities to other nurses and the delegation of nursing care activities to other health care workers. While delegation and assignment are used here in a generic moral sense, it is understood that individual states may have a particular legal definition of these terms.

The nurse must make reasonable efforts to assess individual competency when assigning selected components of nursing care to other healthcare workers. This assessment involves evaluating the knowledge, skills and experience of the individual to whom the care is assigned, the complexity of the assigned tasks, and the health status of the patient. The nurse is also responsible for monitoring the activities of these individuals and evaluating the quality of the care provided. Nurses may not delegate responsibilities such as assessment and evaluation; they may delegate tasks. The nurse must not knowingly assign or delegate to any member of the nursing team a task for which that person is not prepared or qualified. Employer policies or directives do not relieve the nurse of responsibility for making judgments about the delegation and assignment of nursing care tasks.

Nurses functioning in management or administrative roles have a particular responsibility to provide an environment that supports and facilitates appropriate assignment and delegation. This includes providing appropriate orientation to staff, assisting less experienced nurses in developing necessary skills and competencies, and establishing policies and procedures that protect both the patient and nurse from the inappropriate assignment or delegation of nursing responsibilities, activities or tasks.

Nurses functioning in educator or preceptor roles may have a less direct relationship with patients. However, through assignment of nursing care activities to learners they share responsibility and accountability for the care provided. It is imperative that the knowledge and skills of the learner be sufficient to provide the assigned nursing care and that appropriate supervision be provided to protect both the patient and the learner.

5 The nurse owes the same duties to self as to others, including the responsibility to preserve integrity and safety, to maintain competence, and to continue personal and professional growth.

5.1 Moral self-respect

Moral respect accords moral worth and dignity to all human beings irrespective of their personal attributes or life situation. Such respect extends to oneself as well; the same duties that we owe to others we owe to ourselves. Self-regarding duties refer to a realm of duties that primarily concern oneself and include professional growth and maintenance of competence, preservation of wholeness of character, and personal integrity.

5.2 Professional growth and maintenance of competence

Though it has consequences for others, maintenance of competence and ongoing professional growth involves the control of one's own conduct in a way that is primarily self-regarding. Competence affects one's self-respect, self-esteem, professional status, and the meaningfulness of work. In all nursing roles, evaluation of one's own performance, coupled with peer review, is a means by which nursing practice can be held to the highest standards. Each nurse is responsible for participating in the development of criteria for evaluation of practice and for using those criteria in peer and self-assessment.

Continual professional growth, particularly in knowledge and skill, requires a commitment to lifelong learning. Such learning includes, but is not limited to, continuing education, networking with professional colleagues, self-study, professional reading, certification and seeking advanced degrees. Nurses are required to have knowledge relevant to the current scope and standards of nursing practice, changing issues, concerns, controversies, and ethics. Where the care required is outside the competencies of the individual nurse, consultation should be sought or the patient should be referred to others for appropriate care.

5.3 Wholeness of character

Nurses have both personal and professional identities that are neither entirely separate, nor entirely merged, but are integrated. In the process of becoming a professional, the nurse embraces the values of the profession, integrating them with personal values. Duties to self involve an authentic expression of one's own moral point-of-view in practice. Sound ethical decision making requires the respectful and open exchange of views between and among all individuals with relevant interests. In a community of moral discourse, no one person's view should automatically take precedence over that of another. Thus the nurse has a responsibility to express moral perspectives, even when they differ from those of others, and even when they might not prevail.

This wholeness of character encompasses relationships with patients. In situations where the patient requests a personal opinion from the nurse, the nurse is generally free to express an informed personal opinion as long as this preserves the voluntariness of the patient and maintains appropriate professional and moral boundaries. It is essential to be aware of the potential for undue influence attached to the nurse's professional role. Assisting patients to clarify their own values in reaching informed decisions may be helpful in avoiding unintended persuasion. In situations where nurses' responsibilities include care for those whose personal attributes, condition, lifestyle or situation is stigmatized by the community and are personally unacceptable, the nurse still renders respectful and skilled care.

5.4 Preservation of integrity

Integrity is an aspect of wholeness of character and is primarily a self-concern of the individual nurse. An economically constrained health care environment presents the nurse with particularly troubling threats to integrity. Threats to integrity may include a request to deceive a patient, to withhold information, or to falsify records, as well as verbal abuse from patients or coworkers. Threats to integrity may also include an expectation that the nurse will act in a way that is inconsistent with the values or ethics of the profession, or more specifically a request that is in direct violation of the Code of Ethics. Nurses have a duty to remain consistent with both their personal and professional values and to accept compromise only to the degree that it remains an integrity-preserving compromise. An integrity-preserving compromise does not jeopardize the dignity or well-being of the nurse or others. Integrity-preserving compromise can be difficult to achieve, but is more likely to be accomplished in situations where there is an open forum for moral discourse and an atmosphere of mutual respect and regard.

Where nurses are placed in situations of compromise that exceed acceptable moral limits or involve violations of the moral standards of the profession, whether in direct patient care or in any other forms of nursing practice, they may express their conscientious objection to participation. Where a particular treatment, intervention, activity, or practice is morally objectionable to the nurse, whether intrinsically so or because it is inappropriate for the specific patient, or where it may jeopardize both patients and nursing practice, the nurse is justified in refusing to participate on moral grounds. Such grounds exclude personal preference, prejudice, convenience or arbitrariness. Conscientious objection may not insulate the nurse against formal or informal penalty.

The nurse who decides not to take part because of conscientious objection must communicate this decision in appropriate ways. Whenever possible, such a refusal should be made known in advance and in time for alternate arrangements to be made for patient care. The nurse is obliged to provide for the patient's safety, to avoid abandonment, and to withdraw only when assured that alternative sources of nursing care are available to the patient.

Where patterns of institutional behavior or professional practice compromise the integrity of all its nurses, nurses should express their concern or conscientious objection collectively to the appropriate body or committee. In addition, they should express their concern, resist, and seek to bring about a change in those persistent activities or expectations in the practice setting that are morally objectionable to nurses and jeopardize either patient or nurse well being.

6 The nurse participates in establishing, maintaining and improving health care environments and conditions of employment conducive to the provision of quality health care and consistent with the values of the profession through individual and collective action.

6.1 Influence of the environment on moral virtues and values

Virtues are habits of character that predispose persons to meet their moral obligations; that is, to do what is right. Excellences are habits of character that predispose a person to do a particular job or task well. Virtues such as wisdom, honesty and courage are habits or attributes of the morally good person. Excellences such as compassion, patience and skill are habits of character of the morally good nurse. For the nurse, virtues and excellences are those habits that affirm and promote the values of human dignity, well-being, respect, health, independence and other values central to nursing. Both virtues and excellences, as aspects of moral character, can be either nurtured by the environment in which the nurse practices or they can be diminished or thwarted. All have a responsibility to create, maintain, and contribute to environments that support the growth of virtues and excellences and enable nurses to fulfill their ethical obligations.

6.2 Influence of the environment on ethical obligations

All nurses, regardless of role, have a responsibility to create, maintain, and contribute to environments of practice that support nurses in fulfilling their ethical obligations. Environments of practice include observable features, such as working conditions, and written policies and procedures setting out expectations for nurses, as well as less tangible characteristics such as informal peer norms. Organizational structures, role descriptions, health and safety initiatives, grievance mechanisms, ethics committees, compensation systems, and disciplinary procedures all contribute to environments that can either present barriers or foster ethical practice and professional fulfillment.

Environments in which employees are provided fair hearing of grievances, are supported in practicing according to standards of care, and are justly treated allow the realization of the values of the profession and are consistent with sound nursing practice.

6.3 Responsibility for the health care environment

The nurse is responsible for contributing to a moral environment that encourages respectful interactions with colleagues, support of peers, and identification of issues that need to be addressed. Nurse administrators have a particular responsibility to assure that employees are treated fairly and that nurses are involved in decisions related to their practice and working conditions. Acquiescing and accepting unsafe or inappropriate practices, even if the individual does not participate in the specific practice, is equivalent to condoning unsafe practice. Nurses should not remain employed in facilities that routinely violate patient rights or require nurses to severely and repeatedly compromise standards of practice or personal morality.

As with concerns about patient care, nurses should address concerns about the health care environment through appropriate channels. Organizational changes are difficult to accomplish and may require persistent efforts over time. Toward this end, nurses may participate in collective action such as collective bargaining or workplace advocacy, preferably through a professional association such as the state nurses association, in order to address the terms and conditions of employment. Agreements reached through such action must be consistent with the profession's standards of practice, the state law, regulating practice and the Code of Ethics for Nursing. Conditions of employment must contribute to the moral environment, the provision for quality patient care and professional satisfaction for nurses.

The professional association also serves as an advocate for the nurse by seeking to secure just compensation and humane working conditions for nurses. To accomplish this, the professional association may engage in collective bargaining on behalf of nurses. While seeking to assure just economic and general welfare for nurses, collective bargaining, nonetheless, seeks to keep the interests of both nurses and patients in balance.

7 **The nurse participates in the advancement of the profession through contributions to practice, education, administration, and knowledge development.**

7.1 Advancing the profession through active involvement in nursing and in health care policy

Nurses should advance their profession by contributing in some way to the leadership, activities, and the viability of their professional organizations. Nurses can also advance the profession by serving in leadership or mentorship roles or on committees within their places of employment. Nurses who are self-employed can advance the profession by serving as role models for professional integrity. Nurses can also advance the profession through participation in civic activities related to health care or through local, state, national, or international initiatives. Nurse educators have a specific responsibility to enhance students' commitment to professional and civic values. Nurse administrators have a responsibility to foster an employment environment that facilitates nurses' ethical integrity and professionalism, and nurse researchers are responsible for active contribution to the body of knowledge supporting and advancing nursing practice.

7.2 Advancing the profession by developing, maintaining, and implementing professional standards in clinical, administrative, and educational practice

Standards and guidelines reflect the practice of nursing grounded in ethical commitments and a body of knowledge. Professional standards and guidelines for nurses must be developed by nurses and reflect nursing's responsibility to society. It is the responsibility of nurses to identify their own scope of practice as permitted by professional practice standards and guidelines, by state and federal laws, by relevant societal values, and by the Code of Ethics.

The nurse as administrator or manager must establish, maintain, and promote conditions of employment that enable nurses within that organization or community setting to practice in accord with accepted standards of nursing practice and provide a nursing and health care work environment that meets the standards and guidelines of nursing practice. Professional autonomy and self-regulation in the control of conditions of practice are necessary for implementing nursing standards and guidelines and assuring quality care for those whom nursing serves.

The nurse educator is responsible for promoting and maintaining optimum standards of both nursing education and of nursing practice in any settings where planned learning activities occur. Nurse educators must also ensure that only those students who possess knowledge, skills and the competencies that are essential to nursing graduate from their nursing programs.

7.3 Advancing the profession through knowledge development, dissemination, and application to practice

The nursing profession should engage in scholarly inquiry to identify, evaluate, refine and expand the body of knowledge that forms the foundation of its discipline and practice. In addition, nursing knowledge is derived from the sciences and from the humanities. Ongoing scholarly activities are essential to fulfilling a profession's obligations to society. All nurses working alone or in collaboration with others can participate in the advancement of the profession through the development, evaluation, dissemination, and application of knowledge in practice. However, an organizational climate and infrastructure conducive to scholarly inquiry must be valued and implemented for this to occur.

8 **The nurse collaborates with other health professionals and the public in promoting community, national, and international efforts to meet health needs.**

8.1 Health needs and concerns

The nursing profession is committed to promoting the health, welfare, and safety of all people. The nurse has a responsibility to be aware not only of specific health needs of individual patients, but also of broader health concerns such as world hunger, environmental pollution, lack of access to health care, violation of human rights, and inequitable distribution of nursing and health care resources. The availability and accessibility of high-quality health services to all people requires both inter-disciplinary planning and collaborative partnerships among health professionals and others at the community, national, and international levels.

8.2 Responsibilities to the public

Nurses, individually and collectively, have a responsibility to be knowledgeable about the health status of the community and existing threats to health and safety. Through support of and participation in community organizations and groups, the nurse assists in efforts to educate the public, facilitates informed choice, identifies conditions and circumstances that contribute to illness, injury, and disease, fosters healthy life styles, and participates in institutional and legislative efforts to promote health and meet national health objectives. In addition, the nurse supports initiatives to address barriers to health, such as poverty, homelessness, unsafe living conditions, abuse and violence and lack of access to health services.

The nurse also recognizes that health care is provided to culturally diverse populations in this country and in all parts of the world. In providing care, the nurse should avoid imposition of the nurse's cultural values upon others. The nurse should affirm human dignity and show respect for the values and practices associated with different cultures and use approaches to care that reflect awareness and sensitivity.

9 **The profession of nursing, as represented by associations and their members, is responsible for articulating nursing values, for maintaining the integrity of the profession and its practice, and for shaping social policy.**

9.1 Assertion of values

It is the responsibility of a professional association to communicate and affirm the values of the profession to its members. It is essential that the professional organization encourages discourse that supports critical self-reflection and evaluation within the profession. The organization also communicates to the public the values that nursing considers central to social change that will enhance health.

9.2 The profession carries out its collective responsibility through professional associations

The nursing profession continues to develop ways to clarify nursing's accountability to society. The contract between the profession and society is made explicit through such mechanisms as (a) The Code of Ethics for Nurses, (b) the standards of nursing practice, (c) the ongoing development of nursing knowledge derived from nursing theory, scholarship, and research in order to guide nursing actions, (d) educational requirements for practice, (e) certification, and (f) mechanisms for evaluating the effectiveness of professional nursing actions.

9.3 Intraprofessional integrity

A professional association is responsible for expressing the values and ethics of the profession and also for encouraging the professional organization and its members to function in accord with those values and ethics. Thus, one of its fundamental responsibilities is to promote awareness of and adherence to the Code of Ethics and to critique the activities and ends of the professional association itself. Values and ethics influence the power structures of the association in guiding, correcting, and directing its activities. Legitimate concerns for the self-interest of the association and the profession are balanced by a commitment to the social goods that are sought. Through critical self-reflection and self-evaluation, associations must foster change within themselves, seeking to move the professional community towards its stated ideals.

9.4 Social reform

Nurses can work individually as citizens or collectively through political action to bring about social change. It is the responsibility of a professional nursing association to speak for nurses collectively in shaping and reshaping health care within our nation, specifically in areas of health care policy and legislation that affect accessibility, quality, and the cost of health care. Here, the professional association maintains vigilance and takes action to influence legislators, reimbursement agencies, nursing organizations, and other health professions. In these activities, health is understood as being broader than delivery and reimbursement systems, but extending to health-related sociocultural issues such as violation of human rights, homelessness, hunger, violence and the stigma of illness.

APPENDIX D

The ICN Code of Ethics for Nurses

An international code of ethics for nurses was first adopted by the International Council of Nurses (ICN) in 1953. It has been revised and reaffirmed at various times since, most recently with this review and revision completed in 2005.

PREAMBLE

Nurses have four fundamental responsibilities: to promote health, to prevent illness, to restore health and to alleviate suffering. The need for nursing is universal.

Inherent in nursing is respect for human rights, including cultural rights, the right to life and choice, to dignity and to be treated with respect. Nursing care is respectful of and unrestricted by considerations of age, colour, creed, culture, disability or illness, gender, sexual orientation, nationality, politics, race or social status.

Nurses render health services to the individual, the family and the community and co-ordinate their services with those of related groups.

THE ICN CODE

The *ICN Code of Ethics for Nurses* has four principal elements that outline the standards of ethical conduct.

Elements of the Code

1. Nurses and People

The nurse's primary professional responsibility is to people requiring nursing care.

In providing care, the nurse promotes an environment in which the human rights, values, customs and spiritual beliefs of the individual, family and community are respected.

The nurse ensures that the individual receives sufficient information on which to base consent for care and related treatment.

The nurse holds in confidence personal information and uses judgement in sharing this information.

The nurse shares with society the responsibility for initiating and supporting action to meet the health and social needs of the public, in particular those of vulnerable populations.

The nurse also shares responsibility to sustain and protect the natural environment from depletion, pollution, degradation and destruction.

2. Nurses and Practice

The nurse carries personal responsibility and accountability for nursing practice, and for maintaining competence by continual learning.

The nurse maintains a standard of personal health such that the ability to provide care is not compromised.

The nurse uses judgement regarding individual competence when accepting and delegating responsibility.

The nurse at all times maintains standards of personal conduct which reflect well on the profession and enhance public confidence.

The nurse, in providing care, ensures that use of technology and scientific advances are compatible with the safety, dignity and rights of people.

3. Nurses and the Profession

The nurse assumes the major role in determining and implementing acceptable standards of clinical nursing practice, management, research and education.

The nurse is active in developing a core of research-based professional knowledge.

The nurse, acting through the professional organisation, participates in creating and maintaining safe, equitable social and economic working conditions in nursing.

4. Nurses and Co-Workers

The nurse sustains a co-operative relationship with co-workers in nursing and other fields.

The nurse takes appropriate action to safeguard individuals, families and communities when their health is endangered by a co-worker or any other person.

Suggestions for Use of the *ICN Code of Ethics for Nurses*

The *ICN Code of Ethics for Nurses* is a guide for action based on social values and needs. It will have meaning only as a living document if applied to the realities of nursing and health care in a changing society.

To achieve its purpose the *Code* must be understood, internalised and used by nurses in all aspects of their work. It must be available to students and nurses throughout their study and work lives.

Applying the Elements of the *ICN Code of Ethics for Nurses*

The four elements of the *ICN Code of Ethics for Nurses*: nurses and people, nurses and practice, nurses and the profession, and nurses and co-workers, give a framework for the standards of conduct. The following chart will assist nurses to translate the standards into action. Nurses and nursing students can therefore:

- Study the standards under each element of the *Code*.
- Reflect on what each standard means to you. Think about how you can apply ethics in your nursing domain: practice, education, research or management.
- Discuss the *Code* with co-workers and others.
- Use a specific example from experience to identify ethical dilemmas and standards of conduct as outlined in the *Code*. Identify how you would resolve the dilemmas.
- Work in groups to clarify ethical decision making and reach a consensus on standards of ethical conduct.
- Collaborate with your national nurses' association, co-workers, and others in the continuous application of ethical standards in nursing practice, education, management and research.

Element of the Code # 1: NURSES AND PEOPLE		
Practitioners and Managers	**Educators and Researchers**	**National Nurses' Associations**
Provide care that respects human rights and is sensitive to the values, customs and beliefs of all people.	In curriculum include references to human rights, equity, justice, solidarity as the basis for access to care.	Develop position statements and guidelines that support human rights and ethical standards.
Provide continuing education in ethical issues.	Provide teaching and learning opportunities for ethical issues and decision making.	Lobby for involvement of nurses in ethics review committees.
Provide sufficient information to permit informed consent and the right to choose or refuse treatment.	Provide teaching/learning opportunities related to informed consent.	Provide guidelines, position statements and continuing education related to informed consent.
Use recording and information management systems that ensure confidentiality.	Introduce into curriculum concepts of privacy and confidentiality.	Incorporate issues of confidentiality and privacy into a national code of ethics for nurses.
Develop and monitor environmental safety in the workplace.	Sensitise students to the importance of social action in current concerns.	Advocate for safe and healthy environment.

Element of the Code # 2: NURSES AND PRACTICE		
Practitioners and Managers	**Educators and Researchers**	**National Nurses' Associations**
Establish standards of care and a work setting that promotes safety and quality care.	Provide teaching/learning opportunities that foster life long learning and competence for practice.	Provide access to continuing education, through journals, conferences, distance education, etc.
Establish systems for professional appraisal, continuing education and systematic renewal of licensure to practice.	Conduct and disseminate research that shows links between continual learning and competence to practice.	Lobby to ensure continuing education opportunities and quality care standards.
Monitor and promote the personal health of nursing staff in relation to their competence for practice.	Promote the importance of personal health and illustrate its relation to other values.	Promote healthy lifestyles for nursing professionals. Lobby for healthy work places and services for nurses.

Element of the Code # 3: NURSES AND THE PROFESSION		
Practitioners and Managers	**Educators and Researchers**	**National Nurses' Associations**
Set standards for nursing practice, research, education and management.	Provide teaching/learning opportunities in setting standards for nursing practice, research, education and management.	Collaborate with others to set standards for nursing education, practice, research and management.
Foster workplace support of the conduct, dissemination and utilisation of research related to nursing and health.	Conduct, disseminate and utilise research to advance the nursing profession.	Develop position statements, guidelines and standards related to nursing research.
Promote participation in national nurses' associations so as to create favourable socio-economic conditions for nurses.	Sensitise learners to the importance of professional nursing associations.	Lobby for fair social and economic working conditions in nursing. Develop position statements and guidelines in workplace issues.

Element of the Code # 4: NURSES AND CO-WORKERS		
Practitioners and Managers	**Educators and Researchers**	**National Nurses' Associations**
Create awareness of specific and overlapping functions and the potential for inter-disciplinary tensions.	Develop understanding of the roles of other workers.	Stimulate co-operation with other related disciplines.
Develop workplace systems that support common professional ethical values and behaviour.	Communicate nursing ethics to other professions.	Develop awareness of ethical issues of other professions.
Develop mechanisms to safeguard the individual, family or community when their care is endangered by health care personnel.	Instil in learners the need to safeguard the individual, family or community when care is endangered by health care personnel.	Provide guidelines, position statements and discussion fora related to safeguarding people when their care is endangered by health care personnel.

Dissemination of the *ICN Code of Ethics for Nurses*

To be effective the *ICN Code of Ethics for Nurses* must be familiar to nurses. We encourage you to help with its dissemination to schools of nursing, practising nurses, the nursing press and other mass media. The Code should also be disseminated to other health professions, the general public, consumer and policy-making groups, human rights organisations and employers of nurses.

Glossary of Terms Used in the *ICN Code of Ethics for Nurses*

Co-worker	Other nurses and other health and non-health related workers and professionals.
Co-operative relationship	A professional relationship based on collegial and reciprocal actions, and behaviour that aim to achieve certain goals.
Family	A social unit composed of members connected through blood, kinship, emotional or legal relationships.
Nurse shares with society	A nurse, as a health professional and a citizen, initiates and supports appropriate action to meet the health and social needs of the public.
Personal health	Mental, physical, social and spiritual wellbeing of the nurse.
Personal information	Information obtained during professional contact that is private to an individual or family, and which, when disclosed, may violate the right to privacy, cause inconvenience, embarrassment, or harm to the individual or family.
Related groups	Other nurses, health care workers or other professionals providing service to an individual, family or community and working toward desired goals.

APPENDIX E

CNA Joint Statement on Advance Directives: Policy Statement

All persons have the right to make decisions regarding their health care and treatment including the right to request or refuse life-sustaining treatment.

The co-sponsors of this statement agree that all those involved in health care have a duty to uphold the client's right to self-determination.

The autonomy of every individual must be recognized and respected. Arising out of the principle of autonomy is the right to self-determination and therefore the requirement for consent to any intervention. An important issue has been raised by the public in recent years expressing the fear that should they become seriously ill and unable to speak for themselves, they will be subjected to treatments for which they would not wish to give consent.

This statement is intended to promote the principle of client[1] self-determination within health care agencies and facilities, particularly in relation to the treatment and care given in the continuing care sector. It is a guide for the development of policies which will support individual clients in freely expressing their preferences regarding health care and treatment, including the use of life-sustaining procedures,[2] should the individual later become incompetent to make such decisions. Informed consent requires choosing from among recommended options and understanding the possible outcomes.

Documented advance directives[3] are a method for people to express their preferences about health care and treatment. Health care professionals should be aware of the law in their own jurisdictions because each province and territory can and may have legislation governing advance directives. Whether or not advance directives are addressed in legislation, they provide a framework and a focus for discussion that can foster communication between clients and those who need to understand the client's wishes—including family[4] members, significant others, friends, substitute decision-makers[5] and health care providers.[6]

It is recognized that health care agencies and facilities are not the only settings in which advance directives should be discussed. Ideally, the public should be made aware of the opportunity to formulate advance directives before any medical crisis occurs, through health and legal education programs, community health centres and through discussions with their health care professionals. However, it will often be on admission to a health care agency or facility that the subject is first raised.

The presentation of the idea of advance directives and the discussion and documenting of advance directives must occur in a way that is sensitive to the client's needs and fears. Advance directives must never become a requirement for care nor a burden to the client. Advance directives are not intended to replace dialogue but to promote dialogue and record the outcome.

Policies and guidelines cannot cover all possible situations therefore health care agencies and facilities are encouraged to have ethics consultation mechanisms in place to address specific situations.

Guidelines for Establishing Advance Directives Within an Agency/Facility

Forms for documenting advance directives are carefully designed through interdisciplinary collaboration and the involvement of client groups, community groups and the public, drawing on the values and the resources of the community. The agencies and facilities within a community should give full consideration to developing one form or making an agreement to respect the forms coming from other agencies/facilities.

The opportunity to prepare advance directives is offered to all competent[7] clients who are chronically or terminally ill, or who meet other criteria established by the agency/facility, or who request them.

The agency/facility determines the appropriate personnel and the appropriate time frame for preparing advance directives that best suit the setting, the individual clients and their care.

The policies are supported by education and information within the agency/facility which:

a. Enables designated health care providers to offer support to clients in understanding and completing advance directives, and
b. Enables staff to implement the directives.

It is not to be assumed that because an incompetent client does not have advance directives that all possible interventions are desired by the client.

The review of advance directives is initiated by the client or the appropriate personnel at regular intervals (e.g., annually, semi-annually) and with changed circumstances (e.g., following severe illness or prior to surgery).

Effective communication among all relevant parties is crucial to achieving the goals of advance directives. Therefore the client must be asked for permission to communicate the advance directives, and any changes, on a need to know basis, to all persons who will be caring for the client—including health care providers and possibly volunteers, family members, friends and significant others.

In the case of transfer, within or between agencies/facilities, or between the client's home and agencies/facilities, the advance directives are communicated verbally and in writing to the transferring and receiving care givers.

The documents for advance directives are included in the health record of the client.

Guidelines for Discussing Advance Directives With a Client

Clients can make advance directives which a) give instruction about specific treatments and circumstances, and/or b) name a substitute decision-maker.

The advance directives offer the client the opportunity to give instruction regarding desired levels of intervention and particular treatments from a wide range of options available to them (such as, but not limited to: cardiopulmonary resuscitation; transfer to other agencies; admission to intensive care unit; tube feeding and blood transfusion) and to specify wishes for reversible and/or irreversible conditions.

The purpose of advance directives is explained in terms which are understandable to the client and sensitive to the client's situation. This generally includes explaining the possible events that may require health care decisions, and the treatment options and their possible outcomes.

Advance Directives are Open to Change by the Competent Client at Any Time

The agency/facility staff makes clear to the client that supportive care and comfort care will always be offered.

The discussion of advance directives includes finding out whether the client already has an advance directive such as a "living will."[8] If so the facility/agency requests to review the previous document with the objective of understanding the client's wishes and discussing them in the current context. If the agency/facility policy requires more direction or information than is found in the previous document, the agency/facility staff explain their concern and offer to support the client in preparing a revised advance directive.

The discussion of the advance directives makes clear to the client that if she or he becomes incapable of making decisions related to health care that her or his directive will be followed. Only when the directive is not clear or not applicable in light of changed circumstances would it not be specifically followed but would then be used as a guide.

The opportunity for ongoing discussion and consultation with others (e.g., spiritual advisors, family members) is facilitated to support the client in coming to decisions about the treatments for which she or he will give consent. The competent person's advance directives should take priority in cases where family members and/or significant others disagree, but because of the evolving legal status of advance directives, legal advice should be sought in such cases. Consideration by an ethics committee may also be helpful.

All necessary documentation is completed and signed by the client and other health care personnel as may be required by the agency/facility.

A selected list of resources is available from the statement co-sponsors.

Notes

1. Client: In this document client is taken only in the individual sense, i.e., the person receiving health care services, whether in an acute care or long term care setting or at home.

2. Life-sustaining procedures: Treatments which sustain the client's life can range from artificial methods of maintaining hydration and nutrition, to cardiopulmonary resuscitation, blood transfusion and mechanical ventilation. It is most important that vague terms, such as "heroic measures" or "extraordinary means" be avoided in outlining treatment options.

3. Advance directive: There are two basic forms of advance directives—instructional directives and those which name a substitute decision-maker. An advance directive is a document intended to govern the kind of treatment that a competent person will receive if she or he later becomes incompetent. The document can be but is not necessarily a form created by a health care agency/facility.

4. Family: In matters of care giving, family is recognized to be those persons who are identified by the client as providing familial support, whether or not they are biologically related. However, in matters of legal decision-making it must be noted that provincial legislation defining family is not uniform across Canada and may include obligations to recognize family members in priority according to their biological relationship. Health care agencies/facilities should ensure that policies and procedures reflect the legal requirements of their particular jurisdictions.

5. Substitute decision-maker: This is a person designated in an advance directive by the client to make decisions about health care and treatment on the client's behalf. Whether a person is a legally recognized substitute decision-maker depends on provincial legislation, court appointments, regulations and guidelines as and where these exist. Legislation is not uniform across Canada. Health care agencies/facilities should ensure that policies and procedures reflect the legal requirements of their particular jurisdiction.

6. Health care providers: This term is taken to mean all those who are involved in providing care to the client and may include professionals, personal care attendants, home support workers and others. This intention to include all care providers is important because any of these persons may be attending the client alone at the time when the advance directives will need to be implemented and each one will need to know what to do.

7. Competence: Assessing competence can be difficult because it is not always a constant state. A person may be competent to make decisions regarding some aspects of life but not others; as well, competence can be temporal in that a person may be lucid and oriented at certain times of the day and then not at other times. The definition and assessment of competence are governed by the provinces or territories. Health professionals should be aware of the laws (e.g., capacity to consent, age of consent) and facility or agency policies regarding the assessment and documentation of incompetence.

8. Living will: A form of advance directive. A written declaration, made by an individual, intending to govern decisions regarding life-sustaining treatments that the person will receive if she or he later becomes incompetent. "Living will" is a popular term arising from consumer groups and the dying with dignity movement. The fill-in-the-blank forms for living wills have been criticized for using vague terms open to misinterpretation. Health care providers may encounter these forms and should be prepared to incorporate them into their discussions with clients.

Approved by the Board of Directors
September 1994

Glossary

Accountability   The state of being answerable to someone for something one has done.

Active voluntary euthanasia   An act in which the physician both provides the means of death for a patient, such as a lethal dose of medication, and administers it.

Activism   A passionate approach to everyday activities that is committed to seeking a more just social order through critical analysis, provocation, transformation, and rebalancing of power.

Act-utilitarianism   A basic type of utilitarianism that suggests people choose actions that will, in a given circumstance, increase the overall good.

Administrative law   The branch of law that consists mainly of the legal powers granted to administrative agencies by the legislature, and the rules that the agencies make to carry out their powers.

Advance directives   Instructions that indicate which health care interventions to initiate or withhold, or which designate someone who will act as a surrogate in making such decisions, in the event that a person loses decision-making capacity.

Allocative policies   Policies designed to provide net benefits to some distinct group or class of individuals or organizations, at the expense of others, in order to ensure that public objectives are met.

Anonymity   A situation in which even the researcher cannot link information with a particular participant in a study.

Appeals to conscience   Personal and subjective beliefs, founded on a prior judgment of rightness or wrongness, that are motivated by personal sanction, rather than external authority.

Assault   The unjustifiable attempt or threat to touch a person without consent that results in fear of immediately harmful or threatening contact.

Assisted suicide   A situation in which patients receive the means of death from someone, such as a physician, but activate the process themselves.

Authenticity   The quality of being genuine and consistent over time.

Authority   The state of having legitimate power and sovereignty.

Autonomy   An ethical principle that literally means self-governing. It denotes having the freedom to make independent choices.

Axiology   The branch of philosophy that studies the nature and types of values.

Battery   The unlawful touching of another or the carrying out of threatened physical harm including every willful, angry, and violent or negligent touching of another's person, clothes, or anything attached to his or her person or held by him or her.

Belmont Report   Policies developed by the United States National Commission for the Protection of Human Subjects of Biomedical and Behavioral Research (1978) regarding ethical principles for research with human participants in the United States.

Beneficence The ethical principle that requires one to act in ways that benefit another. In research, this implies the protection from harm and discomfort, including a balance between the benefits and risks of a study.

Bullying The act of intimidating another person, through harassment, threats, or coercion, causing them harm.

Cartesian philosophy A widespread belief during the Renaissance related to Descartes' proposal that the universe is a physical thing, and all therein is analogous to machines that can be analyzed and understood, and that the mind and body are separate entities.

Case law Principles of law arising out of judicial opinions and decisions. Also known as common law.

Categorical imperative The Kantian maxim stating that no action can be judged as right which cannot reasonably become a law by which every person should always abide.

Character ethics Theories of ethics, sometimes called virtue ethics, that are related to the concept of innate moral virtue.

Charter of Rights and Freedoms A comprehensive list of the rights, freedoms, and privileges applicable to all Canadian citizens.

Cheating Dishonesty and deception regarding examinations, projects, or papers.

Civil law (Also called private law) The law that determines a person's legal rights and obligations in many kinds of activities involving other people.

Code of nursing ethics Explicit declaration of the primary goals and values of the profession that indicate the profession's acceptance of the responsibility and trust with which it has been invested by society.

Coercion Actual or implied threat of harm or penalty for not participating in a research project, or offering excessive rewards for participation in the project.

Common law A system of law, also known as case law, based largely on previous court decisions. In this system, decisions are based upon earlier court rulings in similar cases, or precedents. Over time, these precedents take on the force of law. This is the basis of the legal system in Canada (except for the province of Quebec, where the legal system is based on French civil law).

Communitarian theories Theories of justice that place the community, rather than the individual, the state, the nation, or any other entity, at the centre of the value system; that emphasize the value of public goods; and that conceive of values as rooted in communal practices.

Compassion A focal virtue combining an attitude of active regard for another's welfare with an imaginative awareness and emotional response of deep sympathy, tenderness, and discomfort at the other person's misfortune or suffering.

Competence A person's ability to make meaningful life decisions. A declaration of incompetence involves legal action with a ruling by a judge that the person is unable to make such life decisions.

Complementary therapies Therapeutic interventions that derive from traditions other than conventional Western medicine which are used by patients with or without the knowledge of conventional medical practitioners.

Confidentiality The ethical principle that requires nondisclosure of private or secret information with which one is entrusted. In research, confidentiality refers to the researcher's assurance to participants that information provided will not be made public or available to anyone other than those involved in the research process without the participant's consent.

Consent A complex legal and ethical notion, arising from autonomy and dignity, which states that persons have the right to decide what can and cannot be done to them. In law, it is often referred to as the right to be free from interference. In health care, it is an absolute necessity to obtain consent from patients or participants in research prior to carrying out any interventions or actions.

Consequentialism A theory of ethics, sometimes called utilitarianism. In these theories, the moral worth of an action or choice is evaluated based on the consequences or outcomes as opposed to the intentions or duties of the moral agent.

Constitutional law A formal set of rules and principles that describe the powers of a government and the rights of the people.

Contract An agreement between two or more people that can be enforced by law.

Contract law A type of law that deals with the rights and obligations of people who make contracts.

Cosmology A branch of philosophy that describes the structure, origin, and processes of the universe.

Covert values Expectations that are not in writing that are often identified only through participation in, or controversies within, an organization or institution.

Criminal Code of Canada It is the formal articulation of all offenses and procedures.

Criminal law A type of law that deals with crimes, or actions considered harmful to society.

Cultural awareness Knowledge about values, beliefs, behaviours, and the like of cultures other than one's own.

Cultural competence Skill in dealing with transcultural issues, which is demonstrated through cultural awareness and cultural sensitivity.

Cultural sensitivity The ability to incorporate a patient's cultural perspective into nursing assessments, and to modify nursing care in order to be as congruent as possible with the patient's cultural perspective.

Culture The total lifeways of a group of interacting individuals, consisting of learned patterns of values, beliefs, behaviours, and customs shared by that group.

Decision-making capacity The ability of a person to understand all information about a health condition, to communicate understanding and choices, and to reason and deliberate; and the possession of personal values and goals that guide the decision.

Declaration of Helsinki   Principles issued by the World Medical Assembly to guide clinical research in 1964; revised in 1975, 1983, 1989, 1996, 2000, and most recently in 2008.

Defamation   Harm that occurs to a person's reputation and good name, diminishes others' value or esteem, or arouses negative feelings toward the person by the communication of false, malicious, unprivileged, or harmful words.

Deontology   Related to the term "duty," deontology is a group of ethical theories based upon the rationalist view that the rightness or wrongness of an act depends upon the nature of the act, rather than the consequences that occur as a result of it.

Discernment   A focal virtue of sensitive insight, acute judgment, and understanding that eventuates in decisive action.

Distributive justice   Application of the ethical principle of justice that relates to fair, equitable, and appropriate distribution in society, determined by justified norms that structure the terms of social cooperation. Its scope includes policies that allot diverse benefits and burdens such as property, resources, taxation, privileges, and opportunities.

Diversity   The experience within nursing of differences among colleagues and patients in areas such as gender, age, socioeconomic position, sexual orientation, health status, ethnicity, race, or culture.

Do not resuscitate (DNR) orders   Written directives placed in a patient's medical chart indicating that cardiopulmonary resuscitation is to be avoided.

Durable power of attorney   Allows a competent person to designate another as a surrogate or proxy to act on her or his behalf in making health care decisions in the event of the loss of decision-making capacity.

Duty to care   A legal principle referring to the obligation imposed on someone to act or refrain from acting in a way that would cause harm to another person.

Egalitarian theories   Theories of justice that promote ideals of equal distribution of social benefits and burdens, and recognize the social obligation to eliminate or reduce barriers that prevent fair equality of opportunity.

Empirical   Knowledge gained through the processes of observation and experience.

Empowerment   A helping process and partnership, enacted in the context of love and respect for self and others, through which individuals and groups are enabled to change situations, and are given skills, resources, opportunities, and authority to do so. It involves creating a vision, taking risks, making choices, and behaving in authentic ways.

Ethical dilemma   Occurs when there are conflicting moral claims.

Ethical principles   Basic and obvious moral truths that guide deliberation and action. Major ethical principles include autonomy, beneficence, nonmaleficence, veracity, confidentiality, justice, fidelity, and others.

Ethical treatment of data Implies integrity of research protocols and honesty in reporting findings.

Ethic of caring An approach to ethical decision making grounded in relationship and mutual responsibility, in which choices are contextually bound and strategies are focused on maintaining connections and not hurting anyone.

Ethic of justice An approach to ethical decision making, based on objective rules and principles in which choices are made from a stance of separateness.

Ethics A formal process for making logical and consistent decisions based upon moral beliefs.

Ethnocentrism Judging behaviours of someone from another culture by the standards of one's own culture.

Eugenics Meaning "good birth," eugenics is based in the belief that some human traits are more desirable for society than others, and that society should weed out what proponents consider to be undesirable traits. Proponents of eugenics advocate policies that encourage so called "genetically superior" people to have children, while discouraging so called "genetically inferior" people from having children, through practices such as forced sterilization.

Euthanasia Causing the painless death of a person in order to end or prevent suffering.

Expertise The characteristic of having a high level of specialized skill and knowledge.

Explicit consent Either verbal or written consent specifically articulating the patient's agreement to a particular treatment or procedure.

External locus of control The belief that forces outside oneself direct or rule one's life, whether these be generalized forces such as fate or other persons who are perceived as more powerful.

External standards of nursing practice Guides for nursing care that are developed by non-nurses, legislation, or institutions.

False imprisonment The unlawful, unjustifiable detention of a person within fixed boundaries, or an act intended to result in such confinement.

Felonies Serious crimes that carry significant fines and jail sentences. Examples of felonies include first- and second-degree murder, arson, burglary, extortion, kidnaping, rape, and robbery.

Fidelity An ethical principle related to the concept of faithfulness and the practice of promise keeping.

Forgery Includes fraud or intentional misrepresentation.

Formalism A term often used to refer to deontology.

Fraud A deliberate deception for the purpose of securing an unfair or unlawful gain.

Full disclosure Indicates that a research participant must be fully informed of the nature of a study, anticipated risks and benefits, time commitment, expectations of the participant and the researcher, and the right to refuse to participate.

Genetic diagnosis A process of biopsy of embryos to determine the presence of genetic flaws and gender prior to implantation.

Genetic engineering The ability to genetically alter organisms for a variety of purposes, particularly to promote their health and strength.

Genetic screening A process for determining whether persons are predisposed to certain diseases, and whether couples have the possibility of giving birth to a genetically impaired infant.

Globalization A set of processes or goals aiming to integrate economic, social, political, and trade systems across boundaries.

Grassroots lobbying Lobbying efforts that involve mobilizing a committed constituency to influence the opinions of policy makers.

Guardian *ad litem* A court appointed guardian for a particular action or proceeding; such a guardian may not oversee all of the person's affairs.

Harassment Unwanted and persistent behaviours, words, or actions directed at another person that causes that person emotional distress or threatens him or her substantially.

Health policies Authoritative decisions focusing on health that are made in the legislative, executive, or judicial branches of government and are intended to direct or influence the actions, behaviours, or decisions of others; their lifestyles and personal behaviours; and improvements in the availability, accessibility, and quality of their health care services.

Human Rights The basic rights, fundamental freedoms and privileges to which all humans are entitled.

Implied consent Consent that is inferred from a person's actions, presence or informed cooperation.

Informed consent A process by which patients are informed of the possible outcomes, alternatives, and risks of treatments and required to give their consent freely. This implies legal protection of a patient's right to personal autonomy by providing the opportunity to choose a course of action, including the right to refuse medical recommendations and to choose from available therapeutic alternatives. *In research*, this refers to consent to participate in a research study after the research purpose, expected commitment, risks and benefits, any invasion of privacy, and ways that anonymity and confidentiality will be addressed have been explained.

Integrity Refers to adherence to moral norms that is sustained over time. Implicit in integrity is trustworthiness and a consistency of convictions, actions, and emotions.

Intentional infliction of emotional distress Also known as "intentional infliction of mental distress" or the "tort of outrage," this is a relatively new tort claim in Canada, allowing for a claim to be made against someone who acts in a heinous, reckless, or extreme way, resulting in emotional distress for another.

Intentional torts Willful or intentional acts that violate another person's rights or property.

Internal locus of control   The belief that one is able to influence or control things that happen in one's life.

Internal standards of nursing practice   Standards of nursing practice that are developed within the profession of nursing.

Invasion of privacy   Includes intrusion on the patient's physical and mental solitude or seclusion, public disclosure of private facts, publicity that places the patient in a false light in the public eye, or appropriation for the defendant's benefit or advantage of the patient's name or likeness.

Involuntary euthanasia   Euthanasia practised without consent. In this case, the person is, for some reason, incapable or unable to consent to euthanasia. The decision should be based on clear ideas about the authentic wishes of the individual, if he/she could consent.

Judicial decisions   Authoritative court decisions that direct or influence the actions, behaviours, or decisions of others.

Justice   An ethical principle that relates to fair, equitable, and appropriate treatment in light of what is due or owed to persons, recognizing that giving to some will deny receipt to others who might otherwise have received these things. *In research*, justice implies the rights of fair treatment and privacy, including anonymity and confidentiality.

Kantianism   A deontological theory of ethics based upon the writings of the philosopher Immanuel Kant.

Law   The system of enforceable principles and processes that governs the behaviour of people in respect to relationships with others and with the government.

Libel   Printed defamation by written words and images that injure a person's reputation or cause others to avoid, ridicule, or view the person with contempt.

Libertarian theories   Theories of distributive justice that propose that the just society protects the rights of property and liberty of each person, allowing citizens to improve their circumstances by their own effort.

Living wills   Legal documents developed voluntarily by persons, giving directions to health care providers related to withholding or withdrawing life support if certain conditions exist.

Lobbying   The art of persuasion—attempting to convince a legislator, a government official, the head of an agency, or an official to comply with a request—whether it is convincing them to support a position on an issue or to follow a particular course of action.

Locus of control   Beliefs about the ability to control events in one's life.

Loyalty   Showing sympathy, care, and reciprocity to those with whom we appropriately identify; working closely with others toward shared goals; keeping promises; making mutual concerns a priority; sacrificing personal interests to the relationship; and giving attention to these over a substantial period of time.

Malpractice   The form of negligence in which any professional misconduct, unreasonable lack of professional skill, or nonadherence to the accepted standard of care causes injury to a patient or client.

Managed care An integrated form of health care delivery and financing that represents attempts to control costs by modifying the behaviour of providers and patients.

Material rules Rules by which distributive justice decisions regarding entitlement are made.

Medical futility Situations in which medical interventions are judged to have no medical benefit, or in which the chance for success is low.

Misdemeanour A criminal offence of a less serious nature than a felony, usually punishable by a fine or short jail sentence, or both.

Misrepresentation of personal performance It includes submitting work that has been taken from another and represented as one's own, allowing someone else to write an exam using your name, or not being forthright with academic records or documents.

Moral development A product of the sociocultural environment in which one lives and develops that reflects the intellectual and emotional process through which one learns and incorporates values regarding right and wrong.

Moral distress The reaction to a situation in which there are moral problems that seem to have clear solutions, yet one is unable to follow one's moral beliefs because of external or institutional restraints. This may be evidenced in anger, frustration, dissatisfaction, and poor performance in the work setting.

Moral integrity A focal virtue that relates to soundness, reliability, wholeness, an integration of character, and fidelity in adherence to moral norms sustained over time.

Moral outrage A state that occurs when someone else in the health care setting performs an act the nurse believes to be immoral. In cases of moral outrage, the nurse does not participate in the act and therefore does not feel responsible for wrong, but feels powerlessness to prevent it.

Moral philosophy The philosophical discussion of what is considered to be good or bad, right or wrong.

Moral thought Individuals' cognitive examination of right and wrong, good and bad.

Moral uncertainty A state that occurs when one senses that there is a moral problem, but is not sure of the morally correct action; when one is unsure what moral principles or values apply; or when one is unable to define the moral problem.

Moral values Preferences or dispositions reflective of right or wrong, should or should not, in human behaviour.

Naturalism A view of moral judgment that regards ethics as dependent upon human nature and psychology.

Negligence The omission to do something that a reasonable person, guided by those ordinary considerations that ordinarily regulate human affairs, would do, or doing something that a reasonable and prudent person would not do.

Noncompliance Denoting an unwillingness on the part of the patient to participate in health care activities that have been recommended by health care providers.

Nonmaleficence An ethical principle related to beneficence that requires one to act in such a manner as to avoid causing harm to another, including deliberate harm, risk of harm, and harm that occurs during the performance of beneficial acts.

Nonvoluntary euthanasia Euthanasia imposed upon someone who does not provide consent.

Nuremberg Code A set of principles for the ethical conduct of research.

Nurse practice acts Legislative statutes within each province that define nursing, describe boundaries of practice, establish standards for nurses, and protect the domain of nursing.

Nursing process A model commonly used for decision making in nursing.

Obligation Being required to do something by virtue of a moral rule, a duty, or some other binding demand, such as a particular role or relationship.

Overt values Values of individuals, groups, institutions, and organized systems that are explicitly communicated through philosophy and policy statements.

Palliative care A comprehensive, interdisciplinary, and total care approach, focusing primarily on comfort and support of patients and families who face illness that is chronic or not responsive to curative treatment.

Partisan Adherence to the ideology of a particular political party.

Paternalism A gender-biased term that literally means acting in a "fatherly" manner, the traditional view of which implies well-intended actions of benevolent decision making, leadership, protection, and discipline, which, in the health care arena, manifest in the making of decisions on behalf of patients without their full consent or knowledge.

Philosophy The intense and critical examination of beliefs and assumptions.

PIPEDA The *Personal Information Protection and Electronic Documents Act* is a federal law addressing the privacy of personal information for all Canadians.

Plagiarism Taking another's ideas or work and presenting them as one's own.

Policies are plans of action that guide actions—of governments, institutions, corporations, communities, etc. Policies often reflect the values and beliefs of the majority or of those directly responsible for creating the policy.

Policy formulation A phase of the policy-making process that includes such actions as agenda setting and the subsequent development of legislation.

Policy implementation A phase of the policy-making process that follows enactment of legislation and includes taking actions and making additional decisions necessary to implement legislation such as rule making and policy operation.

Policy modification A phase of the policy-making process that exists to improve or perfect legislation previously enacted.

Political Relates to the complex process of policy making within the government.

Political issues Those issues that are regulated or influenced by decisions within either the executive, judicial, or legislative branches of government.

Political parties Organized groups with distinct ideology that seek to control government.

Politics   refers to anything that involves groups of persons making decisions or influencing how decisions are made or resources are allocated. The term implies both action and thought.

Power   The ability to do or act; the capability of doing or accomplishing something.

Practical dilemma   A situation in which moral claims compete with nonmoral claims.

Practical imperative   The Kantian maxim requiring that one treat others always as ends and never as a means.

Precedents   Court rulings upon which subsequent rulings in similar cases are based. Over time these precedents take on the force of law.

Principles   Basic and obvious truths that guide deliberation and action.

Private law (Also called civil law)   The law that determines a person's legal rights and obligations in many kinds of activities involving other people.

Profession   A complex, organized occupation preceded by a long training program geared toward the acquisition of exclusive knowledge necessary to provide a service that is essential or desired by society, leading to a monopoly that provides autonomy, public recognition, prestige, power, and authority for the practitioner.

Public law   Law that defines a person's rights and obligations in relation to government, and describes the various divisions of government and their powers.

Quality of life   A subjective appraisal of factors that make life worth living and contribute to a positive experience of living.

Racism   The assumption that members of one race are superior to those of another.

Rationalism   A view of moral judgment that regards truth as necessary, universal, and superior to the information received from the senses; having an origin in the nature of the universe, or in the nature of a higher being.

Regulatory policies   Policies that are designed to influence the actions, behaviours, and decisions of others through directive techniques.

Respect for human dignity   Implies the rights of patients to full disclosure and self-determination regarding participation in research and in making health care choices.

Respect for persons   An attitude by which one considers others to be worthy of high regard.

Right to fair treatment   Assures equitable treatment of participants in the research selection process, during the study, and after the completion of the study.

Right to privacy   The right to be left alone or to be free from unwanted publicity. In research, this is the right of research participants to determine when, where, and what kind of information is shared, with an assurance that information and observations are treated with respect and kept in strict confidence.

Rules or **regulations**   Policies that are established to guide the implementation of laws and programs.

Rule-utilitarianism   A type of utilitarianism that suggests people choose rules that, when followed consistently, will maximize the overall good.

Scope of practice   A description of the procedures, actions, and responsibilities of a health care professional. Also refers to clearly defined parameters or boundaries of duties and commitments.

Self-awareness   Conscious awareness of one's thoughts, feelings, physical, and emotional responses, and insights in various situations.

Sexism   The assumption that members of one sex are superior to those of the other.

Sexual harassment   All unwelcome sexual advances, request for sexual favours, and other conduct of a sexual nature.

Slander   Defamation that occurs when one speaks unprivileged or false words about another.

Spectrum of urgency   A spectrum depicting the degree of urgency in health care decision making, ranging from minor and nonurgent to severe and very urgent.

Spirituality   Concern with, and exploration of, that which is unseen or unknown.

Standards of nursing practice   Written documents outlining minimum expectations for nursing care.

Statutes or **laws**   Legislation that has been enacted by legislative bodies and approved by the executive branch of government.

Statutory (legislative) law   Formal laws written and enacted by federal, provincial/territorial, or local legislatures.

Steadfastness   The quality of remaining loyal or true despite, or in the face of, adversity.

Stereotyping   Expecting all persons from a particular group to behave, think, or respond in a certain way based on preconceived ideas.

Submission of false information   It may include examples such as submitting a false statement such as a medical certificate to avoid completing an assignment or writing an exam, submitting false academic records, or altering official academic documents.

Sympathy   Sharing, in imagination, of others' feelings.

Theory   A proposed explanation for a class of phenomena.

Tort   A wrong or injury that a person suffers because of someone else's action, either intentional or unintentional. The action may cause bodily harm; damage a person's property, business, or reputation; or make unauthorized use of a person's property.

Tri-council policy statement on ethical conduct for research involving humans   Canadian federal guidelines for the ethical conduct of research. The three councils refer to the three major granting agencies in Canada: The Social Sciences and Humanities Research Council (SSHRC), the Canadian Institutes of Health Research (CIHR), and the Natural Sciences and Engineering Research Council (NSERC).

Trustworthiness   A focal virtue that results in recognition by others of one's consistency and predictability in following moral norms.

Unintentional torts Torts that occur when an act or omission causes unintended injury or harm to another person.

Utilitarianism A moral theory which holds that an action is judged as good or bad in relation to the consequence, outcome, or end result derived from it.

Utilitarian theories Theories of distributive justice that distribute resources based on the premise of the greatest good for the greatest number of people. These theories place social good before individual rights.

Utility The property of usefulness in any object, whereby it tends to produce benefit, advantage, pleasure, good, or happiness or prevent mischief, pain, evil, or unhappiness.

Values Ideals, beliefs, customs, modes of conduct, qualities, or goals that are highly prized or preferred by individuals, groups, or society.

Values clarification Refers to the process of becoming more conscious of and naming what one values or considers worthy.

Values conflict Internal or interpersonal conflict that occurs in circumstances in which personal values are at odds with those of patients, colleagues, or the institution.

Veracity Truth telling.

Victim blaming Holding the people burdened by social conditions accountable for their own situations and responsible for needed solutions.

Virtue ethics Theories of ethics, usually attributed to Aristotle, which represent the idea that an individual's actions are based upon innate moral virtue.

Whistleblowing Speaking out about unsafe or questionable practices affecting patient care or working conditions. This should be resorted to only after a person has unsuccessfully used all appropriate organizational channels to right a wrong, and has a sound moral justification for taking this action.

Whistleblowers Persons who alert the public about serious wrongdoing created or concealed within an organization, such as unsafe conditions, incompetence, or professional misconduct.

Index